NEURO-AIDS

NEURO-AIDS

ALIREZA MINAGAR
AND
PAUL SHAPSHAK
EDITORS

Nova Biomedical Books
New York

NOTICE TO THE READER

The Publisher has taken reasonable care in the preparation of this book, but makes no expressed or implied warranty of any kind and assumes no responsibility for any errors or omissions. No liability is assumed for incidental or consequential damages in connection with or arising out of information contained in this book. The Publisher shall not be liable for any special, consequential, or exemplary damages resulting, in whole or in part, from the readers' use of, or reliance upon, this material.

Independent verification should be sought for any data, advice or recommendations contained in this book. In addition, no responsibility is assumed by the publisher for any injury and/or damage to persons or property arising from any methods, products, instructions, ideas or otherwise contained in this publication.

This publication is designed to provide accurate and authoritative information with regard to the subject matter cover herein. It is sold with the clear understanding that the Publisher is not engaged in rendering legal or any other professional services. If legal, medical or any other expert assistance is required, the services of a competent person should be sought. FROM A DECLARATION OF PARTICIPANTS JOINTLY ADOPTED BY A COMMITTEE OF THE AMERICAN BAR ASSOCIATION AND A COMMITTEE OF PUBLISHERS.

Library of Congress Cataloging-in-Publication Data
Neuro-AIDS / Alireza Minagar and Paul Shapshak, editors.
       p. ; cm.
Includes bibliographical references and index.
ISBN 1-59454-610-X
1. Nervous system--Infections. 2. HIV infections. 3. AIDS (Disease) --Complications. 4. AIDS dementia complex.   I. Minagar, Alireza. II. Shapshak, Paul.
[DNLM: 1. AIDS Dementia Complex--etiology. 2. HIV Infections--etiology. 3. AIDS Dementia Complex--complications. 4. Central Nervous System Diseases--complications.   WC 503.3
N494 2006]
RC359.5.N43   2006
616.8--dc22   2006007847

Published by Nova Science Publishers, Inc. ✦New York

Contents

Preface

In chapter I, human immunodeficiency virus-1 (HIV-1) enters the central nervous system (CNS) early in the course of HIV-1 infection and causes a form of subcortical dementia, known as HIV-1 associated dementia (HAD). HAD is perhaps the most significant neurological complication of AIDS and poses a major diagnostic and management challenge to the clinicians. With introduction of highly active anti-retroviral therapy (HAART), the patterns of HIV-1 infection and its CNS complications have changed. Macrophage/microglia are the key cell type that are infected by HIV-1 in the CNS and are mediators of neurodegeneration in pathogenesis of HAD. This chapter mainly addresses clinical features and pathogenesis of HAD.

Chapter II will focus on HIV neuroinvasion---the timing, modes and sites of viral entry into the brain, and the potential impact of antiretroviral therapy on this entry. The question of when HIV enters the brain is particularly important to issues of viral latency and persistence, and the potential for the brain to serve as a significant viral reservoir. Answers to the questions of timing and mode of entry can also help to better delineate the relationship between HIV infection and replication within the brain, and the development of dementia. HIV neuroinvasion during early and late-stage infection, as well as throughout the course of infection, is discussed, along with the potential impact on timing of viral strain specificity, the immune response and compromise of the blood-brain barrier. HIV entry into the brain via cell-free virions and infected leukocytes, particularly monocytes, is considered, with attention to issues pertaining to the blood-brain barrier, the perivascular (Virchow-Robin) space and neuroinvasion in the pediatric setting. Relevant evidence from Simian Immunodeficiency Virus (SIV) model systems is included. Understanding the dynamics and mechanisms of HIV neuroinvasion can help to provide a reasoned foundation for future decisions regarding when and how to treat HIV-associated neurological disease.

As reported in chapter III, HIV-1-associated dementia (HAD) manifests during the late stages of infection by human immunodeficiency virus as a spectrum of neurological and psychiatric symptoms. The disease process is mediated by cellular (cytokine, chemokines and others) and viral neurotoxins produced mainly by brain mononuclear phagocytes (MP; macrophages and microglia) without direct infection of neurons. The prolonged inflammatory state results in the production and release of various factors that can lead to astrocyte dysfunction and neuronal injury when produced in abundance. While the pathogenesis of this neurodegeneration still remains unclear, neuronal damage is induced by the toxins engaging specific neuronal receptors or indirectly through widespread MP/astrocyte inflammatory activities. Cytokines and chemokines play a central role in the generation of this chronic encephalopathy. A chemokine gradient established by brain MP and astrocytes initiate monocyte transendothelial migration, increase the viral reservoir, and provide cellular sources of inflammatory products. Chemokines, cytokines and viral products cause neuronal dysfunction by engaging neural receptors and activating pathways that alter synaptic transmission and neuronal function. Here, we discuss the mechanisms involved in chemokine and cytokine mediated neural compromise and disease progression in HAD.

In certain populations around the world, the HIV pandemic is driven by drug abuse. Mounting evidence suggests that these patient populations may have accelerated and more severe neurocognitive dysfunction as compared to non-drug abusing HIV infected populations. Many drugs of abuse are CNS stimulants, hence it stands to reason that these drugs may synergize with neurotoxic substances released during the course of HIV infection. Clinical and laboratory evidence suggest that the dopaminergic systems are most vulnerable to such combined neurotoxicity although multiple regions of the brain may be involved. Identifying common mechanisms of neuronal injury is critical to developing therapeutic strategies for drug abusing HIV-infected populations. Chapter IV reviews 1) the current evidence for neurodegeneration in the setting of combined HIV infection and use of methamphetamine, cocaine, heroin or alcohol, 2) the proposed underlying mechanisms involved in this combined neurotoxicity, and 3) future directions for research. This manuscript also suggests therapeutic approaches based on our current understanding of the neuropathogenesis of dementia due to HIV infection and drugs of abuse.

As reported in chapter V, HIV-1 associated dementia (HAD) is the most severe and morbid neuronal disorder caused by HIV-1 invasion of the brain. Apparent causative agents are the viral proteins acting as neurotoxins that induce neuronal apoptosis. Part I reviews contributions of viral load determinations on neuropathogenesis of HAD and efficacy tests of AIDS drugs. They serve important roles in elucidation of the mechanisms of pathogenesis and for drug development. Part II goes in detail on polymerase chain reaction (PCR) methods utilized for determination of viral load. These methods include comparative PCR for viral DNA load, competitive reverse transcription PCR for viral structural RNA and regulatory mRNA load, and real-time PCR for viral cDNA load.

As reported in chapter VI, allostasis is the set of intertwined psycho-social and physico-physiological responses that regulate the psychobiological adaptation to change in homeostasis. Homeostatic change is consequential to stimuli, which can include chronic immunological challenges such as infection with human immune deficiency virus (HIV), and the associated pathologies, which signify progression to the acquired immune deficiency syndrome (AIDS). This chapter examines salient aspects of the current state of knowledge of the psychoneuroendocrino-pathology in HIV/AIDS, and it proposes potential avenues for research and clinical breakthrough in the next decade.

Chapter VII informs about stroke in patients with human immunodeficiency virus (HIV) infection and advanced immunosuppression are mainly related to opportunistic infections, cardiac embolism from cardiomyopathy, and probably hypercoagulability. High-activity antiretroviral therapy (HAART) may now considerably limit or effectively halt the progression of immunosuppression. However, the use of protease inhibitors is associated with metabolic derangements -including dyslipidemia, lipodystrophy and insulin resistance- that might result in accelerated atherosclerosis. Therefore, patients receiving HAART may be at risk for premature vascular events, such as cerebral infarctions. In addition, a small vessel arteriopathy has been documented in HIV-infected patients and impaired vasomotor reactivity might compromise cerebral perfusion, especially as these patients age. Future studies should examine if the prevalence and mechanisms of stroke in HIV-infected patients change as the use of effective antiviral treatment continues to grow.

Chapter VIII reviews Varicella zoster virus (VZV) is an exclusively human neurotropic alphaherpesvirus. Primary infection causes chickenpox (varicella), after which virus becomes latent in ganglia along the entire neuraxis. Virus reactivation usually produces shingles (zoster) and other serious neurologic disorders. In HIV+ and AIDS patients of any age, virus reactivation is more frequent, more protracted and dissemination is more common. Neurologic complications due to VZV in AIDS patients have been found to be as high as 59%. Management of VZV infections in HIV-infected patients often requires prolonged antiviral therapy with hospitalization. Despite immunosuppression, most HIV+ and AIDS patients who develop serious neurological complications due to VZV can be treated successfully, if monitored closely and provided with aggressive antiviral therapy early in the course of infection.

As reported in chapter IX, Neuroimaging technology provides a continuously expanding array of techniques to non-invasively study the living nervous system. In patients infected with human immunodeficiency virus (HIV) or acquired immunodeficiency syndrome (AIDS), neurologic complications represent potentially treatable manifestations requiring early and accurate diagnosis. Many of the central nervous system (CNS) complications are associated with significant morbidity or death if left unrecognized. We shall provide an overview of neuroimaging methods and their role in the evaluation of patients with HIV and AIDS related CNS disorders. Emphasis will be placed on structural magnetic resonance imaging (MRI) and functional imaging. Neuroimaging is a key tool in the clinical management of this population such as in the early detection of HIV or opportunistic infections, tumors, or cerebrovascular disorders. Applications of neuroimaging in this population also include the ability to monitor treatment effects. In addition, through a variety of advanced imaging strategies, the underlying neurochemistry, metabolism, and blood flow of lesions can be studied to aid the differential diagnosis of lesions and guide further management. The authors' aim is for this chapter to be useful to trainees and practitioners in the clinical and imaging fields of general medicine, infectious diseases, and clinical neurosciences.

In chapter X, illicit drug users constitute a large proportion of the patient population contracting AIDS. The purpose of our research is to determine the mechanism by which drugs such as opioids attenuate host immune function. The Simian AIDS (SAIDS) model is among the best available animal model systems for studying human AIDS. Using the SAIDS model, we have found that monkeys chronically treated with morphine and infected with simian AIDS virus have a faster rate of viral replication and mutation and a shorter life span than infected monkeys that have not been treated with morphine. Mechanistic studies have shown that opiates modulate simian AIDS progression by (i) stimulating the expression of chemokine receptor CCR5, a co-receptor on immune cells for HIV/SIV entry and (ii) slowing down the apoptosis of SIV-infected cells, permitting the persistence and survival of the virus.

In: Neuro-AIDS
Editors: A. Minagar and P. Shapshak, pp. 1-13

ISBN: 1-59454-610-X
© 2006 Nova Science Publishers, Inc.

Chapter I

HIV-Associated Dementia: Clinical Features and Pathogenesis

Alireza Minagar[1], and Paul Shapshak[2]*

[1]Department of Neurology, Louisiana State University Health Sciences Center, USA;
[2]Dementia/HIV Laboratory, Department of Psychiatry and Behavioral Sciences,
University of Miami Miller School of Medicine , USA.

Abstract

Human immunodeficiency virus-1 (HIV-1) enters the central nervous system (CNS) early in the course of HIV-1 infection and causes a form of subcortical dementia, known as HIV-1 associated dementia (HAD). HAD is perhaps the most significant neurological complication of AIDS and poses a major diagnostic and management challenge to the clinicians. With introduction of highly active anti-retroviral therapy (HAART), the patterns of HIV-1 infection and its CNS complications have changed. Macrophage/microglia are the key cell type that are infected by HIV-1 in the CNS and are mediators of neurodegeneration in pathogenesis of HAD. This chapter mainly addresses clinical features and pathogenesis of HAD.

Keywords: Human immunodeficiency virus-1 (HIV-1); HIV-1 associated dementia (HAD); neurological complication; NeuroAIDS, neurodegeneration

---

* Correspondence concerning this article should be addressed to: Alireza Minagar, MD, Assistant Professor of Neurology, Psychiatry and Anesthesiology, Department of Neurology, Louisiana State University Health Sciences Center, 1501 Kings Highway Shreveport, LA 71130; Tel: (318) 675-4679; Fax: (318) 675-7805; Email: aminag@lsuhsc.edu. Paul Shapshak, PhD, Director, Dementia/HIV Laboratory, Dept. of Psychiatry and Beh Sci Elliot Bldg, 2013, M849, U of Miami Miller Med School, 1800 NW 10th Ave. Miami, FL 33136, cell. 786-325-4478; tel. 305-243-3917; fax: 305-243-5572; pshapsha@med.miami.edu.

Introduction

Direct involvement of the central nervous system (CNS), particularly the brain, occurs in the early phases of the HIV-1 infection (Resnick et al, 1988; Singer et al, 1994;). Indeed, it is believed that HIV enters CNS at or around the time of seroconversion despite the absence of significant clinical symptoms in most patients. HIV-1-associated dementia (HAD) describes a progressive encephalopathy that results from HIV-1-related damage to the CNS and occurs in the absence of the influence of other conditions or pathogens. Thus, it is a diagnosis of exclusion. The terms "HIV dementia", HIV-1-associated dementia", and HIV-associated cognitive/motor complex" are used synonymously although there are possible changes that are occurring in these definitions. The authors review clinical features and pathogenesis of HAD (de la Monte et al, 1987; Goodkin et al, 2000).

Clinical Manifestations

HAD is a subcortical dementia and the usual cortical manifestations such as aphasia, alexia, and agraphia that occur with cortical dementias like Alzheimer's disease are absent (Navia 1986a; Navia 1986b). Instead, patients with HAD present predominantly with disabling cognitive impairment usually accompanied by motor deficits and behavioral abnormalities (Janssen 1991). Initially, the neuropsychological profile of HAD patients demonstrates a prominence of subcortical dementia, characterized by impaired retrieval of recorded memory, impaired manipulation of acquired knowledge, and slowness of psychomotor speed and thought processes (Goodkin et al, 2000).

Neurological examination is frequently normal in the initial stages of HAD and only subtle deficits such as impairments of rapid eye and limb movements and generalized hyper-reflexia may be observed. The term minor cognitive motor disorder (MCMD) is coined to describe these early subtle abnormalities. However, MCMD is usually associated with progression of HAD and further compromise of patient's neurological status. MCMD is a significant finding in AIDS patients since the introduction of highly active anti-retroviral therapy (HAART), MCMD has become a more obvious and more common manifestation of HIV infection of the CNS (McArthur 2003). With further decline of neurological function, patient develops new learning and memory deterioration with further slowing of mental processing and language deficits. Only when the dementing process of HAD has advanced and more global deficits are present, do patients then develop cortical deficits. The clinical manifestations of HAD involve three major areas of CNS activity: cognition, motor function, and behavior. The typical patient presents with apathy, memory loss, depression, slowness of mental activities and withdrawal from usual activities. The initial manifestations of HAD may be subtle and be attributed to psychiatric disorders. Commonly, patients report loss of concentration, loss of libido, poor short term memory, blunting of emotions, loss of self-confidence and social seclusion. Price and Brew have developed a staging system for severity of HAD (Table) (Price 1988). Motor deficits in patients with HAD consist of clumsiness and poorly formed handwriting, tremor, the tendency to drop objects from their hands, and poor balance. Behavioral and neuropsychiatric abnormalities associated with HAD include memory loss with primarily difficulty with retrieving memory and data, generalized slowness of thought process, and loss of the ability to process acquired or new information. In advanced stages, there is a global impairment of intellectual abilities, which is characterized by severe psychomotor retardation and mutism.

Table. Clinical staging of AIDS dementia complex

Stage 0 (Normal)

Normal mental and motor function

Stage 0.5 (Equivocal or subclinical)

Absent, minimal, or equivocal symptoms without impairment of work or capacity to perform activities of daily living. Mild signs (snout response, slowed ocular or extremity movements) may be present. Gait and strength are normal.

Stage 1 (Mild)

Able to perform all but the more demanding aspects of work or activities of daily living, but with unequivocal evidence (signs or symptoms that may include performance of neuropsychological testing) of functional intellectual or motor impairment. Can walk without resistance.

Stage 2 (Moderate)

Able to perform basic activities of self care, but can not work or maintain the more demanding aspects of daily life. Ambulatory, but may require a single support.

Stage 3 (Severe)

Major intellectual incapacity (cannot follow news or personal events, cannot sustain complex conversation, considerable slowing of all outputs), and motor disability (cannot walk unassisted, requiring walker or personal support, usually with slowing and clumsiness of arms as well).

Stage 4 (End stage)

Nearly vegetative. Intellectual and social comprehension and output are at a rudimentary level. Nearly or absolutely mute. Paraparetic or paraplegic with urinary and fecal incontinence.

A few abnormalities, such as slowing and inaccuracy of saccadic and smooth visual pursuit movements and generalized hyper-reflexia, can be detected in the neurological examination of HAD patients in early phases of the disease. With progression of HAD, patients develop facial hypomotility, spasticity of the lower extremities, frontal release signs, tremor, inability to do tandem gait and paraparesis. A large number of these patients develop peripheral neuropathy which is associated with decrease or loss of tendon reflexes. The presence of focal neurological signs indicates development of opportunistic infections rather than HAD. In terminal stages of HAD, patients become bed-bound with abulia, global dementia, mutism, urinary and fecal incontinence, and decorticate posturing.

Risk factors for development of HAD consist of unexplained mania and seizures, pre-existing cognitive impairment, increased age, high plasma viral load (McArthur 1997), elevated CSF levels of β_2-microglobulin, elevated CSF HIV viral load and the presence of the apolipoprotein E (ε4 allele) (Cutler 2004).

Epidemiology

Due to the impact of HAART on the annual incidence of HAD, its epidemiology should be reviewed prior and post HAART. Before development of HAART, the annual incidence of HAD was 7% and cumulative risk of developing HAD during lifetime in HIV-seropositive individuals was 5-20% (McArthur 1993). Introduction of HAART has been associated with significant decrease in the incidence rates of HAD, while in 2003 the incidence rate began to increase, which may indicate failure of HAART in certain patients (McArthur 2004). In addition, since a larger number of AIDS patients are alive today and live under the HAART therapy, the prevalence of HAD is increasing.

Pathogenesis

The pathogenic mechanisms responsible for development of HAD remain only partially understood. Brain atrophy is a common finding in patients with HAD and frequently affects fronto-temporal areas. Neuropathology of HAD reveals multiple small nodules containing lymphocytes, macrophages, microglia which are scattered throughout the brain, more in the white matter and the subcortical gray matter of the basal ganglia, thalamus, and brainstem (de la Monte 1987). These inflammatory nodules are non-specific and may also be observed in the context of other infections such as toxoplasmosis and cytomegalovirus encephalitis. Multinucleated giant cells in HAD, by expression of CD14 and CD15, represent fusion of macrophages (Williams 2001; Fischer-Smith 2001) and their presence correlates with the severity of dementia (Price 1988). Perivascular infiltration of lymphocytes, monocytes, and macrophages is common in HAD and the presence of viral nucleic acid sequences in perivascular multinucleated cells and endothelial cells has been demonstrated (Wiley 1986). HAD neuropathology is characterized by the combination of multinucleated giant cells, microglial nodules, and perivascular inflammation (de la Monte 1987).

Quantitative MRI and morphometric observations have demonstrated abnormalities of the gray matter in frontal and temporal areas of brain with massive neuronal loss (Everall 1991; Wiley 1991; Ketzler 1990). In addition to these abnormalities, Masliah et al (Masliah 1992) described loss of dendritic arborization and synaptic simplifications. Such cortical abnormalities have also been termed diffuse poliodystrophy (Budka 1991). HIV leukoencephalopathy is another neuropathological manifestation of HIV infection of brain which presents with diffuse with mainly subcortical white matter damage, reactive astrocytosis, infiltration of macrophages and formation of multinucleated giant cells with minimal or absent inflammatory infiltrates). The presence of multinucleated giant cells indicates active HIV-1 replication (Budka 1991). HIV encephalitis is a much less common finding and is recognized by the presence of giant multinucleated cells, inflammatory infiltrate, and microglial nodules with subcortical distribution. Lastly, HIV-cerebral vasculitis has been reported but is uncommon (Mizusawa 1988). Brain atrophy and leptomeningeal fibrosis affects, respectively, one half and one third of patients with advanced AIDS. The cerebral atrophy in HAD patients occurs in a fronto-temporal distribution. MRI studies have demonstrated alterations of the gray matter with neuronal loss, mainly in frontal and temporal regions (Ketzler 1990; Everall 1991; Wiley 1991). Other abnormalities such as loss of dendritic arborization and synaptic simplifications have been reported (Masliah 1992).

Activated macrophages and microglia (MØ) serve as vectors for transmission of HIV-1 infection in the human subject and play a significant role in pathogenesis of HAD (Petito 2004). In the CNS, productive infection is confined to monocyte lineage cells. In addition, productive viral infection takes place in the choroid plexus, where the incidence of infection is actually higher than in brain and is present prior to the onset of AIDS and immunosuppression. Restricted or latent infection occurs in astrocytes and neurons. The presence of peri-neuronal CD4+ lymphocytes, as well as activated microglia, support the potential for a trans-receptor mechanism of viral entry whereas intrinsic gene profiles do not appear to participate in conferring selective neuronal vulnerability or resistance to infection (Petito 2004; Gorry 2005).

Productive viral replication within MØ, development of MØ multinucleated giant cell formation, microglial nodules, and infiltration of MØ within the cerebral tissue are among the characteristic features of the brain neuropathology in HAD. Indeed, the number of activated MØ in affected tissue provides the best neuropathological correlation in HAD (Glass 1995). Emergence of specific subsets of MØ, which express CD14/CD16 and CD14/CD69 surface markers with enhanced ability to secrete neurotoxins further support the pivotal role of MØ in pathogenesis of HAD (Pulliam 1997). Activated MØ demonstrate increased penetration through the BBB and secrete a wide range of immune and viral factors which affect neuronal function (Gelbard 1994; McArthur 2003; Tyor 1992). Some of these factors include the HIV proteins such as Tat, gp120, gp 41, Nef, and Rev as well as pro-inflammatory cytokines such as IFN-γ (Shapshak 2004), chemokines, arachidonic acid metabolites, quinolinic acid, TNF-α-related apoptosis-inducing agent, reactive oxygen species, and matrix metalloproteinases (Gendelman 1998; Williams 2002; Minagar 2002). Pulliam et al (Pulliam 2004) performed global gene expression analysis on CD14 (+) monocytes isolated from HIV-1-infected individuals and controls to identify HIV-1-related changes in monocyte phenotype. Monocytes from subjects with high viral load (HVL) had a significant increase in monocytes expressing CD16, CCR5, and MCP-1. There was also an elevation of sialoadhesin, a macrophage marker of chronic inflammation. Expression of proinflammatory cytokine genes IL-1, IL-6, and TNF-α was unchanged in individuals with HIV-1 compared to control CD14 (+) monocytes. Differential gene expression identified by DNA microarray analysis was confirmed with reverse transcription polymerase chain reaction (RT-PCR), while increased protein expression was characterized by immunofluorescence. The authors state that there is a circulating CD14 (+) macrophage hybrid phenotype in subjects with HVL.

In another study and in order to better understand the innate secretary function of infected MØ, Ciborowski et al (Ciborowski 2004) investigated the proteomic profiles of HIV-1-infected monocyte-derived macrophages. The investigators applied a proteomics platform consisting of one dimensional polyacrylamide gel electrophoresis (1-DE), mass spectrometry peptide sequencing, and bioinformatics to monocyte-derived macrophages to uncover the unravel the products of these cells and their relationship to disease. The results indicated that secretion of MMP-9 by the monocyte-derived macrophages was remarkably decreased following viral infection. In addition, a negative correlation between MMP-9 and HIV-1 reverse transcriptase activity was demonstrated by quantitative Western blot analysis. The results of this study lend further support to the role of immunoregulatory activities of MØ in HIV-1 infection. In another attempt to elucidate the role of MØ in pathogenesis of HAD, Albright and Gonzales-Scarano (Albright 2004) isolated two different types of primary human macrophages: microglia and monocyte-derived macrophages (MDM) from brain tissue and whole blood, respectively and performed microarray analysis of differentially regulated macrophage activation genes in the mixed glia (MIX) cultured in starvation conditions (DMEM alone). Transcript levels from these quiescent glia cultures provided a background level of gene expression and allowed for the identification of upregulated macrophage activation genes in the MIX brain cultures upon treatment with an array of soluble activation factors: serum components, cytokines, and growth factors. The investigators found that 914 genes in the MIX cultures and 734 genes in the MDM cultures had a greater than twofold increase in expression. They identified 180 genes with expression that was increased more than twofold in both culture types. In the MIX cultures, over a 100-fold increase in IL-1beta and TIMP1 transcription; Caspase 9, S100A8 and 9, MMP12, IL-8, monocyte chemotactic protein 1 (MCP1), MRC-1, and IL-6 were also upregulated. Activation of starved MDM cultures resulted in fewer upregulated genes compared to MIX cultures. Genes upregulated in both MIX and MDM included CCL2 (MCP1), CCL7, CXCL5, TNFSF14, kinases, and phosphatases. They concluded that the microarray data may provide leads for identifying previously unknown neurotoxins, disease biomarkers, and pathways responsible for the neuronal apoptosis observed in HAD and for the eventual development of therapies for HAD.

The role of HIV-1 regulatory protein Tat in HAD and its effects on MØ has been reviewed (Minghetti 2004). Tat affects the functional state of MØ and these activated MØ play a role in the neuropathology associated with HIV-1 infection. The Tat-activated MØ synthesize potentially neurotoxic molecules, including proinflammatory cytokines and free radicals, and interferes with molecular mechanisms controlling cAMP levels, intracellular [Ca2+], and ion channel expression.

The role of amyloid precursor protein (APP) in pathogenesis of HAD and its expression by circulating MØ has been studied. Vehmas et al (Vehmas, et al. 2004) examined APP surface expression on circulating leukocytes and in brain tissues from normal individuals and HIV-seropositive subjects with cognitive impairment. Most MØ, and a subset of B-lymphocytes, expressed APP, while T-lymphocytes, granulocytes, and natural killer (NK) cells did not. CD14bright/CD16+ monocytes expressed the highest levels, and CD14dim/CD16+ cells were negative, suggesting a relationship with activation. Higher APP+ MØ levels correlated with increased numbers of CD16+ monocytes, but not with the degree of cognitive impairment. In the brain, APP appeared as axonal immunoreactivity and diffuse plaques, and APP+ perivascular macrophages were seen in cases with severe dementia. The authors concluded that APP may facilitate monocyte entry into the brain.

Astrocytes are the other participants in pathogenesis of HAD and accumulating evidence demonstrate the fact that HIV-1 also infects these CD4-negative brain resident cells (Brack-

Werner 1999; Wang 2004). The presence of infected astrocytes has been reported in various areas of brain, scattered throughout the white matter (Anderson 2003; Tornatore 1994). Despite the fact that MØ are the major cells infected by HIV-1, the infection of even a small number of astrocytes with HIV-1 can have dire consequences for neurons. For example, it has been shown that exposure of human fetal astrocytes (HFAs) in culture to HIV-1 causes a decrease in expression of the glutamate transporter EAAT2 and impair glutamate uptake (Wang 2003). In addition, exposure of HFAs to HIV-1 or to viral gp120 or Tat can exert diffuse effects on the cellular gene expression. However, in vitro cultures of astrocytes reveal that only 1% of HFAs permits virus expression and infection of these cells by HIV-1 is very limited (Bencheikh 1999; He 1997). In order to further elucidate the role of HIV-1-expressing astrocytes in pathogenesis of HAD, Kim et al (Kim 2004 infected human fetal astrocytes with pseudotyped HIV-1 and applied Affymetrix oligonucleotide microarrays to assess global changes in cellular gene expression at the peak of virus production. With a twofold change as a cutoff, HIV-1 increased transcription of 266 genes in astrocytes and suppressed expression of 468. The functions of highly expressed genes consisted of interferon-mediated antiviral responses (OAS1, IFIT1), intercellular contacts (SH3, glia-derived nexin), cell homing/adhesion (matrix metalloproteinases), and cell-cell signaling (neuropilin 1 and 2). Interestingly, genes involved in innate immune responses of astrocytes were largely unaffected. The single most significant effect of HIV-1, however, was down-modulation of at least 55 genes involved in control of cell cycle, DNA replication, and cell proliferation, which were overrepresented in these categories with probability scores of 10(-10)-10(-26). The authors concluded that suggest that HIV-1 expression in astrocytes profoundly alters host cell biology, with potential consequences for the physiological function of astrocytes during HIV-1 infection in the brain.

A new interesting component of HAD pathogenesis is acquired neuronal channelopathies. Gelman et al. (Gelman 2004) using Affymetrix HG-U133 chips performed gene expression profiling of the human brain cortex of patients with HAD and the investigators compared messenger RNA transcripts in the middle frontal gyrus from patients with HAD or milder neurocognitive dysfunction with HIV-negative individuals. The analysis was focused on ionic conductance carriers which control membrane excitation. Over-expressed ionic channel genes in brain cortex of patients with HAD included calcium-driven K+; a leak type of K+ channel; an adenosine receptor which modulates cationic current via G proteins; a G protein-coupled serotonin receptor that modulates cyclic-AMP linked current transduction; a G-protein coupled dopamine receptor; a GABA receptor subunit which conducts chloride current. Under-expressed current generators in demented patients included two voltage gated K^+ channels which influence refractory periods, a Na^+ channel subunit which modifies current inactivation and the onset of after hyperpolarization, a neuronal type of voltage sensitive Ca^{+2} channels which controls postsynaptic membrane excitability, a metabotropic glutamate receptor which regulates cationic gating via G protein coupling, a specific Gα protein which transduces cationic current, an NMDA receptor subunit, and a glycine receptor subunit which modulates chloride current. The authors concluded that these channelopathies were indicative of disruption of neuronal excitability which was consistent with some features of HAD, including its potential reversibility after HIV replication is suppressed, the abnormal EEG recordings, the lack of clear cut correlation with neurodegeneration, and the lack of strict correlation with brain inflammation.

HIV Transmission and HAD Genetics

We have previously reviewed the roles chemokines as well as cytokines play in the pathogenesis of HAD (Shapshak et al, 2000). This is a rapidly moving field and several key issues have been raised (Gonzalez et al, 2001; Gonzalez, et al, 2002; Mummidi, et al, 2000, Mummidi, et al. 1998). The major chemokines and chemokine receptors which are involved in pathogenesis of HAD consist of: CXCL8/IL-8 (receptors: CXCR1 and CXCR2), CXCL10/IP10 (receptor: CXCR3, CXCL12/SDF1α/SDF1β (receptor: CXCR4), CCL2/MCP1 (receptor: CXCR4), CCL3/MIP1α (receptors: CCR1 and CCR5), CCL4/MIP1β (receptor: CCR5), CCL5/RANTES (receptors: CCR1, CCR3, and CCR5), CCL7/MCP3 (receptors: CCR1, CCR2, and CCR3), and CX$_3$CL1/Fractalkine (receptor: CX$_3$CR1) (Gonzalez-Scarano 2005; Martin-Garcia 2004).

Single nucleotide polymorphism (SNIP) mapping of immune response-related genes were described world-wide as well as within the USA that impact on disease progression and the risk for HAD. Analysis of CCR5 haplotypes as well as RANTES and MIP-1a and the CC chemokine receptor 5 gene have supported their role in the spread of HIV globally as well as more restricted ethnic groups (Gonzalez et al, 2001; Mummidi et al, 2000). More specifically, there is a spectrum of CCR5 haplotype pairs that associate with altered HIV-1 susceptibility and mother to child transmission (Mangano et al, 2000). Furthermore, these roles impact on brain infection and they must be understood in that context (Martin-Garcia et al, 2002). Thus, HIV-1infectoin and AIDS dementia are affected by specific combinations of haplotypes of mutant MCP-1 alleles that actually link to physiological to infiltration of tissues by HIV-1 strains as well as MCP-1 levels in the patients (Gonzalez et al, 2002).

Diagnosis

Diffusion weighted imaging (DWI) has been recently used to assess changes in the brain white matter diffusion and to determine whether the obtained findings correlate with neuropsychological test performances. Filippi et al (Filippi 2001) reported an increase in mean diffusivity of frontal and parietal white matter in HIV patients. Cloak and colleagues (Cloak 2004) applied DWI, MR spectroscopy, and neuropsychology testing to 11 HIV-seropositive subjects and 14 seronegative subjects. The apparent diffusion coefficient (ADC) was remarkably increased in HIV patients, primarily in the frontal white matter. Diffusivity showed a positive correlation with the glial marker myo-inositol and a negative correlation with cognitive performance. The authors concluded that increased brain water diffusion may indicate increased glial activation or inflammation, which in turn, may contribute to the cognitive impairment in HIV patients.

Differential Diagnosis

The initial stages of HAD can potentially be mistaken as depression, mania, anxiety, opportunistic infections of the CNS, the adverse effects of psychoactive medications, and nutritional deficiencies. It is very important to differentiate HAD from certain common infections among these patients such as CNS toxoplasmosis, neurosyphilis, tuberculous or cryptoccocal meningitis, CMV encephalitis, and CNS lymphoma. In addition, these disorders may coexist with HAD and further complicate the clinical picture.

Diagnostic Work up

Diagnosis of HAD rests upon meticulous neurologic, laboratory, and neuroimaging assessment. A comprehensive neuropsychological examination provides clinicians by the various patterns of cognitive impairment observed in HAD as well as objective assessment of the severity of these cognitive deficits. Since HAD is a subcortical dementia, usually at the initial stages patients' attention, concentration, and language are unimpaired. On the other hand, memory loss, both verbal and non-verbal, as well as slowing of psychomotor speed are prominent features of HAD. Certain features that are useful for diagnosis of HAD include HIV-1 sero-positivity; a history of progressive cognitive and behavioral impairment accompanied by apathy, memory loss, slowness of mental processing; diffuse abnormalities on neurological examination such as slowed rapid eye movements, hyperactive reflexes, hypertonia, and the presence of release signs; abnormal neuropsychological assessment with prominent abnormalities in at least two areas including frontal lobe, motor speed, and non-verbal memory; CSF analysis reveals elevated β-2 microglobulin level, elevated IgG and protein level while other possible co-infections such as neurosyphilis and cryptococcal meningitis have been excluded; abnormal MRI findings which indicate ill-defined areas of hyperintensities involving white matter; absence of depression or any other major psychiatric disorder; absence of any metabolic abnormalities such as septic encephalopathy and hypoxia; and absence of any active CNS opportunistic infections.

References

Albright, A.V., and Gonzalez-Scarano, F., (2004). Microarray analysis of activated mixed glial (microglia) and monocyte-derived macrophage gene expression. *J. Neuroimmunol, 157*, 27-38.

Anderson, C. E., Tomlinson, G. S., Pauly B, Brannan, F. W., Chiswick, A., Brack-Werner, R., Simmonds, P., Bell, J. E., (2003). Relationship of Nef-positive and GFAP-reactive astrocytes to drug use in early and late HIV infection. *Neuropathol. Appl. Neurobiol, 29*:378-388.

Bencheikh, M., Bentsman, G., Sarkissian, N., Canki, M., and Volsky, D. J., (1999). Replication of different clones of human immunodeficiency virus type 1 in primary fetal human astrocytes: enhancement of viral gene expression by Nef. *J. Neurovirol,* 5:115-124.

Brack-Werner, R., (1999). Astrocytes: HIV cellular reservoirs and important participants in neuropathogenesis. *AIDS,;13*:1-22.

Budka, H., Wiley, C. A., Kleihues, P., Artigas, J., Asbury, A. K., Cho, E. S., Cornblath, D. R., Dal Canto, M. C., et al (1991). HIV-associated disease of the nervous system: review of nomenclature and proposal for neuropathology-based terminology. *Brain Pathol,* *1*,143-152.

Ciborowski, P., Enose, Y., Mack, A., Fladseth, M., and Gendelman, H. E., (2004). Diminished matrix metalloproteinase 9 secretion in human immunodeficiency virus-infected mononuclear phagocytes: modulation of innate immunity and implications for neurological disease. *J. Neuroimmunol, 157,* 11-16.

Cloak, C. C., Chang, L., and Ernst. T., (2004). Increased frontal white matter diffusion is associated with glial metabolites and psychomotor slowing in HIV. *J. Neuroimmunol,157,* 147-152.

Cutler, R. G., Haughey, N. J., Tammara, A., McArthur, J. C., et al., (2004). Dysregulation of sphingolipid and sterol metabolism by ApoE4 in HIV dementia. *Neurology, 63,* 626-630.

de la Monte, S. M., Ho, D. D., Schooley, R. T., Hirsch, M. S., and Richardson, E. P, Jr., (1987). Subacute encephalomyelitis of AIDS and its relation to HTLV-III infection. *Neurology, 37,* 562-569.

Everall, I. P., Luthert, P. J., and Lantos, P. L., (1991). Neuronal loss in the frontal cortex in HIV infection. *Lancet, 337,* 1119-1121.

Filippi, C., Ulug, A. M., Lin, D., Heier, L. A., and Zimmerman, R. D., (2001). Diffusion tensor imaging of patients with HIV and normal-appearing white matter on MR images of the brain. *AJNR Am. J. Neurotadiol, 22,* 277-283.

Fischer-Smith, T., Croul, S., Sverstiuk, A. E., Capini, C., L'Heureux, D., et al., (2001). CNS invasion by CD14+/CD16+ peripheral blood-derived monocytes in HIV dementia: perivascular accumulation and reservoir of HIV infection. *J. Neurovirol, 7,* 528-541.

Gelbard, H. A., Nottet, H. S., Swindells, S., Jett, M., Dzenko, K. A., et al., (1994). Platelet-activating factor: a candidate human immunodeficiency virus type 1-induced neurotoxin. *J. Virol, 68,* 4628-4635.

Gelman, B. B., Soukup, V. M., Schuenke, K. W., Keherly, M. J., Holzer, C. 3rd, Richey, F. J., and Lahart, C. J., (2004). Acquired neuronal channelopathies in HIV-associated dementia. *J. Neuroimmunol,157,* 111-119.

Gendelman, H. E., Zheng, J., Coulter, C. L., et al., (1998). Suppression of inflammatory neurotoxins by highly active antiretroviral therapy in human immunodeficiency virus-associated dementia. *J. Infect. Dis,178,*1000-1007.

Glass, J. D., Fedor, H., Wesselingh, S. L., McArthur, J. C., (1995). Immunocytochemical quantitation of human immunodeficiency virus in the brain: correlations with dementia. *Ann. Neurol, 38,* 755-762.

Gonzalez-Scarano, F., and Martin-Garcia, J., (2005). The neuropathogenesis of AIDS. *Nat. Rev. Immunol, 5,* 69-81.

Gonzalez, E., Rovin, B. H., Sen, L., et al., (2002). HIV-1 infection and AIDS dementia are influenced by a mutant MCP-1 allele linked to increased monocyte infiltration of tissues and MCP-1 levels. *Proc. Natl. Acad. Sci U S A, 99*:13795-13800.

Gonzalez, E., Dhanda, R., Bamshad, M., et al., (2001). Global survey of genetic variation in CCR5, RANTES, and MIP-1alpha: impact on the epidemiology of the HIV-1 pandemic. *Proc. Natl. Acad. Sci. U S A,98,*:5199-5204.

Goodkin, K., Shapshak, P., Fujimura, R. K., Tuttle, R. S., et al. (2000). Immune function, brain, and HIV-1 infection, in Goodkin K, and A Visser (eds): *Psychoneuroimmunology: Stress, Mental Disorders and Health,* Washington, DC: American Psychiatric Association Press, Inc., pp. 243-316.

Gorry, P. R., Churchill, M., Crowe, S. M., Cunningham, A. L., and Gabuzda, D., (2005). Pathogenesis of macrophage tropic HIV-1. *Curr. HIV Res,3,* 53-60.

He, J., Chen, Y., Farzan, M., Choe, H., Ohagen, A., Gartner, S., et al. (1997). CCR3 and CCR5 are co-receptors for HIV-1 infection of microglia. *Nature, 385,* 645-649.

Janssen, R. S., Cornbalth, D. R., Epstein, L. G., et al. (2001). Nomenclature and research care definitions for neurological manifestations of human immunodeficiency virus type-1 (HIV-1) infection. *Report from a working group of the American Academy of Neurology AIDS Task Force Neurology, 41,* 778-785.

Ketzler, S., Weis, S., Haug, H., and Budka, H., (1990). Loss of neurons in the frontal cortex in AIDS brains. *Acta Neuropathol. (Berl), 80*:92-94.

Kim, S. Y., Li, J., Bentsman, G., Brooks, A. I., and Volsky, D. J., (2004). Microarray analysis of changes in cellular gene expression induced by productive infection of primary human astrocytes: implications for HAD. *J. Neuroimmunol, 157,* 17-26.

Mizusawa, H., Hirano, A., Llena, J. F., and Shintaku, M., (1988). Cerebrovascular lesions in acquired immune deficiency syndrome (AIDS). *Acta Neuropathol. (Berl),*76, 451-457.

Mangano, A., Kopka, J., Batalla, M., Bologna, R., and Sen, L., (2000). Protective effect of CCR2-64I and not of CCR5-delta32 and SDF1-3'A in pediatric HIV-1 infection. *J. Acquir. Immune. Defic. Syndr,23,*:52-57.

Martin-Garcia, J., Kolson, D. L., and Gonzalez-Scarano, F., (2002). Chemokine receptors in the brain: their role in HIV infection and pathogenesis. *AIDS,16,* 1709-1730.

Masliah, E., Ge, N., Morey, M., DeTeresa, R., Terry, R. D., and Wiley, C. A., (1992). Cortical dendritic pathology in human immunodeficiency virus encephalitis. *Lab. Invest, 66,*285-291.

McArthur, J. C., Hoover, D. R., et al., (1993). Dementia in AIDS patients: incidence and risk factors. Multicenter AIDS Cohort Study. *Neurology, 43,* 2245-2252.

McArthur, J. C., (2004). HIV dementia: an evolving disease. *J Neuroimmunol, 157,* :3-10.

McArthur, J. C., Haughey, N., Gartner, S., et al., (2003). Human immunodeficiency virus-associated dementia: an evolving disease. *J. Neurovirol, 9,*205-221.

McArthur, J. C., (1987). Neurologic manifestations of AIDS. *Medicine, 66,* 407-437.

Minagar, A., Shapshak, P., Fujimura, R., et al., (2002). The role of macrophage/microglia and astrocytes in the pathogenesis of three neurologic disorders: HIV-associated dementia, Alzheimer disease, and multiple sclerosis. *J. Neurol. Sci, 202,* :13-23.

Minghetti, L., Visentin, S., Patrizio, M., et al., (2004). Multiple actions of the human immunodeficiency virus type-1 Tat protein on microglial cell functions. *Neurochem. Res, 29*, 965-978.

Mummidi, S., Ahuja, S. S., Gonzalez, E., et al., (1998). Genealogy of the CCR5 locus and chemokine system gene variants associated with altered rates of HIV-1 disease progression. *Nat. Med, 4,* :786-93.

Mummidi S, Bamshad M, Ahuja SS, et al., (2000). Evolution of human and non-human primate CC chemokine receptor 5 gene and mRNA. Potential roles for haplotype and mRNA diversity, differential haplotype-specific transcriptional activity, and altered transcription factor binding to polymorphic nucleotides in the pathogenesis of HIV-1 and simian immunodeficiency virus. *J. Biol. Chem, 275,*18946-18961.

Navia, B. A., Jordan, B. D., and Price, R. W., (1986a). The AIDS dementia complex: I. Clinical features. *Ann. Neurol, 19,* 517-24.

Navia, B. A., Cho, E. S., Petito, C. K., and Price, R, W., (1986b). The AIDS dementia complex: II. Neuropathology. *Ann. Neurol, 19,* 525-535.

Petito, C. K., (2004). Human immunodeficiency virus type 1 compartmentalization in the central nervous system. *J. Neurovirol, 10 Suppl 1,* 21-24.

Price, R. W., Sidtis, J., and Rosenblum, M., (1988). AIDS dementia complex: some current questions. *Ann. Neurol, 23(suppl),* S27-33.

Pulliam, L., Sun, B., and Rempel, H., (2004). Invasive chronic inflammatory monocyte phenotype in subjects with high HIV-1 viral load. *J. Neuroimmunol,157,* 93-98.

Pulliam, L., Gascon, R,, Stubblebine, M., McGuire, D., and McGrath, M. S., (1997). Unique monocyte subset in patients with AIDS dementia. *Lancet, 349,* 692-695.

Resnick L, Berger JR, Shapshak P, Tourtellotte WW: Early penetration of the blood-brain-barrier by HTLV-III/LAV, *Neurology,* 38, 9-15, 1988.

Shapshak, P., Duncan, R., Minagar, A., Rodriguez de la Vega, P., Stewart, R. V., and Goodkin, K., (2004). Elevated expression of IFN-gamma in the HIV-1 infected brain. *Front Biosci, 9,* 1073-1081.

Shapshak, P., Fujimura, R. K., and Goodkin, K., (2000), Dementia and the Neurovirulence of HIV-1, CNS Spectrums. *Internat. Psych. J, 5,* 31-42.

Singer EJ, Syndulko K, Fahy-Chandon BN, Shapshak P, Resnick L, Schmid P, Conrad AJ, and Tourtellotte WW, Cerebrospinal fluid p24 antigen levels and intrathecal immunoglobulin G synthesis are associated with cognitive disease severity in HIV-1, AIDS, 8, 197-204, 1994.

Tornatore, C., Chandra, R., Berger, J. R., and Major, E. O., (1994). HIV-1 infection of subcortical astrocytes in the pediatric central nervous system. *Neurology, 44,* 481-487.

Tyor, W. R., Glass, J. D., Griffin, J. W., et al., (1992). Cytokine expression in the brain during the acquired immunodeficiency syndrome. *Ann. Neurol, 31,* 349-360.

Vehmas, A., Lieu, J., Pardo, C. A., McArthur, J. C., and Gartner, S., (2004). Amyloid precursor protein expression in circulating monocytes and brain macrophages from patients with HIV-associated cognitive impairment. *J. Neuroimmunol, 157,* 99-110.

Wang Z, Trillo-Pazos G, Kim SY, Canki M, Morgello S, Sharer LR, Gelbard HA, Su, Z. Z., Kang, D. C., Brooks, A. I., et al., (2004). Effects of human immunodeficiency virus type

1 on astrocyte gene expression and function: potential role in neuropathogenesis. *J. Neurovirol, 10 Suppl 1,* 25-32.

Wang Z, Pekarskaya O, Bencheikh M, Chao W, Gelbard HA, Ghorpade A, Rothstein JD, Volsky DJ. Reduced expression of glutamate transporter EAAT2 and impaired glutamate transport in human primary astrocytes exposed to HIV-1 or gp120. *Virology, 312,* 60-73.

Wiley, C. A., Schrier, R. D., Nelson, J. A., Lampert, P. W., and Oldstone, M. B., (1986). Cellular localization of human immunodeficiency virus infection within the brains of acquired immune deficiency syndrome patients. *Proc. Natl. Acad. Sci. U S A, 83,* 7089-7093.

Wiley, C. A., Masliah, E., Morey, M., et al., (1991). Neocortical damage during HIV infection. *Ann. Neurol, 29,* 651-657.

Williams, K. C., and Hickey, W. F., (2002). Central nervous system damage, monocytes and macrophages, and neurological disorders in AIDS. *Annu. Rev. Neurosci, 25,* 537-562.

Williams KC, Corey S, Westmoreland SV, et al., (2001). Perivascular macrophages are the primary cell type productively infected by simian immunodeficiency virus in the brains of macaques: implications for the neuropathogenesis of AIDS. *J. Exp. Med, 193,* 905-915.

In: Neuro-AIDS
Editors: A. Minagar and P. Shapshak, pp. 15-40

ISBN 1-59454-610-X
© 2006 Nova Science Publishers, Inc.

Chapter II

Mechanisms of HIV Entry into the CNS

Suzanne Gartner[*]

Department of Neurology, Johns Hopkins University School of Medicine,
Baltimore, MD, USA.

Abstract

This chapter will focus on HIV neuroinvasion---the timing, modes and sites of viral entry into the brain, and the potential impact of antiretroviral therapy on this entry. The question of when HIV enters the brain is particularly important to issues of viral latency and persistence, and the potential for the brain to serve as a significant viral reservoir. Answers to the questions of timing and mode of entry can also help to better delineate the relationship between HIV infection and replication within the brain, and the development of dementia. HIV neuroinvasion during early and late-stage infection, as well as throughout the course of infection, is discussed, along with the potential impact on timing of viral strain specificity, the immune response and compromise of the blood-brain barrier. HIV entry into the brain via cell-free virions and infected leukocytes, particularly monocytes, is considered, with attention to issues pertaining to the blood-brain barrier, the perivascular (Virchow-Robin) space and neuroinvasion in the pediatric setting. Relevant evidence from Simian Immunodeficiency Virus (SIV) model systems is included. Understanding the dynamics and mechanisms of HIV neuroinvasion can help to provide a reasoned foundation for future decisions regarding when and how to treat HIV-associated neurological disease.

Keywords: HIV, monocyte, macrophage, brain, neuroinvasion

---

[*] Correspondence concerning this article should be addressed to Suzanne Gartner, Johns Hopkins Hospital, Meyer 6-181, 600 N. Wolfe St., Baltimore, MD 21287. Tele: 410-614-4509; FAX: 410-502-6737; Email: sgartne1@jhem.jhmi.edu.

Introduction

HIV infection can lead to the development of neurological disease. Both the central and peripheral nervous systems may be affected. Disease within the brain can result from the systemic consequences of the infection, such as in the case of opportunistic infections and neoplasms associated with immune suppression. Cognitive impairment and/or motor disorders may also develop, and manifest as either mild or severe dysfunction. Interestingly, the course of this cognitive impairment varies considerably, with some afflicted individuals progressing rapidly to a profound level of dementia, while others remain stable with minimal impairment for long periods. The terms minor cognitive-motor disorder (MCMD) and HIV-associated dementia (HAD) are often used to distinguish these clinical entities. Whether these changes in cognition represent a continuum with a shared etiology is unclear. Typically, however, HAD does not present prior to AIDS, suggesting a possible link with systemic events.

This chapter will focus on HIV neuroinvasion---the timing, modes and sites of viral entry into the brain, and the potential impact of antiretroviral (ARV) therapy on this entry. The question of when HIV enters the brain is particularly important to issues of viral latency and persistence, and the potential for the brain to serve as a significant viral reservoir. Moreover, answers to the questions of timing and mode of entry can help to better delineate the relationship between HIV infection and replication within the brain, and the development of dementia. Thus, an accurate understanding of HIV neuroinvasion can also provide critically-needed new insight into the mechanisms of HIV neuropathogenesis.

Timing of Viral Entry

Viral Entry Early in Infection

Considerable evidence indicates that HIV can enter the brain during acute (primary) infection (Carne, Tedder, Smith, Sutherland, Elkington, Daly, Preston, and Craske, 1985; Davis, Hjelle, Miller, Palmer, Llewellyn, Merlin, Young, Mills, Wachsman, and Wiley, 1992; Hardy, Daar, Sokolov, and Ho, 1991; Ho, Rota, Schooley, Kaplan, Allan, Groopman, Resnick, Felsenstein, Andrews, and Hirsch, 1985; Piette, Tusseau, Vignon, Chapman, Parrot, Leibowitch, and Montagnier, 1986; Resnick, Berger, Shapshak, and Tourtellotte, 1988). Early in the epidemic, several groups reported the presence of neurological symptoms, usually in association with systemic features of infection such as fever, myalgia and truncal rash, during seroconversion to HIV (Allworth and Kemp, 1989; Piette et. al., 1986). Acute encephalopathy, including the presence of seizures, was also seen; most of these patients exhibited impairment of cognition and motor function, as well (Allworth and Kemp, 1989; Hardy et. al., 1991). Importantly, in essentially all cases, the neurological symptoms resolved and frequently, this occurred within days of presentation. The kinetics of this resolution suggests an association with the development of an anti-HIV immune response within the CNS, which has been documented in some cases (Goudsmit, de Wolf, Paul, Epstein, Lange, Krone, Speelman, Wolters, Van der Noordaa, Oleske, and et al., 1986), and more definitively in the SIV model system (Smith, Heyes, and Lackner, 1995). Some of the most insightful information regarding neuroinvasion during acute HIV infection comes from a case of accidental inoculation (Davis et. al., 1992). Although the individual received zidovudine within 45 minutes of the infusion error, he experienced acute HIV infection and died 15 days later. Other therapeutic intervention included treatment with dideoxyinosine and interferon-α. HIV DNA was detected in several regions of his post-mortem brain tissue by PCR and the virus was isolated from the parietal lobe (the only region investigated in this way). Interestingly, however, immunostaining for HIV p24 yielded negative results in the brain, although there were rare infiltrating gp41-positive cells present within perivascular and subpial spaces, and also around the site of a past infarction. Since gp41 has been shown to cross-reactive with a nonviral protein associated with macrophage activation (Chen, Susanna, Steindl, Katinger, and Dierich, 1994), the positive staining seen may represent artifact. Mild perivascular cuffing and a mild lymphocytic meningitis were seen during histological evaluation of the brain, but there were no giant cells, glial nodules or white matter abnormalities. The infectious dose of the inoculum was determined to be 600-700 tissue culture infectious doses ($TCID_{50}$). Neurological symptoms were present and progressed; these were thought to reflect hepatic encephalopathy, although the patient, who was 68 years old, had prior evidence of a mild dementia and a history of severe alcoholism. Of relevance, he never developed pharyngitis, myalgia, a rash, generalized lymphadenopathy, headache or any other conditions indicative of a symptomatic primary HIV infection. Clearly, HIV entered the brain of this individual during an asymptomatic acute infection. The paucity of detectable HIV expression, however, is somewhat unexpected and suggests that significant viral replication may not necessarily follow entry into the brain, even during systemic primary infection. This has implications for the issues of viral latency and the mode of viral entry, be it cell-free or cell-associated. These will be discussed in greater detail later.

SIV infection in macaques is an excellent model for both HIV infection and disease, including the development of neurological disease (Chakrabarti, Hurtrel, Maire, Vazeux, Dormont, Montagnier, and Hurtrel, 1991; Hurtrel, Chakrabarti, Hurtrel, Maire, Dormont, and Montagnier, 1991; Mankowski, Clements, and Zink, 2002; Ringler, Hunt, Desrosiers, Daniel, Chalifoux, and King, 1988; Sasseville and Lackner, 1997; Smith et. al., 1995). Several excellent reports have detailed early SIV neuroinvasion (Chakrabarti et. al., 1991; Mankowski et. al., 2002; Smith et. al., 1995). These should not be overlooked by those interested in HIV neuroinvasion, as the processes and events involved appear quite similar. In a study of early SIV infection in rhesus macaques inoculated intravenously with (uncloned) SIVmac251, Chakrabarti and colleagues found that CNS infection was a frequent and early event, and that virus-expressing cells were detectable within the brain as early as 7 days post infection (Chakrabarti et. al., 1991). These cells were mainly CD68+ and located within the perivascular space, bringing the authors to conclude that they were likely blood-derived monocytes which had crossed the blood-brain barrier (BBB). While the virus-expressing cells were confined to the perivascular space (PVS) at day 7, at 1, 2, and 3 months post-inoculation (p.i.) they were also seen beyond the PVS, within macrophages associated with microglial nodules, as well as scattered throughout the brain parenchyma. This could reflect spread of the virus infection or migration of infected cells from the perivascular space into the parenchyma. A similar study by the same group, in which a significantly higher viral inoculum was used yielded comparable results (Hurtrel, Chakrabarti, Hurtrel, and Montagnier, 1993). Here, quantitation of the virus-expressing cells was performed. At day 7, the average number of expressing cells was 8 per 2 cm^2 area, while at day 30, it was only 3 per 2 cm^2 in the same region of brain. In situ hybridization for viral mRNA was performed using probes for both an SIV regulatory (nef) and structural (env) gene and comparison of the two indicated that the low level of virus expression seen was likely not a consequence of a block at the level of viral transcription.

Viral Entry throughout the Course of Infection

In addition to HIV entry into the brain during acute infection, there might also be continual entry of infected monocytes or free virions throughout the course of infection. Monocyte trafficking into the brain occurs at low levels under normal conditions (Hickey, 1999; Hickey, 2001), in the absence of any compromise of the BBB. These cells enter the brain via transendothelial migration and take up residence within the perivascular space, at least initially (Hickey, Vass, and Lassmann, 1992). They act as scavengers and are thought to play a role in immune function (Bechmann, Priller, Kovac, Bontert, Wehner, Klett, Bohsung, Stuschke, Dirnagl, and Nitsch, 2001; Hickey and Kimura, 1988). Their turnover rate is thought to be on the order of 3 months, whereas the resident microglia persist for years (Bechmann et. al., 2001; Hickey et. al., 1992; Unger, Sung, Manivel, Chenggis, Blazar, and Krivit, 1993). Information regarding the level of HIV brain infection during the asymptomatic stage is limited, but that available indicates that the levels are typically low (Bell, Busuttil, Ironside, Rebus, Donaldson, Simmonds, and Peutherer, 1993; Sinclair, Gray, Ciardi, and Scaravilli, 1994). For example, Bell and colleagues performed quantitative DNA PCR on brain tissues from 13 HIV+ asymptomatic subjects who died suddenly. No HIV DNA was detected in 6 of the brains, and only very low levels were seen in the other 7 (Bell et. al., 1993). Similarly, Sinclair et al detected HIV DNA in only two of eight brains specimens taken from asymptomatic individuals (Sinclair et. al., 1994). Moreover, as evidenced by the lack of viral RNA and proteins, HIV expression is typically absent from the brain during the asymptomatic stage (Gray, Lescs, Keohane, Paraire, Marc, Durigon, and Gherardi, 1992; Sinclair et. al., 1994). These low levels could reflect a continual reseeding and/or the persistence of HIV genomes which entered during acute infection. Phylogenetic analyses might provide insight into this question, but more relevant studies are required. Many of the studies of HIV DNA sequences present in brain have been limited to examination of the V3 hypervariable region of the gp160 envelope gene (Chang, Jozwiak, Wang, Ng, Ge, Bolton, Dwyer, Randle, Osborn, Cunningham, and Saksena, 1998; Di Stefano, Wilt, Gray, Dubois-Dalcq, and Chiodi, 1996; Epstein, Kuiken, Blumberg, Hartman, Sharer, Clement, and Goudsmit, 1991). This region is relatively short and tends to be significantly conserved in brain, owing to its relationship to macrophage-tropism, a typical characteristic of HIV brain viruses. Hence, while it can provide important information regarding HIV tissue and cell compartmentalization, it cannot provide the level of subspecies discrimination needed. In an analysis of HIV gag (p17) sequences and sequences spanning the V1-V2 region of env, Hughes and coworkers found that genetic diversity among gag sequences from lymphoid tissues was consistently lower than that present in brain (Hughes, Bell, and Simmonds, 1997). The calculated age of the viral populations in lymphoid tissue ranged from 2.65-5.6 years, compared with 4.1-6.2 years for the populations in brain, leading the authors to conclude that in two of the study subjects, HIV genetic evolution may have occurred early, several years prior to the onset of AIDS. Moreover, in a study of V1-V5 sequences from multiple regions of brain, Shapshak and colleagues observed regional clustering, suggestive of independent evolution of HIV species within different regions of the same brain (Shapshak, Segal, Crandall, Fujimura, Zhang, Xin, Okuda, Petito, Eisdorfer, and Goodkin, 1999). These fndings are intriguing and demonstrate the potential of HIV genetics to help answer questions relating to both timing and mode of viral entry into the brain.

Limited SIV viral genetics studies have also addressed the question of timing of viral entry. Using their SIV rapid progressor model, which features accelerated development of SIV encephalitis and disease progression in general, Clements and colleagues observed "steady-state" levels of viral DNA throughout the first 56 days following inoculation, whereas viral RNA, which was detectable at significant levels at day 10, was absent from the brain at day 21 (Clements, Babas, Mankowski, Suryanarayana, Piatak, Tarwater, Lifson, and Zink, 2002). The authors also examined sequences of the V1 hypervariable region of the envelope gene recovered at day 56 from brain DNA and RNA and from PBMC RNA from a macaque with widespread viral replication and mild SIV encephalitis. The neurovirulent molecular clone, SIV/17E-Fr, predominated in both the brain DNA and RNA, but was not represented among molecular clones recovered from the PBMC RNA. This lack of sequence homology between the brain- and circulating leukocyte-derived viral species suggests that trafficking cells may not be entering the brain during the asymptomatic stage of infection, or near the late stage. However, only PBMC RNA, and not DNA, was examined, so only viral strains actively replicating within the PBMC would be detectable. Reported studies, as well as unpublished work from our laboratory, suggest that circulating monocytes are often quiescently infected (Sonza, Mutimer, Oelrichs, Jardine, Harvey, Dunne, Purcell, Birch, and Crowe, 2001). HIV and SIV replication and particle production in monocyte/macrophages is tightly linked to the state of differentiation of the cell (Schuitemaker, Kootstra, Koppelman, Bruisten, Huisman, Tersmette, and Miedema, 1992; Sonza, Maerz, Deacon, Meanger, Mills, and Crowe, 1996; Triques and Stevenson, 2004), and blood monocytes typically require some level of maturation before they can support active viral replication (Kalter, Nakamura, Turpin, Baca, Hoover, Dieffenbach, Ralph, Gendelman, and Meltzer, 1991; Rich, Chen, Zack, Leonard, and O'Brien, 1992). SIV/17E-Fr replicates well in macaque blood monocytes (Flaherty, Hauer, Mankowski, Zink, and Clements, 1997). Also, monocytes generally represent only about 5-10% of the PBMC population. It is conceivable, therefore, that in contrast to what was found in PBMC RNA, the SIV subspecies present within DNA recovered from circulating purified monocytes might include a predominance of SIV/17E-Fr. This would reflect latent infection of the monocytes. More information is needed, however, to determine if there is low-level seeding of the brain with HIV (or SIV) throughout the asymptomatic stage. Such seeding would more likely be mediated by infected monocytes taking advantage of a normal physiological process.

Viral Entry Late in Infection

Previously, we have proposed that an initial *critical* step towards the development of HIV dementia is an *increase* in the trafficking of blood monocytes into the brain, and that this increase is a consequence of systemic events that occur with, and after, the onset of AIDS (Gartner, 2000). In a study of HIV gp160 sequences recovered from DNA prepared from lymphoid tissues and multiple regions of brain from a patient with HIV dementia, we observed high homology between sequences from brain parenchymal deep white matter and bone marrow, and moreover, sequences recovered from DNA from blood monocytes collected 5 months earlier were even more genetically similar (Liu, Tang, McArthur, Scott, and Gartner, 2000). These findings support the idea that bone marrow-derived monocytes traffic into the brain. They also suggest that bone marrow may be a site of events that ultimately lead to the enhanced trafficking of monocytes into the tissues. We believe that significant neuroinvasion occurs in most infected individuals late in the course of infection, during AIDS. One of the best correlates of HIV dementia is encephalitis (Glass, Fedor, Wesselingh, and McArthur, 1995; Wiley and Achim, 1994). HIV encephalitis is characterized by the presence of macrophage-derived multinucleated giant cells, along with increased numbers of monocyte/macrophages, within the perivascular space. Thus, we reason that while significant neuroinvasion occurs in most infected individuals during AIDS, the process is even more amplified in those who go on to develop HIV encephalitis and cognitive impairment. The AIDS stage of infection is characterized by both functional immune suppression, and immune activation. Our model links neuroinvasion to events occurring outside of the brain during endstage disease. Some, if not most, of these events likely take place within the bone marrow, given that marrow is the site of monocyte production, as well as HIV infection (Weiser, Burger, Campbell, Donelan, and Mladenovic, 1996). Activation of monocytes prior to their exit from marrow, and/or during the short time they spend in the blood, may occur and could serve to prime them for transendothelial migration. This increase in monocyte trafficking is likely not limited to brain. Donaldson et al demonstrated that HIV disease progression---movement from the asymptomatic stage of infection to AIDS---is associated with the appearance of infection in nonlymphoid tissues, including brain (Donaldson, Bell, Ironside, Brettle, Robertson, Busuttil, and Simmonds, 1994). Endstage SIV infection is also characterized by widespread infection of nonlymphoid tissues, the target cell in these being macrophages (Hirsch, Zack, Vogel, and Johnson, 1991). Regardless of whether more of these monocytes are infected than in the pre-AIDS situation, the net result, because of the sheer increase in their numbers, is likely to translate into an increase in the number of infected cells entering the brain. This could explain why HAD typically does not develop until frank AIDS is present (McArthur, Cohen, Selnes, Kumar, Cooper, McArthur, Soucy, Cornblath, Chmiel, Wang, and et al., 1989). Otherwise, it is necessary to explain why, if the virus is responsible, it can take 10-15 years or more from the time of viral entry during acute infection, to the development of detectable disease. It is critically important, however, to avoid assuming that this increase in the level of HIV infection in brain is itself directly responsible for the development of neurological disease, particularly cognitive impairment. Monocyte/macrophage numbers are also increased as a consequence of this enhanced trafficking, and based on what is known about the number of these cells harboring genome, it is likely that most of those invading the brain are not infected. Also, the abundance of macrophages, appears to be a better correlate of HAD than the presence or extent of HIV infection (Glass et. al., 1995; Johnson, Glass, McArthur, and Chesebro, 1996). Ultimately, the infiltration of uninfected monocytes into the brain may prove to be as important to the development of HAD as HIV infection and/or replication.

Role of Strain Specificity in Viral Entry

It is conceivable that the timing of neuroinvasion could depend on the viral strain. In a serial sacrifice study, Smith and colleagues compared SIVmac1A11, a nonpathogenic molecularly cloned strain, with uncloned SIVmac251 and with a molecular clone derived from this swarm (SIVmac239), both pathogenic (Smith et. al., 1995). Animals were followed for up to 23 weeks. SIV was recovered from the plasma of animals inoculated with SIVmac1A11 at weeks 2 and 4, but not later, and was never recovered from the CSF. Also, no intrathecal immune response was detected in the SIVmac1A11 infected animals, nor were neuropathological changes characteristic of brain infection seen. In contrast, based on these same measures, inoculation with SIVmac251 or SIVmac239 resulted in infection of the brain. These findings are somewhat puzzling in that the primary host cell for infection within brain is the macrophage, and while SIVmac1A11 replicates well and induces cytopathicity in both T-lymphocytes and macrophages, SIVmac239 has a limited ability to infect macrophages, at least in vitro. However, the SIV-expressing cells in the brains of the SIVmac239 and SIVmac251 inoculated animals appeared to be macrophages. This could reflect a change in chemokine coreceptor usage during acute infection. The high level of virus replication during this time could likely support the random generation of mutations associated with receptor usage, followed by selection of such mutations. SIVmac1A11 has delayed replication kinetics, relative to SIVmac239, so possibly, the immune response initiated by infection was sufficient to prevent development of the events required for neuroinvasion, most probably, transendothelial migration of infected monocytes into the perivascular space.

Less is known about the genetic and biologic features of HIV strains that can enter the brain early. However, it has been reported that the strains typically transmitted, and therefore present during acute infection, are macrophage-tropic (Zhu, Mo, Wang, Nam, Cao, Koup, and Ho, 1993). Thus, it is likely that the HIV strains entering the brain during acute infection are macrophage-tropic. The factors which determine whether HIV neuroinvasion elicits meningitis or meningoencephalitis are unknown. While the predominant determinants are likely to reside with the host, it is conceivable that viral strain specificity could also play a role. Many of the initial reports demonstrating early HIV neuroinvasion were studies of individuals who experienced symptomatic acute infection (Carne et. al., 1985; Piette et. al., 1986). At present, there is insufficient evidence to determine the frequency of this event in the setting of asymptomatic acute infection. Specific characteristics of HIV strains, including features such as replication kinetics, could impact the potential for neuroinvasion.

Role of the Immune Response in Viral Entry

The immune response may play a role in the timing of HIV neuroinvasion. HIV entry during acute infection would necessarily occur in the absence of a host immune response. This absence could, in a sense, facilitate neuroinvasion since, presumably, both humoral and cellular immune responses could act to some degree as a barrier. The targets---free virions and virus-expressing cells---could effectively be neutralized or destroyed prior to entry into the brain, for example, within the circulation. It is also conceivable that virions and/or infected cells could cross the BBB and be confronted by specific antibody or cytotoxic lymphocytes, particularly within the PVS, and subsequently be eliminated. Immune-mediated clearance has been shown to occur in several virus infections in humans. Also, evidence from the SIV system suggests that the immune response is primarily responsible for diminishing the productive infection in brain (Greco, Westmoreland, Ratai, Lentz, Sakaie, He, Sehgal, Masliah, Lackner, and Gonzalez, 2004; Smith et. al., 1995). This could reflect the elimination of many infected cells from the brain. A decline in the level of viral DNA folllowing acute infection was not seen in the SIV rapid progressor model (Clements et. al., 2002), but this may not be the case in other SIV systems in which the time between acute infection and disease is considerably longer. As noted earlier, the levels of HIV DNA present in brain during the asymptomatic stage are either very low, or undetectable. Presumably, the intrathecal immune response would play the predominant role in this immune control, but the systemic response might also contribute by limiting plasma viremia and infected leukocytes, most probably virus-expressing leukocytes.

One would expect that the immune response could participate in controlling subsequent HIV entry into the brain, particularly during the asymptomatic stage of infection. However, while free virus particles might be neutralized and virus-expressing cells killed, latently infected monocytes could remain free of attack within the circulation and continue to cross the BBB uninterrupted, again making use of a normal physiological process. Once latency is broken and they begin to replicate and express HIV, they could, however, become targets of destruction. The timing of their eradication relative to completion of the viral life cycle is difficult to predict. Potentially, infectious particles could be released at levels sufficient to provide for spread of the infection, prior to eradication of the cell. Equally important are the questions of how long a macrophage can live in the brain and how long HIV latency can be maintained in this cell. The turnover rate for PVM appears to be on the order of 3 months, but it is not clear if these cells leave the brain or die. Resident microglia represent a very stable population with a very low tnrnover rate. Potentially, latently-infected macrophages could persist for months or even longer, thereby evading any immune response and when the response wains, or for whatever reason replication is initiated, then the infection could spread to other cells, some of whom might also establish a latent infection. Thus, there could be a dynamic situation between virus expression and the immune response.

Long-term immunity in the setting of chronic virus infection usually requires occasional low-level virus expression. That is, immunity cannot be maintained indefinitely under conditions of complete viral latency. This is likely to be the case in HIV infection, as well, although the timing and other particulars of the situation may be more complicated, owing to the fact that this infection leads to destruction of the immune system over time. Also, in the case of HIV, as with other lentiviruses, antigenic drift occurs, so that neutralizing antibody is able to remove virus particles bearing envelope proteins that reflect replication of prior members of the quasispecies, but not those species currently being produced (Albert, Abrahamsson, Nagy, Aurelius, Gaines, Nystrom, and Fenyo, 1990; Arendrup, Nielsen, Hansen, Pedersen, Mathiesen, and Nielsen, 1992). Thus, an important question relates to the level of HIV replication within brain during the asymptomatic stage of infection. As noted earlier, for HIV and SIV, the level of virus replication within brain during this stage is minimal.

Timing of Viral Entry and Establishment of Latency

One of the most important questions regarding early HIV neuroinvasion is whether this initial viral entry is able to lead to establishment of a permanent infection within the brain. This has often been assumed to be the case, although evidence is lacking. A persistent infection could be either latent or productive, with virus expression occurring continuously or possibly even sporadically. In the few studies reported, no, or only very low levels, of HIV DNA were detected in brain parenchymal tissues taken from HIV-infected individuals who died during the asymptomatic stage of infection (Bell et. al., 1993; Sinclair et. al., 1994). Although several studies of early SIV infection have examined viral RNA loads, few have assessed viral DNA levels. An exception is in the case of the rapid progressor model developed by Clements and colleagues, in which pig-tailed macaques are simultaneously inoculated intravenously with both a neurovirulent molecular clone and an immunosuppressive viral swarm (Clements et. al., 2002). These animals experience an accelerated course of immune deterioration and more than 90% develop SIV encephalitis. The animals are at the terminal stage of disease by 3 months. It is conceivable that 3 months is too short an interval for macrophages infected during acute infection to drop out. This model is also characterized by the development of low levels of SIV-specifc binding antibody, but no neutralizing antibodies (Mankowski et. al., 2002). Evidence from other SIV infection systems strongly suggests that it is the immune response which curtails and diminishes the initial infection within the brain (Greco, Sakaie, Aminipour, Lee, Chang, He, Westmoreland, Lackner, and Gonzalez, 2002; Smith et. al., 1995). Thus, this lack of a significant response in the rapid progressor model may also help to explain the persisting SIV DNA levels in this system.

One additional very intriguing study of relevance comes from Hurtrel and coworkers, in which they compared intracerebral versus intravenous SIV inoculation of macaques (Hurtrel et. al., 1991). Intravenous, but not intracerebral inoculation led to brain pathology characterized by numerous multinucleated giant cells, glial nodules and areas of demyelination. This suggests that following its direct introduction into the brain parenchyma, sustained spread of the virus infection may not readily occur in the absence of immune suppression. A consistent finding in the IV-inoculated animals was an increase in the number of perivascular macrophages; lymphocytic infiltrates were minimal. These investigators also found that resident microglia were only weakly susceptible to infection. Furthermore, Baskin and colleagues found that intrathecal inoculation of SIV does not result in an increased incidence of brain disease (Baskin, Murphey-Corb, Roberts, Didier, and Martin, 1992) suggesting that the CSF compartment does not provide the virus access to the parenchyma is such a way that sustained infection can result. HIV infection of the brain parenchyma has been reported to be independent of infection of the meninges (Sharer, 1992). However, these processes were shown to occur simultaneously in macaques inoculated intravenously with SIV (Smith et. al., 1995).

Whether the initial entry of HIV into the brain results in establishment of a life-long brain infection is still unknown. Furthermore, although the brain is frequently considered a reservoir for HIV, the ability of this potential reservoir to reseed peripheral lymphoid tissues also remains in question. It is possible that several factors, both viral- and host-derived, converge to determine the final outcome. Obviously, these questions have considerable clinical significance, and their answers could impact the direction of treatment options. Therapeutic targets could include residual virus in brain, as well as the trafficking monocyte population. More studies to address these issues are urgently needed.

Timing of Entry and Compromise of the Blood-Brain Barrier

One final issue of importance regarding the timing of HIV entry into the brain relates to whether compromise of the BBB occurs during neuroinvasion, or is even necessary. The frequency and extent of this compromise is likely to vary, depending on the stage of HIV infection. More frequent and more extensive disruption of this barrier is probable during endstage disease (Goswami, Kaye, Miller, McAllister, and Tedder, 1991), when opportunistic infections may be present, whereas during the asymptomatic stage, the endothelium is more likely to remain unperturbed. Acute infection, particularly that accompanied by meningitis or meningoencephalitis, could be associated with disruption of the BBB. Interestingly, however, in their serial sacrifice study of neuroinvasion during acute and early SIV infection, Smith et al found that BBB integrity was maintained throughout the course of study (up to 23 weeks), as determined by the CSF albumin/serum albumin ratio (Smith et. al., 1995). This method, of course, cannot detect more subtle barrier compromise. In constrast, Stephens et al did detect BBB disruption during acute SIV infection (Stephens, Singh, Kohler, Jackson, Pacyniak, and Berman, 2003), and Andersson and colleagues found evidence of disruption during the asymptomatic stage of HIV infection (Andersson, Hagberg, Fuchs, Svennerholm, and Gisslen, 2001).

Whether BBB disruption facilitates HIV neuroinvasion may also depend on the mode of viral entry. Monocyte transendothelial migration is a normal physiological process, so HIV entering as infected monocytes, particularly latently-infected ones, would not require any alteration of the endothelium. Neuroinflammation, however, involves changes in the BBB, including endothelial cell alterations, and can be characterized by leukocyte infiltration (Lassmann, Schmied, Vass, and Hickey, 1993). Consequently, its presence could permit the entry of greater numbers of HIV-infected monocytes or even infected T-lymphocytes. It seems likely that free HIV particles could enter the brain, along with other serum constituents, at sites of barrier disruption. The subsequent fate of these particles is, however, uncertain. Thus, while compromise of the BBB could facilitate or enhance HIV neuroinvasion, it does not appear to be essential.

Modes and Sites of Viral Entry

As alluded to earlier, HIV could enter the brain as either free virus particles or infected cells. These infected cells could be either monocytes, or CD4+ lymphocytes, the two primary hosts for productive infection. There are a few reports of HIV infection of other types of leukocytes, including CD8+ T-cells and NK-cells, but the significance of these is unclear, and they will not be considered further. While CD4+ lymphocytes could conceivably transport HIV, either as a product of active viral replication, or in a latent form, evidence supporting this possibility is lacking in both studies of humans and SIV-infected macaques. The cells actively expressing HIV or SIV within the brain parenchyma, including within the perivascular space, have been shown in numerous studies to be macrophages (Chakrabarti et. al., 1991; Gosztonyi, Artigas, Lamperth, and Webster, 1994; Hurtrel et. al., 1993; Vazeux, 1991). Moreover, CD4+ lymphocytes are themselves rarely seen in the brains of HIV-infected individuals (Vazeux, 1991), arguing against the possibility that their entry as latently-infected cells is a significant event. The transendothelial migration of infected blood-borne monocytes clearly appears to represent a primary mode of HIV neuroinvasion. As noted above, the infected monocytes could cross the BBB making use of a normal physiological process, and/or take advantage of conditions such as neuroinflammation and/or the presence of opportunistic infections, which could facilitate transendothelial migration. Moreover, alterations integral to the monocytes themselves, such as the presence of a state of cellular activation, could enhance their transmigratory capabilities. The factors and processes which set the stage for monocyte transendothelial migration, and participate in its execution, will be considered here. Similarly, information regarding the mechanisms involved in the movement of HIV particles across the BBB will be discussed. Lastly, some viruses appear to be able to enter the CNS via axonal transport, a classic example being poliovirus (Ohka, Yang, Terada, Iwasaki, and Nomoto, 1998). Although HIV can be detected near peripheral nerves, there is no evidence to suggest that it can travel along nerves to the brain.

Viral Entry, the Blood-Brain Barrier, and the Perivascular Space

The microvascular endothelium that lines blood vessels within the brain differs significantly from that found elsewhere in the body. The brain microvascular endothelial cells, along with other elements, form a diffusion barrier, the BBB, which prevents most substances in the blood from entering into the brain (Ballabh, Braun, and Nedergaard, 2004). A key element of this barrier are the tight junctions which form between endothelial cells and thereby restrict diffusion. Pericytes and the foot processes of astrocytes are also components of the barrier, a primary role for astrocytes being to maintain the tight junctions. Pericytes appear to contribute to structural support, and also play a role in angiogenesis and formation of the tight junctions (Allt and Lawrenson, 2001). Obviously, disruption of the barrier, or perturbation of the endothelial cells, could increase the opportunity for HIV to enter into the brain.

Regardless of whether HIV crosses the BBB in infected cells or as free virions, once it completely traverses the endothelium, it encounters the perivascular space (PVS), formally referred to as the Virchow-Robin space. This is a unique neuroanatomical structure, in that it is contiguous with the subpial space and partially filled with CSF (Esiri and Gay, 1990). Under normal conditions, small numbers of perivascular macrophages reside within these spaces, where they are thought to perform immune surveillance. For the entering virions to be able to establish infection, they must encounter a susceptible target cell and infect it. Given the fragile nature of these particles, and their apparent short half-life, this event most likely must occur within hours of entry. Macrophages are normal residents of the PVS and could readily serve as targets, so there is the potential for entering particles to establish an infection. With the macrophage as host, this infection could be either productive or latent. Within the PVS, however, except during the primary infection, there is also the potential for virions to encounter neutralizing antibody and be eliminated. Similarly, it is possible that subsequent to primary infection, HIV-expressing cells entering into the PVS could encounter cytotoxic T-cells and also be eliminated. Little is known about HIV-specific CTL within the brain, including within the PVS. However, such cells have been detected in CSF, even without in vitro expansion (Jassoy, Johnson, Navia, Worth, and Walker, 1992). The entry of latently-infected cells might represent a particularly attractive strategy for the virus, permitting initial evasion of the immune response, while preserving the potential for virus replication and expression later, when a less hostile microenvironment might be present.

Viral Entry Via Infected Monocytes

Not surprisingly, a number of viruses infect monocytes and macrophages. Monocytes are particularly attractive hosts for viral latency because of their longevity, their generally quiescent nature, their particular roles within the immune response, and their ability to traffic into almost every tissue and organ within the body under normal circumstances. Important to keep in mind is the fact that HIV is a lentivirus, and what characterizes lentiviruses is their ability to infect and replicate in macrophages. Hence, clues to understanding the HIV infection process, as well as HIV pathogenesis, may come from close study of viral systems such as VISNA and Equine Infectious Anemia Virus (EIAV).

In the natural history setting, the incidence of HIV neurological disease appears to be significantly higher in children. Rates ranging from 12-90% have been reported (Belman, Diamond, Dickson, Horoupian, Llena, Lantos, and Rubinstein, 1988; Epstein, Sharer, Oleske, Connor, Goudsmit, Bagdon, Robert-Guroff, and Koenigsberger, 1986; Lobato, Caldwell, Ng, and Oxtoby, 1995; Scott, Hutto, Makuch, Mastrucci, O'Connor, Mitchell, Trapido, and Parks, 1989). Encephalopathy may even be the initial manifestation of the presence of AIDS (Gonzalez del Rey, Randolph, and Hoecker, 1989). HIV DNA has frequently been detected in post-mortem brain tissues from children who died with AIDS (Sei, Saito, Stewart, Crowley, Brouwers, Kleiner, Katz, Pizzo, and Heyes, 1995; Sharer, 1992), with a significant amount present as unintegrated molecules (Shaw, Harper, Hahn, Epstein, Gajdusek, Price,

Navia, Petito, O'Hara, Groopman, and et al., 1985). HIV expression has also been detected in pediatric brains, the productively-infected cells being limited to macrophages and microglial cells (Tornatore, Chandra, Berger, and Major, 1994). In addition, these investigators demonstrated expression of the HIV nonstructural protein, nef, within astrocytes, suggesting HIV infection, but restricted replication, in this cell type. As with HIV encephalopathy in adults, however, there is not a clear correlation between the level of HIV expression, and the presence of neurological disease (Vazeux, Lacroix-Ciaudo, Blanche, Cumont, Henin, Gray, Boccon-Gibod, and Tardieu, 1992).

Although in utero transmission of HIV has been documented, infants usually acquire the infection perinatally (Blanche, Tardieu, Duliege, Rouzioux, Le Deist, Fukunaga, Caniglia, Jacomet, Messiah, and Griscelli, 1990). It is difficult to determine the timing of HIV entry into the brain in these situations, and few studies have attempted to do so. Early in the epidemic, children also acquired HIV infection from blood products or transfusions (Desposito, McSherry, and Oleske, 1988). There are significant differences between the course of HIV infection in children, and these are particularly apparent in the brain, partly owing to the fact that the brain is still developing in children (Mintz, 1996; Wilfert, Wilson, Luzuriaga, and Epstein, 1994). Discussion of these issues is beyond the scope of this chapter. However, relative to the question of the mode of HIV entry into the brain, it may be important to consider the fact that infants and children have significantly higher levels of circulating monocytes compared to adults (Brandt, Levan, Mitelman, Olsson, and Sjogren, 1974; Lugada, Mermin, Kaharuza, Ulvestad, Were, Langeland, Asjo, Malamba, and Downing, 2004). While the absolute monocyte count in adults ranges between 285-500 cells per mm^3, in children it is up to 750 cells per mm^3. Moreover, during the first two weeks of life, absolute counts of 1000-1200 are normal (Brandt et. al., 1974). If, as data from the SIV model suggest, initial entry of the virus into the body is followed by seeding of the bone marrow by day 3 (Mandell, Jain, Miller, and Dandekar, 1995) and consequent trafficking of infected monocytes into the brain soon after, then this normal relative monocytosis in infants may facilitate HIV seeding of the brain. Interestingly, high levels of circulating monocytes, along with low levels of CD8+ T-cells, have been shown to be a predictor of progressive encephalopathy in HIV-infected children (Sanchez-Ramon, Bellon, Resino, Canto-Nogues, Gurbindo, Ramos, and Munoz-Fernandez, 2003). Of course, other unique features of the developing brain may also play a role.

A number of factors have been identified which appear to enhancement monocyte migration across the BBB. These include adhesion molecules (Nottet, Persidsky, Sasseville, Nukuna, Bock, Zhai, Sharer, McComb, Swindells, Soderland, and Gendelman, 1996), chemokines (Persidsky, Ghorpade, Rasmussen, Limoges, Liu, Stins, Fiala, Way, Kim, Witte, Weinand, Carhart, and Gendelman, 1999; Schmidtmayerova, Nottet, Nuovo, Raabe, Flanagan, Dubrovsky, Gendelman, Cerami, Bukrinsky, and Sherry, 1996; Weiss, Downie, Lyman, and Berman, 1998), and HIV products (Lafrenie, Wahl, Epstein, Hewlett, Yamada, and Dhawan, 1996). Interestingly, Koedel and colleagues found that the HIV nef protein, but not Tat, gp120 or gp160, was a chemotractic for leukocytes in vitro (Koedel, Kohleisen, Sporer, Lahrtz, Ovod, Fontana, Erfle, and Pfister, 1999).

Viral Entry Via Cell-Free Virions

Based primarily on studies using in vitro models, a number of molecules have been implicated in the transport of HIV particles across the BBB, typically via perturbation of the BBB. These include cell-derived products (Bobardt, Salmon, Wang, Esko, Gabuzda, Fiala, Trono, Van der Schueren, David, and Gallay, 2004; Borghi, Panzeri, Shattock, Sozzani, Dobrina, and Meroni, 2000), drugs (Fiala, Gan, Zhang, House, Newton, Graves, Shapshak, Stins, Kim, Witte, and Chang, 1998), and HIV-specific proteins (Andras, Pu, Deli, Nath, Hennig, and Toborek, 2003; Cioni and Annunziata, 2002; Sporer, Koedel, Paul, Kohleisen, Erfle, Fontana, and Pfister, 2000). Some of these appear to act by directly perturbing the endothelium, for example, by eliciting neuroinflammation. Others may act in more subtle ways, relying on natural processes to orchestrate the effects. In all of these instances, however, a common consequence could be enhancement of the potential for HIV particle transmigration, and perhaps also cell transmigration. Also, although they lack CD4, the primary receptor for HIV, there is evidence suggesting that endothelial cells themselves can serve as hosts for HIV infection and replication (Moses, Bloom, Pauza, and Nelson, 1993). Endothelial cell infection has also been observed in the SIV system (Mankowski, Spelman, Ressetar, Strandberg, Laterra, Carter, Clements, and Zink, 1994). This infection could promote direct entry of HIV virions into the PVS, the particles being derived from endothelial cells actively replicating and expressing the virus.

Transport of HIV particles through endothelial cells, with subsequent release on the parenchymal side, has also been proposed as a mechanism by which HIV virions can cross the BBB (Banks, Akerstrom, and Kastin, 1998; Liu, Lossinsky, Popik, Li, Gujuluva, Kriederman, Roberts, Pushkarsky, Bukrinsky, Witte, Weinand, and Fiala, 2002). In this case, the particles are taken up from the blood by means of adsorptive endocytosis or macropinocytosis. In an elegant study using human brain microvascular endothelial cells as a model of the BBB, Liu et al demonstrated that this process involves lipid rafts, MAPK signaling and glycosylaminoglycans, and proceeds without any disruption of the endothelial cell tight junctions (Liu et. al., 2002). Importantly, they also found that while most of the virion-containing vesicles went on to fuse with lysosomes which resulted in the degradation of the particles, approximately 1% of the particles found their way to the abluminal side.

Paracellular entry via the endothelial cell tight junctions has also been observed, and suggested as a mode of HIV virion transport across the BBB (Fiala, Looney, Stins, Way, Zhang, Gan, Chiappelli, Schweitzer, Shapshak, Weinand, Graves, Witte, and Kim, 1997). TNF-α appears to participate in this process. HIV Tat-induced apoptosis of the endothelial cells also been proposed as a paracellular route, the consequence of this apoptosis being the creation of perforations within the BBB that can permit virus particle entry (Kim, Avraham, Koh, Jiang, Park, and Avraham, 2003).

Entry Via the Choroid Plexus

The choroid plexus (CP) is a highly vascular structure located within the ventricles of the brain. It is composed of a polarized single epithelial layer overlaying a stroma containing fenestrated capillaries. The epithelial cells are joined by tight junctions located on the apical side and hence, they form a "blood-CSF" barrier. These cells secrete the cerebrospinal fluid and provide selective active transport of micronutrients, metabolites and drugs into the CSF (Spector and Lorenzo, 1974). They also absorb material from the CSF and transport it to the blood, thereby providing a cleansing function (Fishman, 1966; Pappenheimer, Heisey, and Jordan, 1961). Moreover, the CP epithelial cells have been shown to take up virus-sized particles (100nm microspheres) injected into the ventricles, and they also bear Fc receptors (Nathanson and Chun, 1989). The fenestrated capillaries allow the passage into stroma of not only macromolecules, but also, unfortunately, microorganisms, which helps explain why this tissue is a frequent site of microbial infection, including opportunistic infections in AIDS patients (Falangola and Petito, 1993). Immune complexes are also very commonly observed within the CP in patients with AIDS and autoimmune diseases, the likely origin being the bloodstream (Falangola, Castro-Filho, and Petito, 1994). Thus, the CP is not protected by a BBB analogous to that within the brain parenchyma.

Macrophages are present within the CP stroma and these appear to have a more activated phenotype, compared to parenchymal microglial cells (Matyszak, Lawson, Perry, and Gordon, 1992). A distinct population of monocyte-derived macrophages, referred to as epiplexus macrophages, is also present (Ling, 1981; Ling, 1983). These are located on the apical side of the epithelium, and their numbers increase significantly following injury or an inflammatory challenge to the brain (Maxwell, Hardy, Watt, McGadey, Graham, Adams, and Gennarelli, 1992). The migration of blood-derived monocytes to the apical side of the CP epithelium, however, has been shown to be a frequent, ongoing process, even under normal conditions (Ling, 1981). Owing in part to their predilection for macrophages, the CP is an early site of infection for several lentiviruses, including VISNA, CaEV, SIV and FIV, and it appears to play a critical role in maintaining viral persistence within the CNS (Narayan, Wolinsky, Clements, Strandberg, Griffin, and Cork, 1982). The CP has also been shown to be a site of HIV infection. For example, in a study of 25 AIDS cases, Falangola et al found HIV infection within CP in 44% of cases, and determined that the virus-expressing cells were macrophages (Falangola, Hanly, Galvao-Castro, and Petito, 1995). In a separate study, HIV+ cells exhibiting a dendritic morphology and also strongly immunoreactive for HLA-DR were observed, indicating that CP dendritic cells may also be targets for productive infection within this tissue (Hanly and Petito, 1998). Of relevance here, HIV infection may be present within the CP during the asymptomatic stage of infection (Gray et. al., 1992; Petito, Chen, Mastri, Torres-Munoz, Roberts, and Wood, 1999). Whether or not it becomes infected during acute HIV infection is unknown. However, in a serial sacrifice study of SIVmac251-inoculated macaques that were evaluated at seven days and one, two and three months following infection, infected cells were rarely detected within the CP (Hurtrel et. al., 1991). This led the authors to conclude that the CP is not a major site of viral entry during early systemic SIV infection.

Influence of Antiretroviral Therapy on HIV Neuroinvasion

The BBB is designed to tightly control the passage of molecules and other substances from the blood into the brain. The entry into brain of such simple molecules as glucose and amino acids is facilitated by specific transporters. Larger, yet still relatively simple molecules, such as insulin and transferrin, cross the BBB via receptor-mediated endocytosis (Pardridge, Eisenberg, and Yang, 1985). Many pharmacologic agents, including antiretroviral drugs, cross the BBB by means of transport systems. The nucleoside reverse transcriptase inhibitors (NRTIs) use probenecid efflux transport mechanisms, which do restrict brain entry, and the protease inhibitors (PIs) appear to use the efflux transporter, P-glycoprotein and also perhaps multi-drug resistance protein (MRP) (Thomas, 2004; Wynn, Brundage, and Fletcher, 2002). P-glycoprotein appears to severely limit brain uptake of the PIs, in that these drugs cannot be detected in the CSF of patients using them (Thomas, 2004). No transporters for the non-nucleoside reverse transcriptase inhibitors (NNRTIs) have been identified.

The incidence of HAD has declined since the introduction of HAART (Dore, Correll, Li, Kaldor, Cooper, and Brew, 1999; Sacktor, Lyles, Skolasky, Kleeberger, Selnes, Miller, Becker, Cohen, and McArthur, 2001). HAART cocktails typically include a PI. This class of drugs appears to play a predominant role in slowing the course of HIV disease progression and similarly, lowering the incidence of HIV neurological disease. Since the PIs do not appreciably cross the BBB, exactly how they act to prevent or retard the development of dementia is unclear. It would seem that they do not exert their influence on HAD by acting directly to inhibit HIV replication within the brain parenchyma. We have proposed that PIs might act to decrease the activation of monocytes, thereby lowering their ability to traffic into the brain (Gartner and Liu, 2002). This decrease in monocyte trafficking would likely lead to a decrease in monocyte-mediated HIV entry into the brain. How PIs might interfere with monocyte activation is an issue for speculation, but this interference is likely mediated by a series of events that take place within the bone marrow, and involves both HIV replication and immunological responses.

HAART has also dramatically improved the longevity and health of HIV-infected individuals and in many, some degree of immune restoration occurs. However, a small number of patients develops an inflammatory reaction in response to this treatment, or experience reactivation or exacerbation of opportunistic infections (Shelburne, Hamill, Rodriguez-Barradas, Greenberg, Atmar, Musher, Gathe, Visnegarwala, and Trautner, 2002). This condition is referred to as "immune restoration disease" (IRD) or "immune reconstitution inflammatory syndrome" (IRIS). The pathogens most commonly seen in this situation are Mycobacterium avium complex, Mycobacterium tuberculosis, cryptococcus, Herpes zoster and Hepatitis B and C (Crump, Tyrer, Lloyd-Owen, Han, Lipman, and Johnson, 1998; French, Price, and Stone, 2004; King, Perlino, Cinnamon, and Jernigan, 2002). In some cases, these infections extend to the brain, where they can be extremely damaging and difficult to treat. The development of a severe, demyelinating leukoencephalopathy, in the absence of any detectable opportunistic infections, has also been observed in patients on HAART (Langford, Letendre, Marcotte, Ellis, McCutchan, Grant, Mallory, Hansen, Archibald, Jernigan, and Masliah, 2002). High levels of HIV RNA were detected in post-mortem brain tissues recovered from these individuals, and intense perivascular infiltrates with HIV gp41+ macrophages were observed, along with widespread myelin loss, axonal injury, microgliosis and astrocytosis. In a separate report, two cases of encephalopathy in association with HAART were described, one acute and the other a worsening of a pre-existing condition (Miller, Isaacson, Hall-Craggs, Lucas, Gray, Scaravilli, and An, 2004). Both patients died. Autopsies were performed and revealed the presence of massive and diffuse perivascular and intraparenchymal infiltrates of CD8+ lymphocytes within the brain. The patient with pre-existing encephalopathy had classic HIV encephalitis with multinucleated giant cells and HIV p24+ macrophages, but in the other (acute presentation), there was no evidence of replicating HIV. The mechanisms underlying these reactive syndromes are unknown. Likewise, is it not clear if this response can lead to significant enhancement of HIV neuroinvasion. Obviously, opportunistic infections, both at the systemic level and within the brain, could perturb the BBB and lead to HIV entry. More significant, however, could be the enhancement of infected monocytes trafficking into the brain. The limited evidence available supports this possible scenario. Thus, ARV therapy could, in some individuals, facilitate HIV neuroinvasion. Typically, this would be expected in patients with endstage disease, but because the triggers for IRD have not been identified, and since some patients use HAART prior to the presence of clinical AIDS, IRD might possibly arise during the asymptomatic stage of infection. Fortunately, the response can sometimes be controlled by withdrawl of HAART and/or treatment with steroids.

Concluding Remarks

As HIV-infected individuals live longer, their chances of developing ARV resistance mutations will increase. Undoubtedly, new drugs will be developed to attack this problem, but other therapeutic approaches will also be needed. Understanding the dynamics and mechanisms of HIV neuroinvasion can help to provide a reasoned foundation for future decisions regarding when and how to treat HIV-associated neurological disease. If the infection of brain is mediated primarily by transendothelial migration of blood-borne monocytes, and if the initial entry of the virus into the brain is essentially cleared by immune mechanisms and a significant reseeding takes place only after AIDS has developed, then controlling monocyte trafficking may represent an important therapeutic target. More information is needed, however, to determine the validity of these propositions.

References

Albert, J., Abrahamsson, B., Nagy, K., Aurelius, E., Gaines, H., Nystrom, G. and Fenyo, E.M. (1990). Rapid development of isolate-specific neutralizing antibodies after primary HIV-1 infection and consequent emergence of virus variants which resist neutralization by autologous sera. *Aids, 4*, 107-112.

Allt, G. and Lawrenson, J.G. (2001). Pericytes: cell biology and pathology. *Cells Tissues Organs, 169*, 1-11.

Allworth, A.M. and Kemp, R.J. (1989). A case of acute encephalopathy caused by the human immunodeficiency virus apparently responsive to zidovudine. *Med. J. Aust, 151*, 285-286.

Andersson, L.M., Hagberg, L., Fuchs, D., Svennerholm, B. and Gisslen, M. (2001). Increased blood-brain barrier permeability in neuro-asymptomatic HIV-1-infected individuals--correlation with cerebrospinal fluid HIV-1 RNA and neopterin levels. *J. Neurovirol, 7*, 542-547.

Andras, I.E., Pu, H., Deli, M.A., Nath, A., Hennig, B. and Toborek, M. (2003). HIV-1 Tat protein alters tight junction protein expression and distribution in cultured brain endothelial cells. *J. Neurosci. Res, 74*, 255-265.

Arendrup, M., Nielsen, C., Hansen, J.E., Pedersen, C., Mathiesen, L. and Nielsen, J.O. (1992). Autologous HIV-1 neutralizing antibodies: emergence of neutralization-resistant escape virus and subsequent development of escape virus neutralizing antibodies. *J. Acquir. Immune. Defic. Syndr, 5*, 303-307.

Ballabh, P., Braun, A. and Nedergaard, M. (2004). The blood-brain barrier: an overview: structure, regulation, and clinical implications. *Neurobiol. Dis, 16*, 1-13.

Banks, W.A., Akerstrom, V. and Kastin, A.J. (1998). Adsorptive endocytosis mediates the passage of HIV-1 across the blood-brain barrier: evidence for a post-internalization coreceptor. *J. Cell Sci, 111 (Pt 4)*, 533-540.

Baskin, G.B., Murphey-Corb, M., Roberts, E.D., Didier, P.J. and Martin, L.N. (1992). Correlates of SIV encephalitis in rhesus monkeys. *J. Med. Primatol, 21*, 59-63.

Bechmann, I., Priller, J., Kovac, A., Bontert, M., Wehner, T., Klett, F.F., Bohsung, J., Stuschke, M., Dirnagl, U. and Nitsch, R. (2001). Immune surveillance of mouse brain perivascular spaces by blood-borne macrophages. *Eur. J. Neurosci, 14*, 1651-1658.

Bell, J.E., Busuttil, A., Ironside, J.W., Rebus, S., Donaldson, Y.K., Simmonds, P. and Peutherer, J.F. (1993). Human immunodeficiency virus and the brain: investigation of virus load and neuropathologic changes in pre-AIDS subjects. *J. Infect. Dis, 168*, 818-824.

Belman, A.L., Diamond, G., Dickson, D., Horoupian, D., Llena, J., Lantos, G. and Rubinstein, A. (1988). Pediatric acquired immunodeficiency syndrome. Neurologic syndromes. *Am. J. Dis. Child, 142*, 29-35.

Blanche, S., Tardieu, M., Duliege, A., Rouzioux, C., Le Deist, F., Fukunaga, K., Caniglia, M., Jacomet, C., Messiah, A. and Griscelli, C. (1990). Longitudinal study of 94 symptomatic infants with perinatally acquired human immunodeficiency virus infection. Evidence for a bimodal expression of clinical and biological symptoms. *Am. J. Dis. Child, 144*, 1210-1215.

Bobardt, M.D., Salmon, P., Wang, L., Esko, J.D., Gabuzda, D., Fiala, M., Trono, D., Van der Schueren, B., David, G. and Gallay, P.A. (2004). Contribution of proteoglycans to human immunodeficiency virus type 1 brain invasion. *J. Virol, 78*, 6567-6584.

Borghi, M.O., Panzeri, P., Shattock, R., Sozzani, S., Dobrina, A. and Meroni, P.L. (2000). Interaction between chronically HIV-infected promonocytic cells and human umbilical vein endothelial cells: role of proinflammatory cytokines and chemokines in viral expression modulation. *Clin. Exp. Immunol, 120*, 93-100.

Brandt, L., Levan, G., Mitelman, F., Olsson, I. and Sjogren, U. (1974). Trisomy G-21 in adult myelomonocytic leukaemia. An abnormality common to granulocytic and monocytic cells. *Scand. J. Haematol, 12*, 117-122.

Carne, C.A., Tedder, R.S., Smith, A., Sutherland, S., Elkington, S.G., Daly, H.M., Preston, F.E. and Craske, J. (1985). Acute encephalopathy coincident with seroconversion for anti-HTLV-III. *Lancet, 2*, 1206-1208.

Chakrabarti, L., Hurtrel, M., Maire, M.A., Vazeux, R., Dormont, D., Montagnier, L. and Hurtrel, B. (1991). Early viral replication in the brain of SIV-infected rhesus monkeys. *Am. J. Pathol, 139*, 1273-1280.

Chang, J., Jozwiak, R., Wang, B., Ng, T., Ge, Y.C., Bolton, W., Dwyer, D.E., Randle, C., Osborn, R., Cunningham, A.L. and Saksena, N.K. (1998). Unique HIV type 1 V3 region sequences derived from six different regions of brain: region-specific evolution within host-determined quasispecies. *AIDS Res Hum Retroviruses, 14*, 25-30.

Chen, Y.H., Susanna, A., Steindl, F., Katinger, H. and Dierich, M.P. (1994). HIV-1 gp41 shares a common immunologic determinant with normal human blood lymphocytes and monocytes. *Aids, 8*, 130-131.

Cioni, C. and Annunziata, P. (2002). Circulating gp120 alters the blood-brain barrier permeability in HIV-1 gp120 transgenic mice. *Neurosci. Lett, 330*, 299-301.

Clements, J.E., Babas, T., Mankowski, J.L., Suryanarayana, K., Piatak, M., Jr., Tarwater, P.M., Lifson, J.D. and Zink, M.C. (2002). The central nervous system as a reservoir for simian immunodeficiency virus (SIV): steady-state levels of SIV DNA in brain from acute through asymptomatic infection. *J. Infect. Dis, 186*, 905-913.

Crump, J.A., Tyrer, M.J., Lloyd-Owen, S.J., Han, L.Y., Lipman, M.C. and Johnson, M.A. (1998). Military tuberculosis with paradoxical expansion of intracranial tuberculomas complicating human immunodeficiency virus infection in a patient receiving highly active antiretroviral therapy. *Clin. Infect. Dis, 26*, 1008-1009.

Davis, L.E., Hjelle, B.L., Miller, V.E., Palmer, D.L., Llewellyn, A.L., Merlin, T.L., Young, S.A., Mills, R.G., Wachsman, W. and Wiley, C.A. (1992). Early viral brain invasion in iatrogenic human immunodeficiency virus infection. *Neurology, 42*, 1736-1739.

Desposito, F., McSherry, G.D. and Oleske, J.M. (1988). Blood product acquired HIV infection in children. *Pediatr. Ann, 17*, 341-345.

Di Stefano, M., Wilt, S., Gray, F., Dubois-Dalcq, M. and Chiodi, F. (1996). HIV type 1 V3 sequences and the development of dementia during AIDS. *AIDS Res. Hum. Retroviruses, 12*, 471-476.

Donaldson, Y.K., Bell, J.E., Ironside, J.W., Brettle, R.P., Robertson, J.R., Busuttil, A. and Simmonds, P. (1994). Redistribution of HIV outside the lymphoid system with onset of AIDS. *Lancet, 343*, 383-385.

Dore, G.J., Correll, P.K., Li, Y., Kaldor, J.M., Cooper, D.A. and Brew, B.J. (1999). Changes to AIDS dementia complex in the era of highly active antiretroviral therapy. *Aids, 13*, 1249-1253.

Epstein, L.G., Kuiken, C., Blumberg, B.M., Hartman, S., Sharer, L.R., Clement, M. and Goudsmit, J. (1991). HIV-1 V3 domain variation in brain and spleen of children with AIDS: tissue-specific evolution within host-determined quasispecies. *Virology, 180*, 583-590.

Epstein, L.G., Sharer, L.R., Oleske, J.M., Connor, E.M., Goudsmit, J., Bagdon, L., Robert-Guroff, M. and Koenigsberger, M.R. (1986). Neurologic manifestations of human immunodeficiency virus infection in children. *Pediatrics, 78,* 678-687.

Esiri, M.M. and Gay, D. (1990). Immunological and neuropathological significance of the Virchow-Robin space. *J. Neurol. Sci, 100,* 3-8.

Falangola, M.F., Castro-Filho, B.G. and Petito, C.K. (1994). Immune complex deposition in the choroid plexus of patients with acquired immunodeficiency syndrome. *Ann. Neurol, 36,* 437-440.

Falangola, M.F., Hanly, A., Galvao-Castro, B. and Petito, C.K. (1995). HIV infection of human choroid plexus: a possible mechanism of viral entry into the CNS. *J. Neuropathol. Exp. Neurol, 54,* 497-503.

Falangola, M.F. and Petito, C.K. (1993). Choroid plexus infection in cerebral toxoplasmosis in AIDS patients. *Neurology, 43,* 2035-2040.

Fiala, M., Gan, X.H., Zhang, L., House, S.D., Newton, T., Graves, M.C., Shapshak, P., Stins, M., Kim, K.S., Witte, M. and Chang, S.L. (1998). Cocaine enhances monocyte migration across the blood-brain barrier. Cocaine's connection to AIDS dementia and vasculitis? *Adv. Exp. Med. Biol, 437,* 199-205.

Fiala, M., Looney, D.J., Stins, M., Way, D.D., Zhang, L., Gan, X., Chiappelli, F., Schweitzer, E.S., Shapshak, P., Weinand, M., Graves, M.C., Witte, M. and Kim, K.S. (1997). TNF-alpha opens a paracellular route for HIV-1 invasion across the blood-brain barrier. *Mol. Med, 3,* 553-564.

Fishman, R.A. (1966). Blood-brain and CSF barriers to penicillin and related organic acids. *Arch. Neurol, 15,* 113-124.

Flaherty, M.T., Hauer, D.A., Mankowski, J.L., Zink, M.C. and Clements, J.E. (1997). Molecular and biological characterization of a neurovirulent molecular clone of simian immunodeficiency virus. *J. Virol, 71,* 5790-5798.

French, M.A., Price, P. and Stone, S.F. (2004). Immune restoration disease after antiretroviral therapy. *Aids, 18,* 1615-1627.

Gartner, S. (2000). HIV infection and dementia. *Science, 287,* 602-604.

Gartner, S. and Liu, Y. (2002). Insights into the role of immune activation in HIV neuropathogenesis. *J. Neurovirol, 8,* 69-75.

Glass, J.D., Fedor, H., Wesselingh, S.L. and McArthur, J.C. (1995). Immunocytochemical quantitation of human immunodeficiency virus in the brain: correlations with dementia. *Ann. Neurol, 38,* 755-762.

Gonzalez del Rey, J., Randolph, C. and Hoecker, J. (1989). Encephalopathy as a presentation of pediatric AIDS: case report. *Ann. Allergy, 63,* 313-316.

Goswami, K.K., Kaye, S., Miller, R., McAllister, R. and Tedder, R. (1991). Intrathecal IgG synthesis and specificity of oligoclonal IgG in patients infected with HIV-1 do not correlate with CNS disease. *J. Med. Virol, 33,* 106-113.

Gosztonyi, G., Artigas, J., Lamperth, L. and Webster, H.D. (1994). Human immunodeficiency virus (HIV) distribution in HIV encephalitis: study of 19 cases with combined use of in situ hybridization and immunocytochemistry. *J. Neuropathol. Exp. Neurol, 53,* 521-534.

Goudsmit, J., de Wolf, F., Paul, D.A., Epstein, L.G., Lange, J.M., Krone, W.J., Speelman, H., Wolters, E.C., Van der Noordaa, J., Oleske, J.M. and et al. (1986). Expression of human immunodeficiency virus antigen (HIV-Ag) in serum and cerebrospinal fluid during acute and chronic infection. *Lancet, 2*, 177-180.

Gray, F., Lescs, M.C., Keohane, C., Paraire, F., Marc, B., Durigon, M. and Gherardi, R. (1992). Early brain changes in HIV infection: neuropathological study of 11 HIV seropositive, non-AIDS cases. *J. Neuropathol. Exp. Neurol, 51*, 177-185.

Greco, J.B., Sakaie, K.E., Aminipour, S., Lee, P.L., Chang, L.L., He, J., Westmoreland, S., Lackner, A.A. and Gonzalez, R.G. (2002). Magnetic resonance spectroscopy: an in vivo tool for monitoring cerebral injury in SIV-infected macaques. *J. Med. Primatol, 31*, 228-236.

Greco, J.B., Westmoreland, S.V., Ratai, E.M., Lentz, M.R., Sakaie, K., He, J., Sehgal, P.K., Masliah, E., Lackner, A.A. and Gonzalez, R.G. (2004). In vivo 1H MRS of brain injury and repair during acute SIV infection in the macaque model of neuroAIDS. *Magn. Reson. Med, 51*, 1108-1114.

Hanly, A. and Petito, C.K. (1998). HLA-DR-positive dendritic cells of the normal human choroid plexus: a potential reservoir of HIV in the central nervous system. *Hum. Pathol, 29*, 88-93.

Hardy, W.D., Daar, E.S., Sokolov, R.T., Jr. and Ho, D.D. (1991). Acute neurologic deterioration in a young man. *Rev. Infect. Dis, 13*, 745-750.

Hickey, W.F. (1999). Leukocyte traffic in the central nervous system: the participants and their roles. *Semin. Immunol, 11*, 125-137.

Hickey, W.F. (2001). Basic principles of immunological surveillance of the normal central nervous system. *Glia, 36*, 118-124.

Hickey, W.F. and Kimura, H. (1988). Perivascular microglial cells of the CNS are bone marrow-derived and present antigen in vivo. *Science, 239*, 290-292.

Hickey, W.F., Vass, K. and Lassmann, H. (1992). Bone marrow-derived elements in the central nervous system: an immunohistochemical and ultrastructural survey of rat chimeras. *J. Neuropathol. Exp. Neurol, 51*, 246-256.

Hirsch, V.M., Zack, P.M., Vogel, A.P. and Johnson, P.R. (1991). Simian immunodeficiency virus infection of macaques: end-stage disease is characterized by widespread distribution of proviral DNA in tissues. *J. Infect. Dis, 163*, 976-988.

Ho, D.D., Rota, T.R., Schooley, R.T., Kaplan, J.C., Allan, J.D., Groopman, J.E., Resnick, L., Felsenstein, D., Andrews, C.A. and Hirsch, M.S. (1985). Isolation of HTLV-III from cerebrospinal fluid and neural tissues of patients with neurologic syndromes related to the acquired immunodeficiency syndrome. *N. Engl. J. Med, 313*, 1493-1497.

Hughes, E.S., Bell, J.E. and Simmonds, P. (1997). Investigation of the dynamics of the spread of human immunodeficiency virus to brain and other tissues by evolutionary analysis of sequences from the p17gag and env genes. *J. Virol, 71*, 1272-1280.

Hurtrel, B., Chakrabarti, L., Hurtrel, M., Maire, M.A., Dormont, D. and Montagnier, L. (1991). Early SIV encephalopathy. *J. Med. Primatol, 20*, 159-166.

Hurtrel, B., Chakrabarti, L., Hurtrel, M. and Montagnier, L. (1993). Target cells during early SIV encephalopathy. *Res. Virol, 144*, 41-46.

Jassoy, C., Johnson, R.P., Navia, B.A., Worth, J. and Walker, B.D. (1992). Detection of a vigorous HIV-1-specific cytotoxic T lymphocyte response in cerebrospinal fluid from infected persons with AIDS dementia complex. *J. Immunol, 149*, 3113-3119.

Johnson, R.T., Glass, J.D., McArthur, J.C. and Chesebro, B.W. (1996). Quantitation of human immunodeficiency virus in brains of demented and nondemented patients with acquired immunodeficiency syndrome. *Ann. Neurol, 39*, 392-395.

Kalter, D.C., Nakamura, M., Turpin, J.A., Baca, L.M., Hoover, D.L., Dieffenbach, C., Ralph, P., Gendelman, H.E. and Meltzer, M.S. (1991). Enhanced HIV replication in macrophage colony-stimulating factor-treated monocytes. *J. Immunol, 146*, 298-306.

Kim, T.A., Avraham, H.K., Koh, Y.H., Jiang, S., Park, I.W. and Avraham, S. (2003). HIV-1 Tat-mediated apoptosis in human brain microvascular endothelial cells. *J. Immunol, 170*, 2629-2637.

King, M.D., Perlino, C.A., Cinnamon, J. and Jernigan, J.A. (2002). Paradoxical recurrent meningitis following therapy of cryptococcal meningitis: an immune reconstitution syndrome after initiation of highly active antiretroviral therapy. *Int. J. STD. AIDS, 13*, 724-726.

Koedel, U., Kohleisen, B., Sporer, B., Lahrtz, F., Ovod, V., Fontana, A., Erfle, V. and Pfister, H.W. (1999). HIV type 1 Nef protein is a viral factor for leukocyte recruitment into the central nervous system. *J. Immunol, 163*, 1237-1245.

Lafrenie, R.M., Wahl, L.M., Epstein, J.S., Hewlett, I.K., Yamada, K.M. and Dhawan, S. (1996). HIV-1-Tat modulates the function of monocytes and alters their interactions with microvessel endothelial cells. A mechanism of HIV pathogenesis. *J. Immunol, 156*, 1638-1645.

Langford, T.D., Letendre, S.L., Marcotte, T.D., Ellis, R.J., McCutchan, J.A., Grant, I., Mallory, M.E., Hansen, L.A., Archibald, S., Jernigan, T. and Masliah, E. (2002). Severe, demyelinating leukoencephalopathy in AIDS patients on antiretroviral therapy. *Aids, 16*, 1019-1029.

Lassmann, H., Schmied, M., Vass, K. and Hickey, W.F. (1993). Bone marrow derived elements and resident microglia in brain inflammation. *Glia, 7*, 19-24.

Ling, E.A. (1981). Ultrastructure and mode of formation of epiplexus cells in the choroid plexus in the lateral ventricles of the monkey (Macaca fascicularis). *J. Anat, 133*, 555-569.

Ling, E.A. (1983). Scanning electron microscopic study of epiplexus cells in the lateral ventricles of the monkey (Macaca fascicularis). *J. Anat, 137 (Pt 4)*, 645-652.

Liu, N.Q., Lossinsky, A.S., Popik, W., Li, X., Gujuluva, C., Kriederman, B., Roberts, J., Pushkarsky, T., Bukrinsky, M., Witte, M., Weinand, M. and Fiala, M. (2002). Human immunodeficiency virus type 1 enters brain microvascular endothelia by macropinocytosis dependent on lipid rafts and the mitogen-activated protein kinase signaling pathway. *J. Virol, 76*, 6689-6700.

Liu, Y., Tang, X.P., McArthur, J.C., Scott, J. and Gartner, S. (2000). Analysis of human immunodeficiency virus type 1 gp160 sequences from a patient with HIV dementia: evidence for monocyte trafficking into brain. *J. Neurovirol, 6 Suppl 1*, S70-81.

Lobato, M.N., Caldwell, M.B., Ng, P. and Oxtoby, M.J. (1995). Encephalopathy in children with perinatally acquired human immunodeficiency virus infection. Pediatric Spectrum of Disease Clinical Consortium. *J. Pediatr, 126*, 710-715.

Lugada, E.S., Mermin, J., Kaharuza, F., Ulvestad, E., Were, W., Langeland, N., Asjo, B., Malamba, S. and Downing, R. (2004). Population-based hematologic and immunologic reference values for a healthy Ugandan population. *Clin. Diagn. Lab. Immunol, 11*, 29-34.

Mandell, C.P., Jain, N.C., Miller, C.J. and Dandekar, S. (1995). Bone marrow monocyte/macrophages are an early cellular target of pathogenic and nonpathogenic isolates of simian immunodeficiency virus (SIVmac) in rhesus macaques. *Lab. Invest, 72*, 323-333.

Mankowski, J.L., Clements, J.E. and Zink, M.C. (2002). Searching for clues: tracking the pathogenesis of human immunodeficiency virus central nervous system disease by use of an accelerated, consistent simian immunodeficiency virus macaque model. *J. Infect. Dis, 186 Suppl 2*, S199-208.

Mankowski, J.L., Spelman, J.P., Ressetar, H.G., Strandberg, J.D., Laterra, J., Carter, D.L., Clements, J.E. and Zink, M.C. (1994). Neurovirulent simian immunodeficiency virus replicates productively in endothelial cells of the central nervous system in vivo and in vitro. *J. Virol, 68*, 8202-8208.

Matyszak, M.K., Lawson, L.J., Perry, V.H. and Gordon, S. (1992). Stromal macrophages of the choroid plexus situated at an interface between the brain and peripheral immune system constitutively express major histocompatibility class II antigens. *J. Neuroimmunol, 40*, 173-181.

Maxwell, W.L., Hardy, I.G., Watt, C., McGadey, J., Graham, D.I., Adams, J.H. and Gennarelli, T.A. (1992). Changes in the choroid plexus, responses by intrinsic epiplexus cells and recruitment from monocytes after experimental head acceleration injury in the non-human primate. *Acta. Neuropathol. (Berl), 84*, 78-84.

McArthur, J.C., Cohen, B.A., Selnes, O.A., Kumar, A.J., Cooper, K., McArthur, J.H., Soucy, G., Cornblath, D.R., Chmiel, J.S., Wang, M.C. and et al. (1989). Low prevalence of neurological and neuropsychological abnormalities in otherwise healthy HIV-1-infected individuals: results from the multicenter AIDS Cohort Study. *Ann. Neurol, 26*, 601-611.

Miller, R.F., Isaacson, P.G., Hall-Craggs, M., Lucas, S., Gray, F., Scaravilli, F. and An, S.F. (2004). Cerebral CD8+ lymphocytosis in HIV-1 infected patients with immune restoration induced by HAART. *Acta. Neuropathol. (Berl), 108*, 17-23.

Mintz, M. (1996). Neurological and developmental problems in pediatric HIV infection. *J. Nutr, 126*, 2663S-2673S.

Moses, A.V., Bloom, F.E., Pauza, C.D. and Nelson, J.A. (1993). Human immunodeficiency virus infection of human brain capillary endothelial cells occurs via a CD4/galactosylceramide-independent mechanism. *Proc. Natl. Acad. Sci. U S A, 90*, 10474-10478.

Narayan, O., Wolinsky, J.S., Clements, J.E., Strandberg, J.D., Griffin, D.E. and Cork, L.C. (1982). Slow virus replication: the role of macrophages in the persistence and expression of visna viruses of sheep and goats. *J. Gen. Virol, 59*, 345-356.

Nathanson, J.A. and Chun, L.L. (1989). Immunological function of the blood-cerebrospinal fluid barrier. *Proc. Natl. Acad. Sci. U S A, 86,* 1684-1688.

Nottet, H.S., Persidsky, Y., Sasseville, V.G., Nukuna, A.N., Bock, P., Zhai, Q.H., Sharer, L.R., McComb, R.D., Swindells, S., Soderland, C. and Gendelman, H.E. (1996). Mechanisms for the transendothelial migration of HIV-1-infected monocytes into brain. *J. Immunol, 156,* 1284-1295.

Ohka, S., Yang, W.X., Terada, E., Iwasaki, K. and Nomoto, A. (1998). Retrograde transport of intact poliovirus through the axon via the fast transport system. *Virology, 250,* 67-75.

Pappenheimer, J.R., Heisey, S.R. and Jordan, E.F. (1961). Active transport of Diodrast and phenolsulfonphthalein from cerebrospinal fluid to blood. *Am. J. Physiol, 200,* 1-10.

Pardridge, W.M., Eisenberg, J. and Yang, J. (1985). Human blood-brain barrier insulin receptor. *J. Neurochem, 44,* 1771-1778.

Persidsky, Y., Ghorpade, A., Rasmussen, J., Limoges, J., Liu, X.J., Stins, M., Fiala, M., Way, D., Kim, K.S., Witte, M.H., Weinand, M., Carhart, L. and Gendelman, H.E. (1999). Microglial and astrocyte chemokines regulate monocyte migration through the blood-brain barrier in human immunodeficiency virus-1 encephalitis. *Am. J. Pathol, 155,* 1599-1611.

Petito, C.K., Chen, H., Mastri, A.R., Torres-Munoz, J., Roberts, B. and Wood, C. (1999). HIV infection of choroid plexus in AIDS and asymptomatic HIV-infected patients suggests that the choroid plexus may be a reservoir of productive infection. *J. Neurovirol, 5,* 670-677.

Piette, A.M., Tusseau, F., Vignon, D., Chapman, A., Parrot, G., Leibowitch, J. and Montagnier, L. (1986). Acute neuropathy coincident with seroconversion for anti-LAV/HTLV-III. *Lancet, 1,* 852.

Resnick, L., Berger, J.R., Shapshak, P. and Tourtellotte, W.W. (1988). Early penetration of the blood-brain-barrier by HIV. *Neurology, 38,* 9-14.

Rich, E.A., Chen, I.S., Zack, J.A., Leonard, M.L. and O'Brien, W.A. (1992). Increased susceptibility of differentiated mononuclear phagocytes to productive infection with human immunodeficiency virus-1 (HIV-1). *J. Clin. Invest, 89,* 176-183.

Ringler, D.J., Hunt, R.D., Desrosiers, R.C., Daniel, M.D., Chalifoux, L.V. and King, N.W. (1988). Simian immunodeficiency virus-induced meningoencephalitis: natural history and retrospective study. *Ann. Neurol, 23 Suppl,* S101-107.

Sacktor, N., Lyles, R.H., Skolasky, R., Kleeberger, C., Selnes, O.A., Miller, E.N., Becker, J.T., Cohen, B. and McArthur, J.C. (2001). HIV-associated neurologic disease incidence changes:: Multicenter AIDS Cohort Study, 1990-1998. *Neurology, 56,* 257-260.

Sanchez-Ramon, S., Bellon, J.M., Resino, S., Canto-Nogues, C., Gurbindo, D., Ramos, J.T. and Munoz-Fernandez, M.A. (2003). Low blood CD8+ T-lymphocytes and high circulating monocytes are predictors of HIV-1-associated progressive encephalopathy in children. *Pediatrics, 111,* E168-175.

Sasseville, V.G. and Lackner, A.A. (1997). Neuropathogenesis of simian immunodeficiency virus infection in macaque monkeys. *J. Neurovirol, 3,* 1-9.

Schmidtmayerova, H., Nottet, H.S., Nuovo, G., Raabe, T., Flanagan, C.R., Dubrovsky, L., Gendelman, H.E., Cerami, A., Bukrinsky, M. and Sherry, B. (1996). Human immunodeficiency virus type 1 infection alters chemokine beta peptide expression in human monocytes: implications for recruitment of leukocytes into brain and lymph nodes. *Proc. Natl. Acad. Sci. U S A, 93*, 700-704.

Schuitemaker, H., Kootstra, N.A., Koppelman, M.H., Bruisten, S.M., Huisman, H.G., Tersmette, M. and Miedema, F. (1992). Proliferation-dependent HIV-1 infection of monocytes occurs during differentiation into macrophages. *J. Clin. Invest, 89*, 1154-1160.

Scott, G.B., Hutto, C., Makuch, R.W., Mastrucci, M.T., O'Connor, T., Mitchell, C.D., Trapido, E.J. and Parks, W.P. (1989). Survival in children with perinatally acquired human immunodeficiency virus type 1 infection. *N. Engl. J. Med, 321*, 1791-1796.

Sei, S., Saito, K., Stewart, S.K., Crowley, J.S., Brouwers, P., Kleiner, D.E., Katz, D.A., Pizzo, P.A. and Heyes, M.P. (1995). Increased human immunodeficiency virus (HIV) type 1 DNA content and quinolinic acid concentration in brain tissues from patients with HIV encephalopathy. *J. Infect. Dis, 172*, 638-647.

Shapshak, P., Segal, D.M., Crandall, K.A., Fujimura, R.K., Zhang, B.T., Xin, K.Q., Okuda, K., Petito, C.K., Eisdorfer, C. and Goodkin, K. (1999). Independent evolution of HIV type 1 in different brain regions. *AIDS Res. Hum. Retroviruses, 15*, 811-820.

Sharer, L.R. (1992). Pathology of HIV-1 infection of the central nervous system. A review. *J. Neuropathol. Exp. Neurol, 51*, 3-11.

Shaw, G.M., Harper, M.E., Hahn, B.H., Epstein, L.G., Gajdusek, D.C., Price, R.W., Navia, B.A., Petito, C.K., O'Hara, C.J., Groopman, J.E. and et al. (1985). HTLV-III infection in brains of children and adults with AIDS encephalopathy. *Science, 227*, 177-182.

Shelburne, S.A., 3rd, Hamill, R.J., Rodriguez-Barradas, M.C., Greenberg, S.B., Atmar, R.L., Musher, D.W., Gathe, J.C., Jr., Visnegarwala, F. and Trautner, B.W. (2002). Immune reconstitution inflammatory syndrome: emergence of a unique syndrome during highly active antiretroviral therapy. *Medicine (Baltimore), 81*, 213-227.

Sinclair, E., Gray, F., Ciardi, A. and Scaravilli, F. (1994). Immunohistochemical changes and PCR detection of HIV provirus DNA in brains of asymptomatic HIV-positive patients. *J. Neuropathol. Exp. Neurol, 53*, 43-50.

Smith, M.O., Heyes, M.P. and Lackner, A.A. (1995). Early intrathecal events in rhesus macaques (Macaca mulatta) infected with pathogenic or nonpathogenic molecular clones of simian immunodeficiency virus. *Lab. Invest, 72*, 547-558.

Sonza, S., Maerz, A., Deacon, N., Meanger, J., Mills, J. and Crowe, S. (1996). Human immunodeficiency virus type 1 replication is blocked prior to reverse transcription and integration in freshly isolated peripheral blood monocytes. *J. Virol, 70*, 3863-3869.

Sonza, S., Mutimer, H.P., Oelrichs, R., Jardine, D., Harvey, K., Dunne, A., Purcell, D.F., Birch, C. and Crowe, S.M. (2001). Monocytes harbour replication-competent, non-latent HIV-1 in patients on highly active antiretroviral therapy. *Aids, 15*, 17-22.

Spector, R. and Lorenzo, A.V. (1974). Specificity of ascorbic acid transport system of the central nervous system. *Am. J. Physiol, 226*, 1468-1473.

Sporer, B., Koedel, U., Paul, R., Kohleisen, B., Erfle, V., Fontana, A. and Pfister, H.W. (2000). Human immunodeficiency virus type-1 Nef protein induces blood-brain barrier disruption in the rat: role of matrix metalloproteinase-9. *J Neuroimmunol, 102*, 125-130.

Stephens, E.B., Singh, D.K., Kohler, M.E., Jackson, M., Pacyniak, E. and Berman, N.E. (2003). The primary phase of infection by pathogenic simian-human immunodeficiency virus results in disruption of the blood-brain barrier. *AIDS Res. Hum. Retroviruses, 19,* 837-846.

Thomas, S.A. (2004). Anti-HIV drug distribution to the central nervous system. *Curr. Pharm. Des, 10,* 1313-1324.

Tornatore, C., Chandra, R., Berger, J.R. and Major, E.O. (1994). HIV-1 infection of subcortical astrocytes in the pediatric central nervous system. *Neurology, 44,* 481-487.

Triques, K. and Stevenson, M. (2004). Characterization of restrictions to human immunodeficiency virus type 1 infection of monocytes. *J. Virol, 78,* 5523-5527.

Unger, E.R., Sung, J.H., Manivel, J.C., Chenggis, M.L., Blazar, B.R. and Krivit, W. (1993). Male donor-derived cells in the brains of female sex-mismatched bone marrow transplant recipients: a Y-chromosome specific in situ hybridization study. *J. Neuropathol. Exp. Neurol, 52,* 460-470.

Vazeux, R. (1991). AIDS encephalopathy and tropism of HIV for brain monocytes/macrophages and microglial cells. *Pathobiology, 59,* 214-218.

Vazeux, R., Lacroix-Ciaudo, C., Blanche, S., Cumont, M.C., Henin, D., Gray, F., Boccon-Gibod, L. and Tardieu, M. (1992). Low levels of human immunodeficiency virus replication in the brain tissue of children with severe acquired immunodeficiency syndrome encephalopathy. *Am. J. Pathol, 140,* 137-144.

Weiser, B., Burger, H., Campbell, P., Donelan, S. and Mladenovic, J. (1996). HIV type 1 RNA expression in bone marrows of patients with a spectrum of disease. *AIDS Res. Hum. Retroviruses, 12,* 1551-1558.

Weiss, J.M., Downie, S.A., Lyman, W.D. and Berman, J.W. (1998). Astrocyte-derived monocyte-chemoattractant protein-1 directs the transmigration of leukocytes across a model of the human blood-brain barrier. *J. Immunol, 161,* 6896-6903.

Wiley, C.A. and Achim, C. (1994). Human immunodeficiency virus encephalitis is the pathological correlate of dementia in acquired immunodeficiency syndrome. *Ann. Neurol, 36,* 673-676.

Wilfert, C.M., Wilson, C., Luzuriaga, K. and Epstein, L. (1994). Pathogenesis of pediatric human immunodeficiency virus type 1 infection. *J. Infect. Dis, 170,* 286-292.

Wynn, H.E., Brundage, R.C. and Fletcher, C.V. (2002). Clinical implications of CNS penetration of antiretroviral drugs. *CNS Drugs, 16,* 595-609.

Zhu, T., Mo, H., Wang, N., Nam, D.S., Cao, Y., Koup, R.A. and Ho, D.D. (1993). Genotypic and phenotypic characterization of HIV-1 patients with primary infection. *Science, 261,* 1179-1181.

In: Neuro-AIDS
Editors: A. Minagar and P. Shapshak, pp. 41-79

ISBN: 1-59454-610-X
© 2006 Nova Science Publishers, Inc.

Chapter III

The Relevance of Chemokines and Cytokines to the Pathogenesis of HIV-1 Associated Dementia

N. Erdmann[1,2], Y. Huang[1,2] and J. Zheng[1,2,3],*

[1]The laboratory of Neurotoxicology at the Center for Neurovirology and
Neurodegenerative Disorders, [2]Dept. Pharmacology and Experimental Neuroscience,
[3]Dept. of Pathology and Microbiology, University of Nebraska Medical Center,
Omaha, NE 68198-5880. USA.

Abstract

HIV-1-associated dementia (HAD) manifests during the late stages of infection by human immunodeficiency virus as a spectrum of neurological and psychiatric symptoms. The disease process is mediated by cellular (cytokine, chemokines and others) and viral neurotoxins produced mainly by brain mononuclear phagocytes (MP; macrophages and microglia) without direct infection of neurons. The prolonged inflammatory state results in the production and release of various factors that can lead to astrocyte dysfunction and neuronal injury when produced in abundance. While the pathogenesis of this neurodegeneration still remains unclear, neuronal damage is induced by the toxins engaging specific neuronal receptors or indirectly through widespread MP/astrocyte inflammatory activities. Cytokines and chemokines play a central role in the generation of this chronic encephalopathy. A chemokine gradient established by brain MP and astrocytes initiate monocyte transendothelial migration, increase the viral reservoir, and provide cellular sources of inflammatory products. Chemokines, cytokines and viral products cause neuronal dysfunction by engaging neural receptors and activating pathways that alter synaptic transmission and neuronal function. Here, we discuss the

* Correspondence concerning this article should be addressed to J. Zheng Laboratory of Neurotoxicology, Center for Neurovirology and Neurodegenerative Disorders, 985880 Nebraska Medical Center, Omaha, NE 68198-5880. Phone: 402-559-5656; Fax: 402-559-3744; Email: jzheng@unmc.edu.

mechanisms involved in chemokine and cytokine mediated neural compromise and disease progression in HAD.

Keywords: HIV-1 associated dementia, astrocytes, microglia, neurons, chemokines, cytokines.

Abbreviations

AIDS	acquired immune deficiency syndrome
HIV	human immunodeficiency virus
CI	cognitive impairment
BBB	blood-brain-barrier
CNS	central nervous system
TNF-α	tumor necrosis factor alpha
IL-1β	interleukin-1 beta
GFAP	glial fibrillary acidic protein
FKN	fractalkine
GRO-α	growth-related oncogene α
HAD	HIV-1 associated dementia
ART	antiretroviral therapy
HIVE	HIV-1 encephalitis
IL-8	interleukin-8
IP-10	interferon gamma inducible protein 10
LTP	long term potentiation
MAP-2	microtubule associated protein-2
MCP-1	monocyte chemotactic protein-1
MDM	monocyte-derived macrophages
MIP-1α/β	macrophage inhibitory proteins-one alpha and –one beta
MP	mononuclear phagocytes
NF	neurofilament
NMDA	N-methyl D-aspartate
NSE	neuronal specific enolase
PAF	platelet activating factor
RANTES	the regulated upon activation normal T cell expressed and secreted
RT	reverse transcriptase
SCID	severe combined immunodeficiency
SDF-1α	stromal derived factor-1 alpha

Introduction

The ability to respond to pathogenic insult is vital to the survival of an organism, and this response must be rapid, robust yet controlled. Such a response requires extensive coordination and is thus reliant upon the intercommunication of various systems and effectors. The principle system in this synchronized response is the immune system, and the signals orchestrating effector cells throughout the body are primarily cytokines. Cytokines are small glycosylated proteins that exist as either membrane-bound or secreted factors, targeting specific receptors throughout the body. Their function, although not exclusively, revolves around the immune system, facilitating its various roles including surveillance, recruitment, activation, development and the influence of apoptotic or survival pathways. Cytokines constitute a relatively redundant family of intercellular messengers that often cause similar effects by acting upon promiscuous receptors. Cytokines act via these receptors on target cells with high affinity and are thus extremely potent, often having effects at picomolar and sometimes even femtomolar concentrations. As a consequence, the production of cytokines is tightly regulated and often strictly localized.

Over 200 different human cytokines have now been identified. Most cytokines are single polypeptide chains, although they may form multimers in biological fluids; for example, tumor necrosis factor (TNF)-alpha circulates as a homotrimer, while IL-12 and IL-23 act as heterodimers. As an exceptionally large and diverse group of factors, cytokines are consequently very difficult to classify. While many factors share structural similarities or have functional homologues, most generalizations are riddled with exceptions. Below, is an effort to help provide a foundation for thinking about these factors and their role in the brain.

Type I Family

Despite a lack in amino acid sequence homology, Type I cytokines and receptors share similar three-dimensional structure; an extracellular region containing four α helices is a characteristic motif of the receptors. Members of this family include Interleukin-2 (IL-2), IL-3, IL-4, IL-5, IL-6, IL-7, IL-9, IL-12, granulocyte-colony stimulating factor (G-CSF), granulocyte macrophage-colony stimulating factor (GM-CSF) and brain-derived neurotrophic factor (BDNF). Among them IL-2, IL-3, IL-4, IL-7 are T cell growth factors; IL-2, IL-6, IL-12 are pro-inflammatory cytokines; G-CSF and GM-CSF are hematopoietic cytokines important for survival and differentiation of hematopoietic lineages.

Type II Family

Type II cytokines include IL-10, IL-19, IL-20, IL-22, and interferons (IFN-α, -β, -ϵ, -κ, -ω, -δ, -τ and -γ). Functions of this group include induction of cellular antiviral states, modulation of inflammatory responses, inhibition or stimulation of cell growth, production or inhibition of apoptosis, as well as affecting many immune mechanisms (Pestka et al., 2004; Renauld, 2003). Notably, IL-10 is a potent anti-inflammatory, immunomodulatory cytokine; the IFN system is an important contributor to innate immunity with IFN-γ serving as a potent pro-inflammatory cytokine.

TNF Family

TNF family is comprised of at least 19 type II transmembrane proteins that have partial homology in extracellular domains. Members of this superfamily are typically homotrimers and include TNF-α, TNF-β, Fas ligand (FasL), CD40 ligand (CD40L), TNF-Related Apoptosis-Inducing Ligand (TRAIL), and nerve growth factor (NGF). This receptor superfamily is subdivided into three groups. The first group includes those with conserved intracellular 'death domains' that activate the caspase cascade and induce apoptosis, e.g. TNF receptor type I (TNF-R1), Fas, TRAIL receptor 1 (TRAIL R-1), TRAIL receptor 2 (TRAIL R-2), death receptor (DR)3 and DR6. The second group includes those with one or more TRAF (TNF receptor associated factor)-interacting motifs (Tims) in their cytoplasmic tails, e.g. TNF-R2, CD 40, and CD 27. Activation of these receptors lead to recruitment of TRAF family members, and activation of multiple signal transduction pathways such as nuclear factor κB (NF-κB), Jun N-terminal Kinase (JNK), P38, extracellular signal-related kinase (ERK) and phosphoinositide3-kinase (PI-3K). The third subset of the TNF receptor family does not contain functional intracellular domains or motifs but still may compete with other receptors for binding and are thus regarded as "decoy receptors". e.g. TRAIL-R3, TRAIL R4 (Dempsey et al., 2003).

IL-1 Family

The IL-1 family is also called the immunoglobulin superfamily. The receptors in this family include both transmembrane and soluble proteins with immunoglobulin-like structure. There are four primary members of the IL-1 family: IL-1α, IL-1β, IL-18, and IL-1Ra. IL-1 ligands (IL-1α and IL-1β, collectively referred to as IL-1) are potent pro-inflammatory cytokines that induce genes associated with inflammation and autoimmune disease. IL-1Ra, on the other hand, is the specific receptor antagonist for IL-1α and IL-1β.

TGF-β Family

Transforming Growth Factor Beta (TGF-β) is the prototypical member of this family, but at least 50 proteins are classified TGF-β members including TGF-β, activins, inhibins, bone morphogenetic proteins (BMPs) and glial cell line-derived neurotrphoic factor (GDNF). TGF-β family receptors have characteristic cysteine-rich extracellular domains, kinase domains, GS domains, and a serine/threonine-rich tail (type II receptors). TGF-β has numerous functions including regulation of neuronal survival, orchestration of repair processes, as well as anti-inflammation. The role of TGF-β in the suppression of adaptive immune responses may be important and will be discussed later in this chapter.

Chemokine Family

Chemokine receptors are a unique family of G-protein coupled receptors and will be discussed in length later due to their profound impact on HIV-1 associated dementia.

All the above families are imperative for homeostatic functions as well as the orchestration of response to pathogenic insult by the immune system. As investigations carry on, this large family will likely see the emergence of newly discovered cytokines, and the family and sub-families of cytokine receptors will continue to change and expand.

CNS Cell Types and Cytokines

The central nervous system (CNS), once thought to be an immune privileged environment, has been shown to interact with the immune system, and cytokines mediate this communication. Normally, CNS cytokine expression levels are minimal (John M. Petitto, 2003); however, during inflammatory states, lymphocytes, monocytes and macrophages migrate into the CNS and produce various factors. As the primary immunocompetent cells in the CNS, macrophage and microglia are major producers and targets of cytokines. Cytokines from macrophage and microglia regulate the intensity and duration of the immune response by stimulating/inhibiting activation, proliferation, differentiation and migration of multiple cell types of the immune system. Macrophage and microglia are the major cellular source for the pro-inflammatory cytokines IL-1α, IL-1β and TNF-α (McGeer and McGeer, 1995; Mrak et al., 1995). Such factors can contribute to the disease process when not appropriately regulated in a chronic disease state. Direct injection of IL-1 into the CNS results in local inflammatory responses and neural degeneration (Wright and Merchant, 1992). Further, macrophage and microglia may be activated by those cytokines to generate more pro-inflammatory cytokines such as IL-6 in an autocrine or paracrine manner (Basu et al., 2004). Interestingly, microglia and astrocytes also produce IL-10 and TGF-β, which have been shown to inhibit the inflammatory response as well as apoptosis in cells of neuronal origin (Prehn et al., 1994). Due to their paradoxical roles, the response of macrophage and microglia to cytokines is dependent upon the presence of different cytokine profiles within the local microenvironment.

Neurons are not major producers of cytokines, however, they are directly regulated by their activity. Cytokines released by macrophages/microglia have been proposed to modulate neuronal survival and death. TNF-α and TRAIL have been shown to bind to death receptors on neurons and cause neuronal apoptosis both *in-vitro* and *in-vivo* (Miura et al., 2003a; Ryan et al., 2004; Shi et al., 1998). Perhaps more importantly, the secondary products of inflammation, primarily from macrophage and microglia, such as glutamate (Jiang et al., 2001), platelet-activating factor (Gelbard et al., 1994; Nishida et al., 1996; Perry et al., 1998), arachidonic acid (Nottet et al., 1995), quinolinic acid (Heyes et al., 1998; Kerr et al., 1995) and nitric oxide (Adamson et al., 1996) are responsible for neural injury and dropout. Conversely, another product of macrophage activation, TGF-β, has been shown to inhibit apoptosis in cells of neuronal origin (Prehn et al., 1994). Stimulation of microglia with immune activators such as LPS leads to the induction of NGF secretion and enhances BDNF production (Nakajima et al., 2001). Such neurotrophins help in the survival of neurons (Allsopp et al., 1998; Park et al., 1998). Additionally, cytokine and neuron interactions may have activity beyond neuronal survival and death; there is evidence of a cytokine circuit in the CNS, possibly responsible for the regulation of diverse neuronal functions such as learning, memory (John M. Petitto, 2003) and thermoregulation (Kluger, 1991).

As the major cell type in the CNS, astrocytes are believed to be vital in the homeostatic maintenance of the microenvironment. HIV can non-productively infect astrocytes (Canki et al., 1997), and this infection occurs via a CD4 independent mechanism possibly involving novel astrocyte surface molecules and HIV gp120 (Ma et al., 1994). Astrocytes may also serve as a reservoir for HIV-1 and allow persistence of latent infection for years (Messam and Major, 2000). HIV-1 viral protein gp-120, as well as pro-inflammatory cytokines, can activate astrocytes and exacerbate neuronal dysfunction (Eddleston and Mucke, 1993; Kaul et al., 2001; Wyss-Coray et al., 1996). For example, the pro-inflammatory cytokine IL-1β induces astrocyte production of Fas ligand (FasL) through the NF-κB pathway. FasL may then interact with Fas in neurons, activating the caspase cascade and causing neuronal death in HAD (Ghorpade et al., 2003). In addition, IL-1 also activates human fetal astrocytes to produce IL-8, M-CSF, G-CSF, and GM-CSF, which can then influence the differentiation and activation of microglia (Aloisi et al., 1992; Lee et al., 1993).

Cytokines and Neuroimmunology

Cytokines are an important element in the brain's immune function, serving to traffic leukocytes, maintain immune surveillance, and recruit inflammatory factors; however, CNS inflammation is unique due to the presence of a nonfenestrated cerebrovascular endothelium known as the blood brain barrier. In the normal physiological state, only activated T-cells cross the barrier and enter the CNS scanning for antigen (Glabinski and Ransohoff, 1999). A restricted inflammatory process is initiated upon encountering foreign antigen, inducing the production of recruitment factors. Upon recruitment, monocytes and lymphocytes cross through the blood brain barrier to mount immune responses in the CNS. Recruitment is dependent upon the presence of chemotactic factors produced within the CNS that facilitate the crossing of the blood brain barrier. This inflammatory state is highly regulated and usually self-limited. Avoidance of uncontrolled activation, release of toxic factors, edema and other effects of robust inflammation is critical to maintenance of the vulnerable microenvironment in the CNS.

Dysregulation of the inflammatory process can lead to a disease process within the CNS. Continual activation and recruitment of effector cells may establish a positive feedback loop that perpetuates inflammatory processes and can ultimately lead to neuronal injury and dropout. Similar yet distinct processes occur in multiple CNS disorders such as Multiple Sclerosis, Parkinson's disease, Alzheimer disease, and stroke. One underlying similarity in each disease state is the cytokine driven inflammatory response. A distinct, but fundamentally related CNS disease process is HIV-1 Associated Dementia (HAD). HIV infection notoriously attacks the immune system in the periphery, but also can lead to a viral induced dementia. The mechanism has yet to be fully elucidated, but cytokines have been shown to play a significant role in disease progression.

HIV usually enters the brain shortly after initial infection, likely catching a ride from peripherally infected monocytes across the blood brain barrier (Koenig et al., 1986). Brain macrophages and microglia, unlike other cellular residents in the CNS, are able to sustain a productive infection within the brain (Eilbott et al., 1989). Thus, while the rest of the body typically experiences a surge in viral load followed by a gradual reduction, the isolated CNS maintains a low, but sustained level of virus. The disease process in the brain progresses somewhat independently from the remainder of the body. Although neurons are not infected by HIV-1, a dementia specific to HIV has been described. Typically manifesting during later stages of disease, the dementia includes a spectrum of neurological impairments including forgetfulness, apathy, hallucinations, delirium, coma, and ultimately death (McArthur, 1987; Navia et al., 1986). The dementia, referred to as HAD previously affected 20-30% of those with advanced HIV. This number has since decreased with the advent of Anti-Retroviral Therapy (ART) in developed countries to around 10% (Dore et al., 1997; Sacktor et al., 2001). However, ART cannot completely protect from or reverse HAD (Dore et al., 1997). Both the number of newly infected individuals and life expectancies continue to rise, and thus the prevalence of HAD has increased as well, making this dementia the most common type for those under the age of 40 (Ellis et al., 1997). Accordingly, HAD is an important effect of HIV infection.

HAD is the clinical consequence of neuronal damage and death. HAD is itself a diagnosis of exclusion and is usually only apparent in the late stages of AIDS, despite early CNS inoculation with virus. The pathologic correlate to HAD, HIV encephalitis (HIVE), is characterized by activated macrophage and microglia, as well as damage of neuronal dendrites and axons and apoptotic neurons. However, neuronal injury and death is the result of indirect complications from the infection. Because viral products are produced and released in the CNS, particularly by macrophage and microglia undergoing productive infection, neuronal death can be induced through two paths that are not mutually exclusive. Neurotoxicity is mediated directly by viral proteins such as gp120, or indirectly through the immune response elicited in the brains of HAD patients. The predominant cause of neuronal toxicity is an indirect mechanism instigated by macrophage, microglia and astrocyte generated toxins (Kaul et al., 2001). The production of virus and toxins by glial and phagocytic cells within the CNS establishes a positive feedback loop driven by cytokines. Damaged macrophages and neurons recruit immune cells to the initial site of infection. The congregating immune cells, MP in particular, fail to eliminate the insult but produce additional toxins, factors, and eventually virus. Macrophage derived neurotoxic products are amplified within the brain as a consequence of productive viral infection and immune activation (Ryan et al., 2002).

In HAD, immune cells are recruited to the site of viral infection, and cytokines are believed to drive this inflammatory response. As a result of HIV-1 infection, the host produces an array of factors including cytokines and proteases yet is unable to clear the infection. The difficulty in eradicating HIV-1 infection prolongs the immune response leading to a chronic inflammatory state. Chronic inflammation is both a friend and foe; on one hand, these responses are essential in limiting viral spread; yet on the other, excessive inflammation is detrimental to resident cells such as neurons.

Cytokines in Neurodegeneration and Neurotoxicity During HAD

Cytokines have been implicated as contributors towards a number of neurodegenerative diseases. Interest in the role of cytokines during HAD increased when a study demonstrated HAD involved an inflammatory process. How HIV-1 infection leads to neuronal injury and/or loss has been and remains the focus of much investigation. During HIV-1 infection, macrophage and microglia are productively infected (Fischer-Smith et al., 2004; Meltzer et al., 1990; Wiley et al., 1986), and once infected become the major cytokine producer in the CNS (Griffin, 1997).

Two distinct models have been proposed as mechanisms in HAD pathogenesis. The first is the direct neuronal injury model, where viral proteins (gp120, tat and Vpr) directly interact with neurons causing neuronal injury through various mechanisms. The role of cytokines in this model has been controversial. On one hand, cytokines like TNF-α have a synergistic apoptotic effect with viral proteins tat (Shi et al., 1998) and gp120 (Kast, 2002). However, other cytokines inhibit the effects of viral proteins on neurons. For example, TGF-β1 prevents gp120-induced neuronal apoptosis by restoring calcium homeostasis (Scorziello et al., 1997); BDNF and IL-10 can inhibit gp-120 mediated cerebellar granule cell death by preventing gp120 internalization and caspase 3 activation *in vitro* (Bachis et al., 2001; Bachis et al., 2003). The second model, referred to as the indirect neuronal injury model, proposes that neurons die as bystanders when excessive local concentrations of soluble pro-inflammatory and neurotoxic factors are released by infected MP and astrocytes. Studies have supported this notion including the observation that viral protein levels do not correlate with neuronal injury (Petito et al., 1994), while neuronal apoptosis correlates well with microglial activation (Adle-Biassette et al., 1995; Glass et al., 1993). Furthermore, studies have shown that cognitively impaired patients have elevated levels of inflammatory markers and activators in contrast to HIV patients without CNS impairment (Sippy et al., 1995; Tyor et al., 1992). Proinflammatory cytokines such as TNF-alpha and IL-1 beta are key molecules in this model. The contribution of different cytokine families to HAD is summarized in table 1 and will be discussed below (see table 1).

Table 1. Role of cytokines in HIV-1 associated dementia

Cytokines classification	Cell source	Effects in the brain	Expression in HAD *	Reference
Type I family				
IL-6	Macrophage/microglia /Astrocyte	Proinflammation	Increase?	(Merrill and Chen, 1991), (Perrella et al., 1992b),(Griffin, 1997), (Gallo et al., 1991)
GM-CSF	Astrocyte	Macrophage defferentiation	Increase	(Perrella et al., 1992b)
IL-4	T-cell	Inhibition of IL-1, IL-6 production Activation of monocytes-macrophages	Decrease	(Wesselingh et al., 1993)
BDNF	Neuron, Astrocyte, Oligodentrocytes	Neuron survival/CNS development	Increase	(Soontornniyomkij et al., 1998), (Boven et al., 1999)
Type II family				
IL-10	Macrophage/microglia	Anit-inflammation	Increase	(Gallo et al., 1994)
IFN-α/β	Macrophage/microglia	Anti-viral	Increase	(Perrella et al., 1992a), (Perrella et al., 2001)
IFN-γ	Macrophage/microglia T-cells	Proinflammation	Increase	(Shapshak et al., 2004)
TNF family				
TNF-α	Macrophage/microglia	Proinflammation	Increase	(Grimaldi et al., 1991)
TRAIL	Macrophage/microglia	Apoptosis	Increase	(Ryan et al., 2004)
NGF	Neuron/astrocytes/microglia/ macrophage	Neuron survival/CNS development	Increase	(Boven et al., 1999)
IL-1 family				
IL-1 α	Macrophage/microglia/Astrocyte	Proinflammation	Increase	(Perrella et al., 1992a)
IL-1 β	Macrophage/microglia/Astrocyte	Proinflammation	Increase?	(Wesselingh et al., 1993), (Gallo et al., 1991)
TGF-β family				
TGF-β	Macrophage/microglia/Astrocyte	Anit-inflammation	Decrease?	(Perrella et al., 2001), (Johnson and Gold, 1996)

* May reflect the protein levels in CSF or protein/RNA levels in vulnerable brain regions. Question mark indicates the variation of reports.

Type I Cytokines

Elevated levels of IL-6, IL-2 and decreased levels of IL-4 have been reported in both CSF and brain sections of HAD patients (Griffin, 1997; Perrella et al., 1992a; Wesselingh et al., 1993). These factors are directly related to the inflammatory state of brain. The activation of a TH1 immune response by infected macrophages results in the synthesis of cytokines such as IL-2 and IL-6 that activate macrophage and coordinate the immune response towards HIV-1. IL-2 induces T-cell proliferation and potentiates the release of other cytokines. IL-3 and GM-CSF stimulate the production of new macrophages by acting on hematopoietic stem cells in bone marrow. New macrophages are recruited to the site of infection by TNF-α and other cytokines on the vascular endothelium that signal macrophages to leave the bloodstream and enter the tissue. Within this family of cytokines, IL-6 may be the most potent inducer of the inflammatory response. In a transgenic animal model, overexpression of IL-6 in the CNS has been reported to have a similar neurological disorder with neurodegenerative diseases (Campbell et al., 1993). The inflammatory response in HAD is coordinated primarily by macrophage to prevent HIV-1 dissemination. On the other hand, many inflammatory signals have been shown to increase HIV replication. IL-2 and GM-CSF are both potent stimulators of HIV-1 replication in activated CD4+ T cells, and GM-CSF increases HIV-1 replication in macrophage cultures (Perno et al., 1990). The activity of type I cytokines during HIV-1 infection promotes the inflammatory response in an effort to eliminate virus, however in the CNS during HAD, type I cytokine mediated inflammation results in neuronal damage as well as causing proliferation of HIV.

Type II Cytokines

Type II cytokines are key to the balance of inflammation and regulation of response in HAD. IL-10 down-regulates the expression of proinflammatory cytokines and up-regulates the expression of the anti-inflammatory agent IL-1Ra. Increased levels of IL-10 in the CSF have been reported in individuals with HIV-1 encephalitis (Gallo et al., 1994). In a recent study in an HAD SCID mouse model, mRNA levels of IL-10 were increased five-fold as compared to uninfected controls, and this change is concurrent with down-regulation of proinflammatory cytokines (IL-1β and IL-6) (Poluektova et al., 2004). Moreover, pretreatment with IL-10 attenuated the neurobehavioral damage induced by HIV-1 gp120 in an in-vivo animal study (Barak et al., 2002). Increased type II immunomodulatory cytokines are possibly an active attempt to control inflammation and maintain or regain balance in CNS microenvironments.

IFNs are considered a sub-family of type II cytokines because of their similar receptor structure to IL-10. IFNs profoundly affect HIV-1 replication in various in-vitro systems. IFN-α and IFN-β are induced by HIV-1 infection and suppress HIV replication at multiple steps of the viral life cycle in macrophage (Gendelman et al., 1992; Gessani et al., 1994). IFN-γ enhances HIV-1 replication in CD4+ T cells in an autocrine manner, while in macrophage culture IFN-γ enhances HIV-1 replication when added prior to infection but inhibits replication when added post-infection. Although levels of IFN-γ have been shown to be elevated in HAD patients (Shapshak et al., 2004), its ultimate role is unclear. IFN-γ shapes the T-cell response and activates MP perhaps limiting viral spread, yet IFN-γ also synergistically enhances the effect of CD40L activation of macrophage. Interferons are known to target infected cells for cell-mediated elimination, but the ultimate role of interferons in HAD pathogenesis is still unclear (Benveniste, 1992).

TNF Superfamily

Among the pro-inflammatory cytokines, TNF-α is the most studied. Elevated levels of TNF-α mRNA is seen in brain tissue collected from HAD patients (Wesselingh et al., 1993). Studies have shown that TNF-α levels in vulnerable brain regions correlate with neurologic disease severity in HIV patients (Gelbard, 1999). During HAD, microglia, macrophages and monocytes show increased expression of TNF-α and TNF receptors (Tyor et al., 1992), an effect promoted by both IFN-γ and IL-1. ART treated HAD patients have a marked decrease in soluble TNF-α levels in the cerebrospinal fluid; this drop in TNF-α coincides with decreased viral load and marked improvement in the neurological function of patients (Gendelman et al., 1998). TNF-α may promote neuronal demise through various mechanisms. Increased BBB permeability and recruitment of activated immune cells facilitates viral invasion of the CNS. Synergy of TNF-α, viral proteins and excitotoxic glutamate activates glia to produce neurotoxins or leads to neuronal apoptosis directly (see review (Saha and Pahan, 2003)). The effects of TNF-α are complex; differing experimental systems or approaches have also shown TNF-α to assume a neuroprotective role.

TRAIL, another member of this family, is not normally expressed in the CNS. However, in HIV-1 infection and HAD, TRAIL-expressing macrophages infiltrate the brain. Numerous CNS cells including MP and neurons express TRAIL-receptors and may be targeted by TRAIL for apoptosis. Neurons, microglia, macrophages and astrocytes, may be induced to express TRAIL upon interaction with immune activators such as IFN-γ or LPS, (Cantarella et al., 2003; Genc et al., 2003; Lee et al., 2003). The regulation of TRAIL by these factors, along with its ability to induce neuronal apoptosis, suggests that TRAIL may be involved in the pathogenesis of HAD (Ryan et al., 2004). HIV-1-infected macrophages expressing TRAIL may initiate neuronal injury through two possible means. Firstly, TRAIL is capable of binding to at least four unique cell surface receptors; all four of these receptors, but not TRAIL itself, have been found in normal human brain. TRAIL expressed on macrophages or the soluble form of TRAIL could interact directly with death receptors (TRAIL Receptor 1 and 2) on neurons initiating apoptosis. Evidence from *in-vitro* studies support this conclusion (Ryan et al., 2004). A similar observation was recently demonstrated in a murine model using human peripheral blood mononuclear cell (PBMC)-transplanted nonobese diabetic (NOD)-severe combined immunodeficiency (SCID)-hu-PBMC-NOC-SCID-mice (Miura et al., 2003b). In this work, LPS was administered to HIV-1-infected hu-PBMC-NOC-SCID-mice to induce infiltration of HIV-1-infected human cells into the perivascular region of the brain. The apoptotic neurons frequently colocalize with HIV-1 infected macrophages expressing TRAIL. Administration of a neutralizing antibody against human TRAIL but not human TNF-α or Fas ligand blocks neuronal apoptosis in the HIV-1-infected brain, suggesting a significant role for TRAIL in MP mediated neuronal apoptosis (Miura et al., 2003b). Secondly, TRAIL may mediate macrophage-macrophage interactions resulting in apoptosis of HIV-1 infected macrophage. The subsequent increase of glutamate together with decreased glutamate uptake by astrocytes, results in excess extracellular glutamate. The presence of high levels of glutamate in the vicinity of neurons causes excitotoxicity and neuronal loss (Huang et al., 2004).

IL-1 Family

IL-1 is rapidly produced upon HIV-1 infection within the CNS. The induction of IL-1 has been shown to be associated with HAD (Zhao et al., 2001). IL-1 in this case serves as a very upstream signal for multiple proinflammatory cytokines, notably TNF-α and IL-6, initiating and amplifying inflammation in the brain, which is responsible for the global activation of macrophage and microgila (Aloisi et al., 1992; Chung and Benveniste, 1990; Lee et al., 1993). Direct injections of IL-1 into the CNS result in local inflammatory responses and neural degeneration (Wright and Merchant, 1992). IL-1 β directly activates HIV-1 replication in a monocytic cell line by transcriptional and post–transcriptional mechanisms independent of NF-κB. IL-1 also synergistically enhances HIV-1 replication with multiple cytokines including IL-4 and IL-6 (Kedzierska et al., 2003).

TGF-β Family

TGF-β is expressed in the brain by astrocytes, MP and oligodendrocytes, and has been shown to exert multiple effects on neurons and glial cells both *in vitro* and *in vivo*. Effects of TGF-β include cell cycle control, differentiation, extracellular matrix formation, hematopoesis, and chemotaxis. Importantly in the CNS, TGF-β has a key role in regulating neuron survival and repair processes. TGF-β has also been shown to play a role in several varieties of CNS pathology including ischemia, excitotoxicity and neurodegenerative diseases such as multiple sclerosis. In mild HAD, the cerebral levels of TGF-β have an inverse correlation to IFN-α and HIV RNA; while in the severe form of HAD, TGF-β is undetectable (Perrella et al., 2001). In specific culture conditions, TGF-β has neurotrophic effects similar to BDNF and NGF, but a change in conditions can shift the effect of TGF-β towards neurotoxicity (Prehn and Miller, 1996). Other members of the TGF-β family such as GDNF and BMPs also show neurotrophic potency.

Molecular Mechanisms of Cytokine Activity in HAD

Specific knowledge of signaling through cytokine receptors has increased tremendously over the past decade. Multiple signaling pathways have been observed for various cytokines. Cytokines influence neuronal survival via two pathways: the direct and indirect pathway. In the direct pathway, cytokines directly interact with receptors on neurons to either promote apoptotic or survival pathways. For example, TNF-α, Fas-L and TRAIL trigger the neuronal extrinsic pathway and cause apoptosis. In the indirect pathway, cytokines act on the other cell types in the CNS and secondary products then influence neuron survival. The ultimate outcome of each individual neuron may depend upon many factors within the local cytokine network. To better understand the molecular mechanisms involved in cytokine-induced neurodegeneration in HAD, we will discuss the molecular signaling of neuronal survival and cell death (see Figure 1).

The signaling events leading to apoptosis can be divided into two distinct pathways, involving either the mitochondria (intrinsic) or death receptors (extrinsic) (for reviews, see (Green, 2003; Green and Reed, 1998)). The mitochondrial pathway is initiated through various stress signals that damage mitochondria. BCL-2 family proteins, including the anti-apoptotic members, i.e. BCL-2 and BCL-XL, and pro-apoptotic members, i.e. Bax, Bak, play a critical role in this pathway (Danial and Korsmeyer, 2004; Green, 2003; Gross et al., 1999; Wang, 2001). The BH3–only BCL-2 family proteins, such as Bid, Bad, Bim, and PUMA, serve as sentinels to these stress signals. Once activated, BH3-only proteins translocate to the outer membrane of mitochondria, where they trigger the oligomerization and activation of both Bax and Bak. In turn, Bax and Bak cause the release of cytochrome c (cyto c) and other apoptogenic factors, including second mitochondrial-derived activator of caspase (SMAC), Htr2, apoptosis inducing factor (AIF), and endonuclease G (EndoG) (Green and Reed, 1998). Cyto c then binds the cytosolic adaptor protein, Apaf-1, mediating the formation of the apoptosis complex "apoptosome", which is composed of cyto c, Apaf-1, and procaspase-9 (Figure 2). Such complexes lead to the activation of caspase-9, which further processes and activates the effector caspases, pro-caspase-3, 6, or 7. Effector caspases then cleave death substrates and complete apoptosis.

The death receptor pathway is initiated through interaction with death receptors and the recruitment of cytoplasmic proteins to specific regions in the intracellular domains of these receptors. The receptor adaptor protein complex then binds pro-caspase 8 and forms a death-inducing signaling complex (DISC) that subsequently releases active caspase 8. Active caspase 8 then activates a caspase cascade and eventually leads to apoptosis of the cell.

Many cytokines influence the activation of apoptotic pathways. TRAIL signaling is one of the paradigms in the TNF superfamily of cytokines. TRAIL interacts directly with death receptors on neurons initiating neuronal apoptosis through activation of the caspase cascade. Fas ligand (FasL), another member of the TNF family, also has similar apoptotic effects towards neurons. In HAD, the increase of death inducing cytokines such as TRAIL has been reported (Ryan et al., 2004).

In contrast to the apoptotic pathway, growth factors and some cytokines bind to cell surface receptors and lead to the activation of survival pathways such as the PI3Kinase (PI3K) pathway and Ras- or PKC-dependent MAP kinase pathway. Activated PI3K leads to downstream Akt phosphorylation and activation. Notably, Akt activation converges with death receptor mediated RIP activation on the activation of the IKK complex and the resulting IKB degradation (Figure 1). IKB degradation releases active NF-κB that leads to transcription of genes necessary for cell survival. Similarly, activation of MAP kinase will lead to nuclear translocation of MAPK together with other transcription factors and co-activators and initiate the transcription of a variety of survival genes (Figure 1).

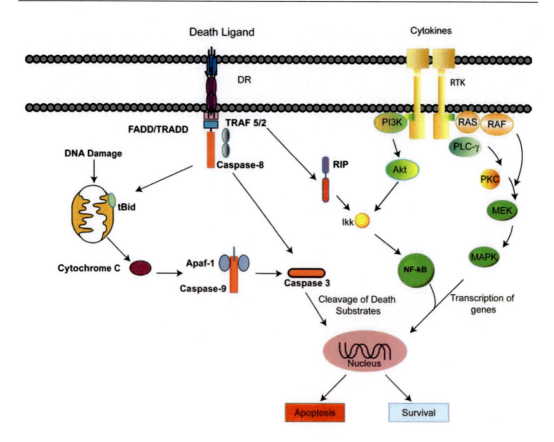

Figure 1. A schematic diagram illustrating cytokine-mediated cell death and survival signaling pathways. The death receptor pathway involves the intrinsic or extrinsic pathway, initiated through death receptors and the recruitment of cytoplasmic proteins to form a death-inducing signaling complex (DISC) that subsequently releases active caspase 8. Active caspase 8 can then activate two distinct pathways: direct activation of caspase 3 or indirect activation of caspase 3 through the mitochondria. In the mitochondrial dependant pathway, Bid is translocated to the outer membrane of the mitochondria, where it triggers the oligomerization and activation of both Bax and Bak. In turn Bax and Bak cause the release of cyto c. Cyto c then binds to the Apaf-1, mediating the formation of the apoptosome and the activation of caspase-9, which further activates the effector caspases, pro-caspase-3, 6, or 7. Effector caspases then cleave death substrates and complete apoptosis. In the survival pathway, activation of cell surface receptor leads to the activation of the PI3Kinase (PI3K) pathway and Ras- or PKC-dependent MAP kinase pathway. Activated PI3K leads to downstream Akt phosphorylation and activation. Notably, Akt activation converges with death receptor mediated RIP activation towards the activation of the IKK complex and resulting in IKB degradation. IKB degradation releases active NF-κB leading to transcription of genes necessary for cell survival. Similarly, activation of MAP kinase will lead to nuclear translocation of MAPK together with other transcription factors and co-activators and initiate the transcription of a variety of survival genes.

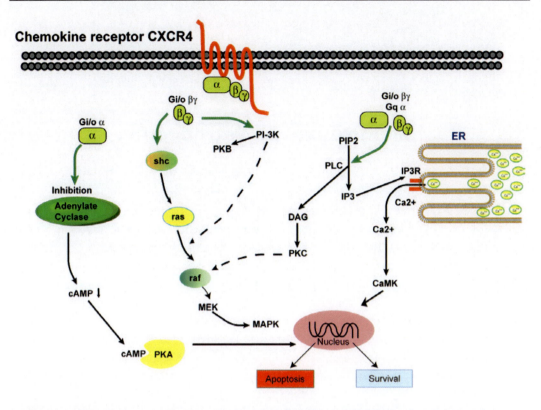

Figure 2. A schematic diagram illustrating chemokine mediated signaling pathways. Chemokine activity is mediated by activating a family of seven transmembrane G-protein coupled receptors (GPCR). GPCRs interact with and signal through heterotrimeric guanine-nucleotide-binding regulatory proteins (G-proteins). Upon stimulation by a ligand, GPCRs undergo a conformational change that leads to activation of the G-protein by GDP-GTP exchange, followed by uncoupling of the G-protein from the receptor. Using SDF-1/CXCR4 interaction as an example, upon activation, G-proteins trigger a cascade of signaling events involving the inhibition of adenylate cyclase activity leading to decreased cytosolic cAMP levels; the activation of phosphalipase C leading to transient increases in cytosolic inositol triphosphate (IP$_3$) and [Ca^{2+}] levels; and the stimulation of MAP kinase phosphorylation which are major components of pro-survival or death signaling pathways in cells and regulate various cellular functions. Other signaling pathways may also be activated and how these signal transduction pathways are linked to chemokine mediated changes in cellular function awaits elucidation.

Neurons constantly receive survival and apoptotic signals from the extracellular environment, influencing the lifespan of each individual cell. In HAD, there is little evidence supporting disruption of survival signals. Various cytokines such as BDNF or NGF increase and may be a compensatory mechanism of the CNS (Boven et al., 1999; Soontornniyomkij et al., 1998). IL-1 β from the IL-1 family or IL-6 from the Type I cytokine family can activate the NFκB pathway, thus potentially promoting survival of neurons. Interestingly, IL-1, TNF and even TRAIL signaling pathways also converge on NIK activation of the IKK complex and the resulting IKB degradation, and NF κB activation. IL-6 also activates the Ras-dependent MAPK pathway. Regarding IL-1β, the activation of NFκB and MAPK initiates transcription of a variety of genes for either survival or the inflammatory response, dependent upon cell type (Srinivasan et al., 2004).

Cytokines are clearly critical to the outcome of neurons and brain function during HIV infection. The various families of cytokines greatly influence the survival of neurons and ultimately brain function. However, because of the unique dependence of HIV infection upon chemokine receptors, the role of chemokines will be discussed at length below.

Chemokines: An Introduction

First discovered in 1987 (Walz et al., 1987; Yoshimura et al., 1987), chemokines entail a group of secreted proteins within the family of cytokines that by definition relate to the induction of migration. These "chemotactic cytokines" are produced by and target a wide variety of cells, but primarily address leukocyte chemoattraction and trafficking immune cells to locations throughout the body via a gradient. There are two general categories of biological activity for chemokines, the maintenance of homeostasis and the induction of inflammation (Moser and Loetscher, 2001). Homeostatic chemokines are involved in roles such as immune surveillance and the navigation of cells through hematopoesis, and are typically expressed constitutively. Inflammatory chemokines are produced in states of infection or following an inflammatory stimulus, and by targeting cells of the innate and adaptive immune system, facilitate an immune response. As is common in biological systems, there are exceptions to categorizations and some factors play dual roles. Within the past several years the links between chemokines, chemokine receptors, and HIV pathogenesis have been shown to be clear and significant (Cocchi et al., 1995; Deng et al., 1996; Dragic et al., 1996; Feng et al., 1996; Michael, 2002; Rizzardi et al., 2002). Chemokine receptors play a critical role, particularly in the early stages of HIV cell entry both in protective and liable capacities. Chemokine receptors CCR5 and CXCR4 are the major co-receptors for viral entry into CD4+ cells (Cocchi et al., 1995; Deng et al., 1996; Dragic et al., 1996; Feng et al., 1996), whereas the presence of chemokines can sometimes help prevent infection. These observations have elicited intense interest in chemokine biology.

Chemokines primarily target leukocytes and help orchestrate the immune system and its response to various stimuli. The factors target key players such as neutrophils, B cells, T cells, macrophages, dendritic cells as well as basophils, eosinophils, and others. The expression of these factors plays critical roles in the development of immune cells. For instance, the proper progression through lymphopoeisis (Cacalano et al., 1994), maturation of T-cells in the thymus (Annunziato et al., 2001), or recruitment of cells to immune tissue for surveillance (Forster et al., 1996) are examples of processes reliant upon chemokine activity. Chemokines also participate in the immune response itself, affecting cell migration, activation and tissue homeostasis.

While produced most often by immune cells, chemokines are also expressed by cells within the brain including endothelial cells, neurons, astrocytes, microglia and oligodendrocytes where they regulate the migration, recruitment, accumulation, and activation of leukocytes in the brain (Wu et al., 2000). Some chemokines such as stromal derived factor-1 alpha (SDF-1α, CXCL12) and fractalkine (FKN, CX3CL1) are constitutively produced in the brain and likely play an important role in central nervous system (CNS) homeostasis and development. Others, such as macrophage inhibitory proteins-one alpha and –one beta (MIP-1α, CCL3 and MIP-1β, CCL4), monocyte chemotactic protein-1 (MCP-1, CCL2), and the regulated upon activation normal T cell expressed and secreted (RANTES, CCL5), are induced by inflammatory stimuli. These chemokines are likely involved in the pathogenesis of a variety of neurodegenerative diseases, where inflammation plays a role in pathogenesis, such as HAD.

The inflammatory response manifest in the brain during HIV-1 infection of the nervous system leads to the development of a chemo-attractant gradient resulting in the formation of multinucleated giant cells in HIVE (Williams et al., 2002). This enables inflammatory monocyte-derived macrophages (MDM) to enter the brain, become infected and expand the sources of neurotoxic secretory factors that lead to the pathological and clinical aspects of disease (Gendelman et al., 1997). Moreover, chemokine receptors are critical for infection in perivascular macrophages and microglia. Studies have shown chemokines and their receptors play a more direct role in the neuropathogenesis of HIV-1 infection. It is now clear that neurons, glia and neural stem cells express chemokine receptors and the interactions of HIV-1 gp120 with neuronal chemokine receptors leads to apoptosis of neurons (Bezzi et al., 2001; Bonavia et al., 2003; Cotter et al., 2002; Hesselgesser et al., 1998; Kaul et al., 2001; Peng et al., 2004; Ryan et al., 2002; Tran and Miller, 2003). These effects may be manipulated by chemokines that act on the same receptors. The presence of chemokine receptors on neural cells also supports the notion that chemokines modulate neuronal physiological functions. Thus, chemokine receptors might have a crucial role in the balance between neuronal protection and injury.

Structure and Classification of Chemokines and their Receptors

Chemokines are 67 to 127 amino acids or 8-11 kd in size and are often translated as propeptides that are then processed during secretion to their active form. Additional processing may occur in the extracellular environment, enhancing, eliminating or changing the effect of signal receptor interactions. Chemokine activity is mediated by activating a family of seven transmembrane G-protein coupled receptors (GPCR). GPCRs interact with and signal through heterotrimeric guanine-nucleotide-binding regulatory proteins (G-proteins). Upon stimulation by a ligand, GPCRs undergo a conformational change that leads to activation of the G-protein by GDP-GTP exchange, followed by uncoupling of the G-protein from the receptor. Upon activation, G-proteins trigger a cascade of signaling events that regulate various cellular functions (Devi, 2000) (Figure 2).

Chemokine receptors are classified into four families based on the number and position of the N-terminal-conserved cysteine residues within the receptor binding domain including: α-chemokine receptors (such as CXCR2 and CXCR4); β-chemokine receptors (such as CCR5, CCR4, CCR3 and CCR2); γ- chemokine receptor (XCR1) and δ- chemokine receptors (CX3CR1) (Cotter et al., 2002; Gabuzda et al., 1998; Hesselgesser and Horuk, 1999; Klein et al., 1999; Miller and Meucci, 1999; van der Meer et al., 2000).

CXC chemokines are further separated into two groups based upon the presence or absence of a specific three amino acid sequence found adjacent to the CXC. The Glu-Leu-

Arg residues constitute the ELR motif, and if present, the CXC chemokine is considered to be ELR(+). The general function of ELR(+) chemokines revolves around neutrophils inducing chemotaxis and promoting angiogenesis (Strieter et al., 1995). Chemokines in this group include CXCL1, CXCL2, CXCL3, CXCL5, CXCL6, CXCL7, CXCL8, CXCL15; unlike ELR(–) members, these factors interact primarily with neutrophils via CXCR1 and CXCR2 receptors. In contrast, ELR(-) chemokines attract lymphocytes and monocytes with little affinity for neutrophils. This subgroup including CXCL4, CXCL9, CXCL10, CXCL11, CXCL12, CXCL13, CXCL14 and CXCL16 has a wider variety of activities, but generally have angiostatic properties and induce chemotaxis in mononuclear cells.

CC chemokines target primarily mononuclear cells and serve in both homeostatic and inflammatory capacities. The family can be divided into five functional groups; allergenic, pro-inflammatory, HCC, developmental and homeostatic. The developmental and homeostatic factors are, as expected, constitutively produced, whereas the other groups contain largely inducible signals. Allergenic CC chemokines target eosinophils, basophils and mast cells accounting for their name, and are both potent attractors and stimulants of histamine release. Both inflammatory and HCC subgroups are participants in inflammation but are separated because of phylogenetics.

CX3CL1 (Fractalkine, FKN) is the lone member of the CX3C subfamily with three intervening residues between the first two cysteines. FKN, the ligand for CX3CR1, is a 373-amino acid, multi-domain molecule found in a wide variety of tissues, including liver, intestine, kidney, and brain. Structural components of FKN include a 76-amino acid chemokine domain (CD) at the N-terminus, which is important in the binding, adhesion, and activation of its target cells (Goda et al., 2000; Harrison et al., 2001; Haskell et al., 2000; Mizoue et al., 1999; Mizoue et al., 2001). FKN has a 241-amino acid mucin-like stalk, which extends the chemokine domain away from the cell surface facilitating adherence of CX3CR1-expressing cells (Fong et al., 2000). FKN also has an 18-amino acid stretch of hydrophobic residues that spans the cell membrane, and an extended carboxyl-terminus that anchors it to the cell surface (Cook et al., 2001; Hoover et al., 2000; Lucas et al., 2001), thus allowing a membrane form as well as a shed soluble form targeting monocytes and T cells (Bazan et al., 1997). The final chemokine member is XCL1 (Lymphotactin), the only representative of the C family. The chemokine targets CD4+ and CD8+ lymphocytes, but does not act on monocytes, and acts through a unique receptor, XCR1. Although having some homology to ligands CCL3 and CCL8, XCL1 lacks the first and third cysteines characteristic of the CC and CXC chemokines.

The brain is a permanent home to cells including astrocytes, neurons, endothelial cells, and microglia, all expressing unique combinations of chemokines and chemokine receptors. Recruited immune cells such as monocytes or macrophage also inhabit the CNS and produce chemokine ligands as well as expressing additional chemokine receptors. Both macrophage and microglia have extensive chemokine expression profiles in addition to multiple receptors. Astrocytes were at one time thought to simply provide support to neurons and have few other interactions within the CNS environment. That view has evolved in part due to the chemokine expression profile of astrocytes. Neurons also generate and receive input from chemokine signals. These expression profiles are summarized in table 2.

Table 2. Chemokines and their Receptor Expressions in CNS

Cell Type	Ligands	Chemokine Receptors	
Mon ocyte s/Ma croph age	MCP-1, MIP-1α/β, RANTES, IL-8, IP-10	CCR2, CCR3, CCR4, CCR5, CXCR4, CX3CR1	(Bernasconi et al., 1996; Cinque et al., 1998; Collman et al., 2000; Gabuzda et al., 2002; Kelder et al., 1998)
Micr oglia	MIP-1α/β, RANTES, MCP-1,3, IL-8, IP-10	CCR2, CCR3, CCR4, CCR5, CXCR3, CXCR4, CX3CR1	(Bernasconi et al., 1996; Cinque et al., 1998; Kelder et al., 1998)
Astro cytes	MCP-1, MIP-1α/β, RANTES, SDF-1α, IL-8, IP-10, FKN	CCR2, CCR3, CCR4, CCR5, CXCR4	(Conant et al., 1998; Zheng et al., 2000b; Zheng et al., 1999b)
Neur ons	FKN, MCP-1	CXCR4, CX3CR1, CXCR2, CCR5, DARC	(Coughlan et al., 2000; Zheng et al., 2000b)
Endo theliu m	IL-8, FKN, IP-10, MGSA, MIG, MCP-1,3,4	DARC, CXCR4, CCR5,	(Gabuzda et al., 2002)

Chemokines have critical developmental and homeostatic functions within the CNS. Factors such as SDF-1 and FKN are constitutively expressed. Multiple chemokines have critical developmental and regenerative roles in the CNS and have been shown to have neural stem cell and progenitor cell (NPC) interactions. NPC are widely thought to provide a reservoir to replace neurons or glia under conditions of brain injury or disease (Gage, 2000; Horner and Gage, 2000). Studies have documented that SDF-1/CXCR4 signaling regulates migration of NPC in the cerebellum (Ma et al., 1998; Zou et al., 1998), dentate gyrus (Bagri et al., 2002; Lu et al., 2001), and cortex (Peng et al., 2004; Stumm et al., 2003). It was recently reported that the recruitment of CXCR4-positive progenitor cells to regenerating tissue is mediated by hypoxic gradients via the transcription factor hypoxia-inducible factor-1 (HIF-1)-induced expression of SDF-1 (Ceradini et al., 2004). This indicates the significant involvement of SDF-1/CXCR4 interaction in tissue damage and repair. Neural progenitor cells have been shown to have active roles in neurodegenerative processes including HAD, and the communications provided by chemokines likely play critical roles in their proliferation and migration throughout the CNS. As the role of this cell population is further elucidated, the chemokine interactions may prove to be critical in brain homeostasis as well as repair in normal and disease states.

HIV-1, Co-Receptors and HIV-1 Associated Dementia

As previously discussed, chemokines are important players in the development and maintenance of an immune response to foreign insult. In some circumstances however, chemokines play a more central role in the pathogenesis of the disease process. Studies have shown multiple viruses including herpesvirus, poxvirus, retrovirus, and lentivirus take advantage of the chemokine system, posing as analogs, to presumably gain a survival advantage by avoiding or altering immune detection and elimination (Murphy, 2001). Another manipulation of chemokine immune defense first described in 1996, is HIV's use of a chemokine co-receptor in human infection (Feng et al., 1996). Initially, HIV was assumed to rely solely on the CD4 surface protein found on T-cells and macrophages for entry into host cells (CD4 as an HIV receptor is reviewed in (Sattentau and Weiss, 1988)). However, CD4 alone did not accurately predict the cell interactions of HIV. This eventually led to the breakthrough revealing that chemokine GPCRs mediated viral membrane fusion with human host cells.

Each HIV strain has different specificities and interactions with various chemokine receptors, but the two primary coreceptors are CCR5 and CXCR4. Macrophage or M-tropic viral strains utilize CCR5 for infection; T-cell or T tropic viral strains rely upon CXCR4. There is another viral subset, dual tropic or R5X4 strains that employ both coreceptors. Further, additional receptors have been shown to have more limited viral interactions including CCR2, CCR3, CCR8, CX3CR1 and others, but the pathophysiological relevance has yet to be determined (Gabuzda and Wang, 2000).

The co-receptor requirement is a result of receptor ligand interactions between the chemokine GPCRs and the HIV coat protein gp120. Virus-cell interactions characteristically begin with gp120 binding CD4, inducing a conformational change in gp120. This change alters the affinity of gp120 for a coreceptor, either CCR5 or CXCR4 resulting in a trimolecular interaction between gp120, CD4 and the coreceptor (Berger et al., 1999; Berson and Doms, 1998; Dimitrov et al., 1998). The multi-molecular interaction then permits fusion of HIV viral membrane to the host cell, permitting entry and consequent integration into the host DNA.

Chemokines and Their Receptors in HAD

Neurons express both chemokines and chemokine receptors, and although not infected by HIV, neurons do express the coreceptors CXCR4 (Zhang et al., 1998) and CCR5 (Rottman et al., 1997). Similar to cells infected by HIV, the neuron coreceptors have affinity for HIV envelope protein gp120, irregardless of CD4. Many groups have since shown neuronal toxicity mediated by viral proteins, particularly gp120 (Chen et al., 2002; Garden et al., 2004; Hesselgesser et al., 1998; Kaul and Lipton, 1999; Ohagen et al., 1999; Zheng et al., 1999b). Upon interaction with coreceptors, gp120 induces signaling cascades that may play a role in promoting apoptosis. Blocking of these cascades can block neuronal death in some cases. Interestingly, different viral strains induce varying levels of neuronal toxicity (Gabuzda and Wang, 1999; Zheng et al., 1999a).

In contrast to HIV-1 coreceptors, some chemokine ligands have the ability to reduce or ablate neuron toxicity. High levels of chemokines RANTES, MIP-1α, and others have been shown to reduce neuron death (Kaul and Lipton, 1999; Meucci et al., 1998), while SDF-1, at higher concentrations may actually promote neuronal death (Hesselgesser et al., 1998; Kaul and Lipton, 1999; Zheng et al., 1999b). The mechanism is not yet completely understood, but may rely upon simple competitive inhibition, receptor expression changes on the cell surface, or another unknown mechanism.

Fractalkine

A more convoluted picture surrounds different chemokines' ability to reduce toxicity via indirect paths. Some chemokine ligands such as FKN have been suggested to promote survival in neurons. When cleaved as a soluble protein, FKN is chemotactic for monocytes and lymphocytes (Chapman et al., 2000b; Imai et al., 1997; Tong et al., 2000). Studies show that regulation of neuronal FKN RNA is not responsive to excitotoxic stimuli. However, analysis at the protein level reveals FKN is cleaved rapidly from cultured neurons in response to the same stimuli (Chapman et al., 2000a; Erichsen et al., 2003; Zheng et al., 2000a). Thus, FKN induces chemotaxis by providing a chemotactic gradient to direct cell migration. However, it is not certain if this mechanism requires signal transduction or receptor mediated G protein activation (Chapman et al., 2000b; Haskell et al., 1999; Haskell et al., 2000; Shiraishi et al., 2000). FKN levels are higher in the CSF of cognitively impaired HIV patients than in infected subjects without cognitive impairment (Erichsen et al., 2003). Moreover, FKN can affect the chemotaxis of primary monocytes across an artificial blood brain barrier, and is neuroprotective to cultured neurons (Meucci et al., 2000; Tong et al., 2000). Thus, this neuronal chemokine may serve as a damage signal to recruit macrophages and microglia to the site of injury (Erichsen et al., 2003; Jung et al., 2000; Tong et al., 2000; Zheng et al., 2000a; Zujovic et al., 2000). Subsequent chemokine-MP interactions can initiate inflammatory responses through the production of chemokines/cytokines or protective responses through the production of neurotrophins (Cotter et al., 2002; Kaul et al., 2001; Xiao and Link, 1998).

MCP-1

Despite some association of chemokines and neuroprotection, there are also detrimental effects of chemokine function during HAD pathogenesis. Shown to be expressed in the brains of HAD patients (Conant et al., 1998), MCP-1 (CCL2) is a potent chemoattractant for monocytes and may help fuel the positive feedback loop of inflammation in the HAD brain. MCP-1 recruits monocytic phagocytes to sites of inflammation as was evidenced by a study using a mouse system with elevated levels of MCP-1 resulting in increased phagocytic cells at lesion sites (Fuentes et al., 1995). A high level of MCP-1 in CSF versus plasma was shown to be predictive of dementia development in monkeys (Zink et al., 2001). While clearly possessing chemotactic properties, the ability of MCP-1 to recruit phagocytes through the BBB was further elucidated with a study showing changes in BBB permeability in the presence of MCP-1 (Song and Pachter, 2004). Increased levels of MCP-1 was shown to result in initial protection from infection, however, upon successful HIV-1 infection, increased MCP-1 was shown to lead to increased susceptibility to the development of HAD (Gonzalez et al., 2002).

IP-10

Interferon gamma inducible protein 10, IP-10 or CXCL10, is a CXC chemokine. As indicated by its name, IP-10 is highly induced by interferon as well as other factors, yet is also produced constitutively throughout the body. IP-10 targets multiple subtypes of activated T-cells and macrophages for migration. IP-10 has been found in very high levels in CSF as well as shown to recruit cells into the CNS in the setting of HAD. While clearly a player in recruitment and inflammation, IP-10's role has also been shown to include cytotoxic effects towards neurons (van Marle et al., 2004) and may stimulate HIV-1 replication in macrophage (Lane et al., 2003).

IL-8

An endogenous ligand for CXCR2, IL-8 is secreted in high levels by HIV-1 infected lymphocytes and macrophages. Although expressed constitutively, immune activation potentiates IL-8 production from infected or uninfected macrophage by agents such as LPS or CD40L (Zheng et al., 2000b). IL-8 levels are increased in the CSF of HAD patients, more so than those lacking cognitive symptoms, supporting the role of IL-8 in HAD (Zheng et al., 2001).

SDF-1

Chemokines have also been shown to have a neuromodulatory capacity, in some cases decreasing excitation and avoiding toxicity. A complicated example is the effect of SDF-1 on glutamate toxicity and uptake, specifically as regulated through astrocytes. SDF-1 (CXCL12) is a member of the C-X-C chemokine subfamily and is the only known physiological ligand for CXCR4 (Rossi and Zlotnik, 2000). SDF-1 is a potent chemoattractant for resting lymphocytes, monocytes, and CD34-positive hematopoietic progenitor cells (Kim and Broxmeyer, 1999). CXCR4 is upregulated in HIV and SIV encephalitis, experimental allergic encephalitis (EAE), and brain tumors (Jiang et al., 1998; Sanders et al., 1998; Vallat et al., 1998; Westmoreland et al., 1998). SDF-1 transcripts are predominantly expressed by oligodendrocytes, astrocytes and neurons in the neocortex, hippocampus and cerebellum (Gleichmann et al., 2000; Stumm et al., 2003). SDF-1 has been shown to be upregulated in the brain of patients with HIVE (Langford et al., 2002; Rostasy et al., 2003; Zheng et al., 1999b). Studies conducted in different settings have shown SDF-1 to promote neuronal survival, reducing glutamate toxicity (Meucci et al., 1998). While another study has shown SDF-1 to increase neuronal death by increasing the release of glutamate and TNF-alpha from glial cells (Bezzi et al., 2001). This may be due to experimental variation or a concentration dependent effect of SDF-1 and glutamate regulation. Recently, it was suggested that SDF-1 could be cleaved to SDF-1 (5-67) and mediate direct neurotoxicity (Zhang et al., 2003).

Therapeutic Avenues Through Chemokines and Their Receptors

In AIDS, like all viral infections, an interplay exists between host immune defenses and viral function. Variation among host phenotype, response and combinations thereof often provides immunity or at least resistance to infection for some individuals. In line with this prediction, human HLA variants have been shown to modify disease progression in HIV infection (reviewed in (Tang and Kaslow, 2003)). Separate from immune system modification is structural alterations preventing infection. Critical to this discussion was the identification of chemokine coreceptor polymorphisms providing almost complete resistance. Homozygosity for CCR5-delta32, a null allele resulting from a 32bp deletion was identified in Caucasian populations in seronegative individuals with repeat exposures. Other coreceptor alleles for CXCR4 and CCR5 have since been identified that also provide some HIV resistance. Because HIV requires coreceptors for the induction of productive viral infection, and naturally occurring alleles have been shown to effectively limit HIV entry, potential therapies may rely upon exploitation of CXCR4 and CCR5.

While naturally occurring resistance is effective for a few fortunate individuals, protecting a population from infection requires development of therapeutic intervention. As discussed, multiple coreceptors for HIV-1 have been identified, and the ability of HIV to mutate presents a great hurdle in the development of effective therapeutic receptor antagonists. Another layer of complexity is the potential side effects of blocking one or multiple chemokine receptors that have homeostatic and inflammatory roles. Despite the inherent difficulties, multiple approaches have been studied and some are now being tested in clinical trials. Small molecule inhibitors, monoclonal antibodies and modified chemokine ligands are all related but distinct approaches to limiting HIV entry (reviewed in (Shaheen and Collman, 2004)). Another approach to block initial HIV infection may be delivering siRNAs targeting the receptors for knockdown (Zhou et al., 2004).

Some chemokine ligands inherently disrupt viral pathogenesis or provide protection against cell death during the disease process. Ligands of HIV coreceptors, such as SDF-1 and RANTES, have been shown to block infection of cells in different systems (Bleul et al., 1996; Lederman et al., 2004). Similarly, ligands to coreceptors have been shown to block HIV envelope protein induced toxicity to neurons (Alkhatib et al., 1996; Meucci and Miller, 1996). The mechanism may be simple blocking or internalization of receptors, or may rely upon the signaling downstream of chemokine interaction.

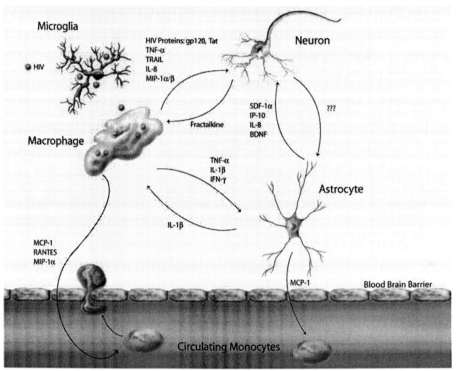

Figure 3. Proposed interaction of cells within the CNS during HIV infection. Mononuclear phagocytic cells, microglia and macrophage, are productively infected by HIV leading to activation and production of multiple secreted factors. Inflammatory processes lead to the amplification of immune response through the recruitment of additional cells. Viral proteins and cytokines interact with receptors on other cell types including neurons and astrocytes, causing physiologic changes and altered expression profiles that combine to lead to eventual neuronal dropout. The evolution of inflammation within the CNS is a complex process involving communication between different cell types. Improper regulation of such factors leads to chronic inflammation and eventual cell death.

Conclusion

HIV-1 invasion of the CNS initiates an inflammatory response mediated and amplified by cytokines. The role of cytokines is complex, particularly in the CNS, due to the overlapping, synergizing and antagonizing effects of various factors. Classifying any individual factor or family of factors as beneficial or detrimental oversimplifies the interactions between various cell types and the signaling cascades initiated by cytokines (Figure 3). Instead, cytokines need to be considered as a balanced network, where subtle modifications can shift cells towards different outcomes such as death, proliferation, migration, induction of inflammation or inhibition of immune responses. Prolonged inflammation has profound changes in the cytokine network and the cells they target, consequently altering the outcome of cell populations. The CNS is a unique environment that is exquisitely sensitive to cytokines, and the dysregulation that is rampant during HIV-1 infection permanently transforms brain function. Cytokine activity and the profile of factors present in the brain eventually determine the outcome of HIV-1 infection and the fate of neurons. The understanding of cytokine function and how the expression or activity of cytokines can be manipulated may provide the key to diagnosing or treating HIV infection within the brain.

Acknowledgments

This work was supported in part by research grants by the National Institutes of Health: R01 NS 41858, P20 RR15635 and P01 NS043985 (JZ). We kindly acknowledge Drs. Howard E. Gendelman, Yuri Persidsky, Anuja Ghorpade, Robin Cotter, Lisa Ryan, Xu Luo and Hui Peng for valuable suggestion and critics of this work. Shelley Herek, David Erichsen, Alicia Lopez, Li Wu, Clancy McNalley, Jianxing Zhao, Douglas Niemann and Mike Bauer provided technical support for this work. Julie Ditter, Robin Taylor, Myhanh Che, Nell Ingraham, Theresa Grutel, Lesley Gendelman and Connie Curro provided outstanding administrative support.

References

Adamson, D. C., Wildemann, B., Sasaki, M., Glass, J. D., McArthur, J. C., Christov, V. I., Dawson, T. M., and Dawson, V. L. (1996). Immunologic No Synthase: Elevation in Severe AIDS Dementia and Induction by HIV-1 gp41. *Science 274*, 1917-1926.

Adle-Biassette, H., Levy, Y., Colombel, M., Poron, F., Natchev, S., Keohane, C., and Gray, F. (1995). Neuronal apoptosis in HIV infection in adults. *Neuropathol. App. Neurobiol. 21*, 218-227.

Alkhatib, G., Combadiere, C., Broder, C. C., Feng, Y., Kennedy, P. E., Murphy, P. M., and Berger, E. A. (1996). CC CKR5: a RANTES, MIP-1alpha, MIP-1beta receptor as a fusion cofactor for macrophage-tropic HIV-1. *Science 272*, 1955-1958.

Allsopp, T. E., Scallan, M. F., Williams, A., and Fazakerley, J. K. (1998). Virus infection induces neuronal apoptosis: A comparison with trophic factor withdrawal. *Cell. Death. Differ. 5*, 50-59.

Aloisi, F., Care, A., Borsellino, G., Gallo, P., Rosa, S., Bassani, A., Cabibbo, A., Testa, U., Levi, G., and Peschle, C. (1992). Production of hemolymphopoietic cytokines (IL-6, IL-8, colony- stimulating factors) by normal human astrocytes in response to IL-1 beta and tumor necrosis factor-alpha. *J. Immunol. 149*, 2358-2366.

Annunziato, F., Romagnani, P., Cosmi, L., Lazzeri, E., and Romagnani, S. (2001). Chemokines and lymphopoiesis in human thymus. *Trends. Immunol. 22*, 277-281.

Bachis, A., Colangelo, A. M., Vicini, S., Doe, P. P., De Bernardi, M. A., Brooker, G., and Mocchetti, I. (2001). Interleukin-10 prevents glutamate-mediated cerebellar granule cell death by blocking caspase-3-like activity. *J. Neurosci. 21*, 3104-3112.

Bachis, A., Major, E. O., and Mocchetti, I. (2003). Brain-derived neurotrophic factor inhibits human immunodeficiency virus-1/gp120-mediated cerebellar granule cell death by preventing gp120 internalization. *J. Neurosci. 23*, 5715-5722.

Bagri, A., Gurney, T., He, X., Zou, Y. R., Littman, D. R., Tessier-Lavigne, M., and Pleasure, S. J. (2002). The chemokine SDF1 regulates migration of dentate granule cells. *Development. 129*, 4249-4260.

Barak, O., Goshen, I., Ben-Hur, T., Weidenfeld, J., Taylor, A. N., and Yirmiya, R. (2002). Involvement of brain cytokines in the neurobehavioral disturbances induced by HIV-1 glycoprotein120. *Brain Res. 933*, 98-108.

Basu, A., Krady, J. K., and Levison, S. W. (2004). Interleukin-1: a master regulator of neuroinflammation. *J. Neurosci. Res. 78*, 151-156.

Bazan, J., Bacon, K., Hardiman, G., Wang, W., Soo, K., Rossi, D., Greaves, D., Zlotnik, A., and Schall, T. (1997). A new class of membrane-bound chemokine with a CX3C motif. *Nature 385*, 640-644.

Benveniste, E. N. (1992). Inflammatory cytokines within the central nervous system:sources, function and mechanisms of action. *Am. J. Physiol. (Cell Physiol) 263*:32, C1-C16.

Berger, E. A., Murphy, P. M., and Farber, J. M. (1999). Chemokine receptors as HIV-1 coreceptors: roles in viral entry, tropism, and disease. *Annu. Rev. Immunol. 17*, 657-700.

Bernasconi, S., Cinque, P., Peri, G., Sozzani, S., Crociati, A., Torri, W., Vicenzi, E., Vago, L., Lazzarin, A., Poli, G., and Mantovani, A. (1996). Selective elevation of monocyte chemotactic protein-1 in the cerebrospinal fluid of AIDS patients with cytomegalovirus encephalitis. *J. Infect. Dis. 174*, 1098-1101.

Berson, J. F., and Doms, R. W. (1998). Structure-function studies of the HIV-1 coreceptors. *Semin. Immunol. 10*, 237-248.

Bezzi, P., Domercq, M., Brambilla, L., Galli, R., Schols, D., De Clercq, E., Vescovi, A., Bagetta, G., Kollias, G., Meldolesi, J., and Volterra, A. (2001). CXCR4-activated astrocyte glutamate release via TNFalpha: amplification by microglia triggers neurotoxicity. *Nat Neurosci 4*, 702-710.

Bleul, C. C., Farzan, M., Choe, h., Parolin, C., Clark-Lewis, I., Sodroski, J., and Springer, T. A. (1996). The lymphocyte chemoattractant SDF-1 is a ligand for LESTR/fusin and blocks HIV-1 entry. *Nature 382*, 829-833.

Bonavia, R., Bajetto, A., Barbero, S., Pirani, P., Florio, T., and Schettini, G. (2003). Chemokines and their receptors in the CNS: expression of CXCL12/SDF-1 and CXCR4 and their role in astrocyte proliferation. *Toxicol. Lett. 139*, 181-189.

Boven, L. A., Middel, J., Portegies, P., Verhoef, J., Jansen, G. H., and Nottet, H. S. (1999). Overexpression of nerve growth factor and basic fibroblast growth factor in AIDS dementia complex. *J. Neuroimmunol. 97*, 154-162.

Cacalano, G., Lee, J., Kikly, K., Ryan, A. M., Pitts-Meek, S., Hultgren, B., Wood, W. I., and Moore, M. W. (1994). Neutrophil and B cell expansion in mice that lack the murine IL-8 receptor homolog. *Science 265*, 682-684.

Campbell, I. L., Abraham, C. R., Masliah, E., Kemper, P., Inglis, J. D., Oldstone, M. B., and Mucke, L. (1993). Neurologic disease induced in transgenic mice by cerebral overexpression of interleukin 6. *Proc. Natl. Acad. Sci. U S A 90*, 10061-10065.

Canki, M., Potash, M. J., Bentsman, G., Chao, W., Flynn, T., Heinemann, M., Gelbard, H., and Volsky, D. J. (1997). Isolation and long-term culture of primary ocular human immunodeficiency virus type 1 isolates in primary astrocytes. *J. Neurovirol. 3*, 10-15.

Cantarella, G., Uberti, D., Carsana, T., Lombardo, G., Bernardini, R., and Memo, M. (2003). Neutralization of TRAIL death pathway protects human neuronal cell line from beta-amyloid toxicity. *Cell Death Differ. 10*, 134-141.

Ceradini, D. J., Kulkarni, A. R., Callaghan, M. J., Tepper, O. M., Bastidas, N., Kleinman, M. E., Capla, J. M., Galiano, R. D., Levine, J. P., and Gurtner, G. C. (2004). Progenitor cell trafficking is regulated by hypoxic gradients through HIF-1 induction of SDF-1. *Nat. Med. 10*, 858-864.

Chapman, G. A., Moores, K., Harrison, D., Campbell, C. A., Stewart, B. R., and Strijbos, P. J. (2000a). Fractalkine Cleavage from Neuronal Membranes Represents an Acute Event in the Inflammatory Response to Excitotoxic Brain Damage. *J. Neurosci. (Online) 20*, RC87.

Chapman, G. A., Moores, K. E., Gohil, J., Berkhout, T. A., Patel, L., Green, P., Macphee, C. H., and Stewart, B. R. (2000b). The role of fractalkine in the recruitment of monocytes to the endothelium. *Eur. J. Pharmacol. 392*, 189-195.

Chen, W., Sulcove, J., Frank, I., Jaffer, S., Ozdener, H., and Kolson, D. L. (2002). Development of a human neuronal cell model for human immunodeficiency virus (HIV)-infected macrophage-induced neurotoxicity: apoptosis induced by HIV type 1 primary isolates and evidence for involvement of the Bcl-2/Bcl-xL-sensitive intrinsic apoptosis pathway. *J. Virol. 76*, 9407-9419.

Chung, I. Y., and Benveniste, E. N. (1990). Tumor necrosis factor-alpha production by astrocytes. Induction by lipopolysaccharide, IFN-gamma, and IL-1 beta. *J. Immunol. 144*, 2999-3007.

Cinque, P., Vago, L., Mengozzi, M., Torri, V., Ceresa, D., Vicenzi, E., Transidico, P., Vagani, A., Sozzani, S., Mantovani, A., et al. (1998). Elevated cerebrospinal fluid levels of monocyte chemotactic protein-1 correlate with HIV-1 encephalitis and local viral replication. *Aids 12*, 1327-1332.

Cocchi, F., DeVico, A. L., Garzino-Demo, A., Arya, S. K., Gallo, R. C., and Lusso, P. (1995). Identification of RANTES, MIP-1alpha, and MIP-1beta as the major HIV-suppressive factors produced by CD8+ T cells. *Science 270*, 1811-1815.

Collman, R. G., Yi, Y., Liu, Q. H., and Freedman, B. D. (2000). Chemokine signaling and HIV-1 fusion mediated by macrophage CXCR4: implications for target cell tropism. *J. Leukoc. Biol. 68*, 318-323.

Conant, K., Garzino-Demo, A., Nath, A., McArthur, J. C., Halliday, W., Power, C., Gallo, R. C., and Major, E. O. (1998). Induction of monocyte chemoattractant protein-1 in HIV-1

Tat-stimulated astrocytes and elevation in AIDS dementia. *Proc. Natl. Acad. Sci. USA.* *95*, 3117-3121.

Cook, D. N., Chen, S. C., Sullivan, L. M., Manfra, D. J., Wiekowski, M. T., Prosser, D. M., Vassileva, G., and Lira, S. A. (2001). Generation and analysis of mice lacking the chemokine fractalkine. *Mol. Cell. Biol. 21*, 3159-3165.

Cotter, R., Williams, C., Ryan, L., Erichsen, D., Lopez, A., Peng, H., and Zheng, J. (2002). Fractalkine (CX3CL1) and brain inflammation: Implications for HIV-1-associated dementia. *J. Neurovirol. 8*, 585-598.

Coughlan, C. M., McManus, C. M., Sharron, M., Gao, Z., Murphy, D., Jaffer, S., Choe, W., Chen, W., Hesselgesser, J., Gaylord, H., et al. (2000). Expression of multiple functional chemokine receptors and monocyte chemoattractant protein-1 in human neurons [In Process Citation]. *Neuroscience 97*, 591-600.

Danial, N. N., and Korsmeyer, S. J. (2004). Cell death: critical control points. *Cell 116*, 205-219.

Dempsey, P. W., Doyle, S. E., He, J. Q., and Cheng, G. (2003). The signaling adaptors and pathways activated by TNF superfamily. *Cytokine Growth Factor Rev. 14*, 193-209.

Deng, H., Liu, R., Ellmeier, W., Choe, S., Unutmaz, D., Burkhart, M., Di Marzio, P., Marmon, S., Sutton, R. E., Hill, C. M., et al. (1996). Identification of a major co-receptor for primary isolates of HIV-1. *Nature 381*, 661-666.

Devi, L. A. (2000). G-protein-coupled receptor dimers in the lime light. *Trends Pharmacol. Sci. 21*, 324-326.

Dimitrov, D. S., Xiao, X., Chabot, D. J., and Broder, C. C. (1998). HIV coreceptors. *J. Membr. Biol. 166*, 75-90.

Dore, G. J., Hoy, J. F., Mallal, S. A., Li, Y., Mijch, A. M., French, M. A., Cooper, D. A., and Kaldor, J. M. (1997). Trends in incidence of AIDS illnesses in Australia from 1983 to 1994: the Australian AIDS cohort. *J. Acquir. Immune. Defic. Syndr. Hum. Retrovirol. 16*, 39-43.

Dragic, T., Litwin, V., Allaway, G. P., Martin, S. R., Huang, Y., Nagashima, K. A., Cayanan, C., Maddon, P. J., Koup, R. A., Moore, J. P., and Paxton, W. A. (1996). HIV-1 entry into CD4+ cells is mediated by the chemokines receptor CC-CKR-5. *Nature 381*, 667-673.

Eddleston, M., and Mucke, L. (1993). Molecular profile of reactive astrocytes--implications for their role in neurologic disease. *Neuroscience 54*, 15-36.

Eilbott, D. J., Peress, N., Burger, H., LaNeve, D., Orenstein, J., Gendelman, H. E., Seidman, R., and Weiser, B. (1989). Human immunodeficiency virus type 1 in spinal cords of acquired immunodeficiency syndrome patients with myelopathy: expression and replication in macrophages. *Proc. Natl. Acad. Sci. U S A 86*, 3337-3341.

Ellis, R. J., Deutsch, R., Heaton, R. K., Marcotte, T. D., McCutchan, J. A., Nelson, J. A., Abramson, I., Thal, L. J., Atkinson, J. H., Wallace, M. R., and Grant, I. (1997). Neurocognitive impairment is an independent risk factor for death in HIV infection. San Diego HIV Neurobehavioral Research Center Group. *Arch. Neurol. 54*, 416-424.

Erichsen, D., Lopez, A. L., Peng, H., Niemann, D., Williams, C., Bauer, M., Morgello, S., Cotter, R. L., Ryan, L. A., Ghorpade, A., et al. (2003). Neuronal injury regulates fractalkine: relevance for HIV-1 associated dementia. *J. Neuroimmunol. 138*, 144-155.

Feng, Y., Broder, C. C., Kennedy, P. E., and Berger, E. A. (1996). HIV-1 entry cofactor: functional cDNA cloning of a seven-transmembrane, G protein-coupled receptor [see comments]. *Science 272*, 872-877.

Fischer-Smith, T., Croul, S., Adeniyi, A., Rybicka, K., Morgello, S., Khalili, K., and Rappaport, J. (2004). Macrophage/microglial accumulation and proliferating cell nuclear antigen expression in the central nervous system in human immunodeficiency virus encephalopathy. *Am. J. Pathol. 164*, 2089-2099.

Fong, A. M., Erickson, H. P., Zachariah, J. P., Poon, S., Schamberg, N. J., Imai, T., and Patel, D. D. (2000). Ultrastructure and function of the fractalkine mucin domain in CX(3)C chemokine domain presentation. *J. Biol. Chem. 275*, 3781-3786.

Forster, R., Mattis, A. E., Kremmer, E., Wolf, E., Brem, G., and Lipp, M. (1996). A putative chemokine receptor, BLR1, directs B cell migration to defined lymphoid organs and specific anatomic compartments of the spleen. *Cell 87*, 1037-1047.

Fuentes, M., Durham, S., Swerdel, M., Letwin, A., Barton, D., Megill, J., Bravo, R., and Lira, L. (1995). Controlled recruitment of monocytes and macrophages to specific organs through transgenic expression of monocyte chemoattractant protein-1. *J. Immunol. 155*, 5769-5776.

Gabuzda, D., He, J., Ohagen, A., and Vallat, A. (1998). Chemokine receptors in HIV-1 infection of the central nervous system. *Immunol. 10*, 203-213.

Gabuzda, D., and Wang, J. (1999). Chemokine receptors and virus entry in the central nervous system. *J. Neurovirol. 5*, 643-658.

Gabuzda, D., and Wang, J. (2000). Chemokine receptors and mechanisms of cell death in HIV neuropathogenesis. *J. Neurovirol. 6 Suppl. 1*, S24-32.

Gabuzda, D., Wang, J., and Gorry, P. (2002). HIV-1-Associated Dementia. In *Chemokines and the nervous system*, R. M. Ransohoff, K. Suzuki, A. E. I. Proudfoot, W. F. Hickey, and J. K. Harrison, eds. (Amsterdam, Elservier Science), pp. 345-360.

Gage, F. H. (2000). Mammalian neural stem cells. *Science 287*, 1433-1438.

Gallo, P., Laverda, A. M., De Rossi, A., Pagni, S., Del Mistro, A., Cogo, P., Piccinno, M. G., Plebani, A., Tavolato, B., and Chieco-Bianchi, L. (1991). Immunological markers in the cerebrospinal fluid of HIV-1-infected children. *Acta Paediatr. Scand. 80*, 659-666.

Gallo, P., Sivieri, S., Rinaldi, L., Yan, X. B., Lolli, F., De Rossi, A., and Tavolato, B. (1994). Intrathecal synthesis of interleukin-10 (IL-10) in viral and inflammatory diseases of the central nervous system. *J. Neurol. Sci. 126*, 49-53.

Garden, G. A., Guo, W., Jayadev, S., Tun, C., Balcaitis, S., Choi, J., Montine, T. J., Moller, T., and Morrison, R. S. (2004). HIV associated neurodegeneration requires p53 in neurons and microglia. *Faseb. J. 18*, 1141-1143.

Gelbard, H., Nottet, H., Dzenko, K., Jett, M., Genis, P., White, R., Wang, L., Choi, Y.-B., Zhang, D., Lipton, S., et al. (1994). Platelet-activating factor: a candidate human immunodeficiency virus type-1 infection neurotoxin. *J. Virol. 68*, 4628-4635.

Gelbard, H. A. (1999). Neuroprotective strategies for HIV-1-associated neurologic disease. *Ann. N Y Acad. Sci. 890*, 312-313.

Genc, S., Kizildag, S., Genc, K., Ates, H., Atabey, N., and Kizyldag, S. (2003). Interferon gamma and lipopolysaccharide upregulate TNF-related apoptosis-inducing ligand expression in murine microglia. *Immunol. Lett. 85*, 271-274.

Gendelman, H. E., Baca, L. M., Kubrak, C. A., Genis, P., Burrous, S., Friedman, R. M., Jacobs, D., and Meltzer, M. S. (1992). Induction of IFN-alpha in peripheral blood mononuclear cells by HIV- infected monocytes. Restricted antiviral activity of the HIV-induced IFN. *J. Immunol. 148*, 422-429.

Gendelman, H. E., Persidsky, Y., Ghorpade, A., Limoges, J., Stins, M., Fiala, M., and Morrisett, R. (1997). The neuropathogenesis of the AIDS dementia complex. *Aids 11*, S35-45.

Gendelman, H. E., Zheng, J., Coulter, C. L., Ghorpade, A., Che, M., Thylin, M., Rubocki, R., Persidsky, Y., Hahn, F., Reinhard, J., Jr., and Swindells, S. (1998). Suppression of inflammatory neurotoxins by highly active antiretroviral therapy in human immunodeficiency virus-associated dementia. *J. Infect. Dis. 178*, 1000-1007.

Gessani, S., Puddu, P., Varano, B., Borghi, P., Conti, L., Fantuzzi, L., Gherardi, G., and Belardelli, F. (1994). Role of endogenous interferon-beta in the restriction of HIV replication in human monocyte/macrophages. *J. Leukoc. Biol. 56*, 358-361.

Ghorpade, A., Holter, S., Borgmann, K., Persidsky, R., and Wu, L. (2003). HIV-1 and IL-1 beta regulate Fas ligand expression in human astrocytes through the NF-kappa B pathway. *J. Neuroimmunol. 141*, 141-149.

Glabinski, A. R., and Ransohoff, R. M. (1999). Chemokines and chemokine recptors in CNS pathology. *J. Neurovirol. 5*, 3-12.

Glass, J. D., Wesselingh, S. L., Selnes, O. A., and McArthur, J. C. (1993). Clinical neuropathologic correlation in HIV-associated dementia. *Neurology 43*, 2230-2237.

Gleichmann, M., Gillen, C., Czardybon, M., Bosse, F., Greiner-Petter, R., Auer, J., and Muller, H. W. (2000). Cloning and characterization of SDF-1gamma, a novel SDF-1 chemokine transcript with developmentally regulated expression in the nervous system. *Eur. J. Neurosci. 12*, 1857-1866.

Goda, S., Imai, T., Yoshie, O., Yoneda, O., Inoue, H., Nagano, Y., Okazaki, T., Imai, H., Bloom, E. T., Domae, N., and Umehara, H. (2000). CX3C-chemokine, fractalkine-enhanced adhesion of THP-1 cells to endothelial cells through integrin-dependent and -independent mechanisms. *J. Immunol. 164*, 4313-4320.

Gonzalez, E., Rovin, B. H., Sen, L., Cooke, G., Dhanda, R., Mummidi, S., Kulkarni, H., Bamshad, M. J., Telles, V., Anderson, S. A., et al. (2002). HIV-1 infection and AIDS dementia are influenced by a mutant MCP-1 allele linked to increased monocyte infiltration of tissues and MCP-1 levels. *Proc. Natl. Acad. Sci. U S A 99*, 13795-13800.

Green, D. R. (2003). The suicide in the thymus, a twisted trail. *Nat. Immunol. 4*, 207-208.

Green, D. R., and Reed, J. C. (1998). Mitochondria and Apoptosis. *Science 281*, 1309-1311.

Griffin, D. E. (1997). Cytokines in the brain during viral infection: clues to HIV-associated dementia. *J. Clin. Invest. 100*, 2948-2951.

Grimaldi, L. M., Martino, G. V., Franciotta, D. M., Brustia, R., Castagna, A., Pristera, R., and Lazzarin, A. (1991). Elevated alpha-tumor necrosis factor levels in spinal fluid from HIV-1- infected patients with central nervous system involvement [see comments]. *Ann. Neurol. 29*, 21-25.

Gross, A., McDonnell, J. M., and Korsmeyer, S. J. (1999). BCL-2 family members and the mitochondria in apoptosis. *Genes Dev. 13*, 1899-1911.

Harrison, J. K., Fong, A. M., Swain, P. A., Chen, S., Yu, Y. R., Salafranca, M. N., Greenleaf, W. B., Imai, T., and Patel, D. D. (2001). Mutational analysis of the fractalkine chemokine domain: Basic amino acid residues differentially contribute to CX3CR1 binding, signaling, and cell adhesion. *J. Biol. Chem. 8*, 8.

Haskell, C. A., Cleary, M. D., and Charo, I. F. (1999). Molecular uncoupling of fractalkine-mediated cell adhesion and signal transduction. Rapid flow arrest of CX3CR1-expressing cells is independent of G-protein activation. *J. Biol. Chem. 274*, 10053-10058.

Haskell, C. A., Cleary, M. D., and Charo, I. F. (2000). Unique role of the chemokine domain of fractalkine in cell capture. Kinetics of receptor dissociation correlate with cell adhesion. *J. Biol. Chem. 275*, 34183-34189.

Hesselgesser, J., and Horuk, R. (1999). Chemokine and chemokine receptor expression in the central nervous system. *J. Neurovirol. 5*, 13-26.

Hesselgesser, J., Taub, D., Baskar, P., Greenberg, M., Hoxie, J., Kolson, D. L., and Horuk, R. (1998). Neuronal apoptosis induced by HIV-1 gp120 and the chemokine SDF-1alpha mediated by the chemokine receptor CXCR4. *Curr. Biol. 8*, 595-598.

Heyes, M. P., Saito, K., Lackner, A., Wiley, C. A., Achim, C. L., and Markey, S. P. (1998). Sources of the neurotoxin quinolinic acid in the brain of HIV-1- infected patients and retrovirus-infected macaques. *Faseb. J. 12*, 881-896.

Hoover, D. M., Mizoue, L. S., Handel, T. M., and Lubkowski, J. (2000). The crystal structure of the chemokine domain of fractalkine shows a novel quaternary arrangement. *J. Biol. Chem. 275*, 23187-23193.

Horner, P. J., and Gage, F. H. (2000). Regenerating the damaged central nervous system. *Nature 407*, 963-970.

Huang, Y., Zhao, J., Ryan, L. A., Lopez, A., Peng, H., Herek, S., and Zheng, J. (2004). TRAIL Induce Apoptosis and Production of Glutamate in HIV-1 Infected Macrophage: Linkage to HIV-1 Associated Dementia. Paper presented at: 11th Conference on Retroviruses and Opportunistic Infections (San Francisco, CA).

Imai, T., Hieshima, K., Haskell, C., Baba, M., Nagira, M., Nishimura, M., Kakizaki, M., Takagi, S., Nomiyama, H., Schall, T. J., and Yoshie, O. (1997). Identification and molecular characterization of fractalkine receptor CX3CR1, which mediates both leukocyte migration and adhesion. *Cell 91*, 521-530.

Jiang, Y., Salafranca, M., Adhikari, S., Xia, Y., Feng, L., Sonntag, M., deFiebre, C., Pennel, N., Streit, W., and Harrison, J. (1998). Chemokine receptor expression in cultured glia and rat experimental allergic encephalomyelitis. *J. Neuroimmunol. 86*, 1-12.

Jiang, Z., Piggee, C., Heyes, M. P., Murphy, C., Quearry, B., Bauer, M., Zheng, J., Gendelman, H. E., and Markey, S. P. (2001). Glutamate is a mediator of neurotoxicity in secretions of activated HIV- 1-infected macrophages. *J. Neuroimmunol. 117*, 97-107.

John M. Petitto, M. J. T., Zhi Huang, Ray D. Beck, Jr. and David A. Hartemink (2003). *Cytokines effects on Learning and memory. In Cytokines and mental health*, Z. Kronfol, ed. (Kluwer Academic Publishers), pp. 211-224.

Johnson, M. D., and Gold, L. I. (1996). Distribution of transforming growth factor-b isoform in human immunodeficiency virus-1 encephalitis. *Human pathology. 27*, 643-649.

Jung, S., Aliberti, J., Graemmel, P., Sunshine, M. J., Kreutzberg, G. W., Sher, A., and Littman, D. R. (2000). Analysis of fractalkine receptor CX(3)CR1 function by targeted deletion and green fluorescent protein reporter gene insertion. *Mol. Cell. Biol. 20*, 4106-4114.

Kast, R. E. (2002). Feedback between glial tumor necrosis factor-alpha and gp120 from HIV-infected cells helps maintain infection and destroy neurons. *Neuroimmunomodulation 10*, 85-92.

Kaul, M., Garden, G. A., and Lipton, S. A. (2001). Pathways to neuronal injury and apoptosis in HIV-associated dementia. *Nature 410*, 988-994.

Kaul, M., and Lipton, S. A. (1999). Chemokines and activated macrophages in HIV gp120-induced neuronal apoptosis. *Proc. Natl. Acad. Sci. U S A. 96*, 8212-8216.

Kedzierska, K., Crowe, S. M., Turville, S., and Cunningham, A. L. (2003). The influence of cytokines, chemokines and their receptors on HIV-1 replication in monocytes and macrophages. *Rev. Med. Virol. 13*, 39-56.

Kelder, W., McArthur, J. C., Nance-Sproson, T., McClernon, D., and Griffin, D. E. (1998). b-Chemokines MCP-1 and RANTES Are Selectively Increased in Cerebrospinal Fluid of Patients with Human Immunodeficiency Virus-Associated Dementia. *Ann. Neurol. 44*, 831-835.

Kerr, S., Armati, P., and Brew, B. (1995). Neurocytotoxicity of quinolinic acid in human brain cultures. *J. Neurovirol. 1*, 375-380.

Kim, C. H., and Broxmeyer, H. E. (1999). Chemokines: signal lamps for trafficking of T and B cells for development and effector function. *J. Leukocyte. Biol. 65*, 6-14.

Klein, R., Williams, K., Alvarez-Hernandez, X., Westmoreland, S., Force, T., Lackner, A., and Luster, A. (1999). Chemokine receptor expression and signaling in macaque and human fetal neurons and astrocytes: implications for the neuropathogenesis of AIDS. *J. Immunol. 163*, 1636-1646.

Kluger, M. J. (1991). Fever: role of pyrogens and cryogens. *Physiol. Rev. 71*, 93-127.

Koenig, S., Gendelman, H. E., Orenstein, J. M., Canto, M. C. D., Pezeshkpour, G. H., Yungbluth, M., Janotta, F., Aksamit, A., Martin, M. A., and Fauci, A. S. (1986). Detection of AIDS virus in macrophages in brain tissue from AIDS patients with encephalopathy. *Science 233*, 1089-1093.

Lane, B. R., King, S. R., Bock, P. J., Strieter, R. M., Coffey, M. J., and Markovitz, D. M. (2003). The C-X-C chemokine IP-10 stimulates HIV-1 replication. *Virology 307*, 122-134.

Langford, D., Sanders, V. J., Mallory, M., Kaul, M., and Masliah, E. (2002). Expression of stromal cell-derived factor 1alpha protein in HIV encephalitis. *J. Neuroimmunol. 127*, 115-126.

Lederman, M. M., Veazey, R. S., Offord, R., Mosier, D. E., Dufour, J., Mefford, M., Piatak, M., Jr., Lifson, J. D., Salkowitz, J. R., Rodriguez, B., et al. (2004). Prevention of vaginal SHIV transmission in rhesus macaques through inhibition of CCR5. *Science 306*, 485-487.

Lee, J., Shin, J. S., Park, J. Y., Kwon, D., Choi, S. J., Kim, S. J., and Choi, I. H. (2003). p38 mitogen-activated protein kinase modulates expression of tumor necrosis factor-related apoptosis-inducing ligand induced by interferon-gamma in fetal brain astrocytes. *J. Neurosci. Res. 74*, 884-890.

Lee, S., Liu, W., Dickson, D., Brosnan, C., and Berman, J. (1993). Cytokine production by human fetal microglia and astrocytes: differential induction by lipopolysaccharide and IL-1B. *J. Immunol. 150*, 2659-2667.

Lu, L., Su, W. J., Yue, W., Ge, X., Su, F., Pei, G., and Ma, L. (2001). Attenuation of morphine dependence and withdrawal in rats by venlafaxine, a serotonin and noradrenaline reuptake inhibitor. *Life Sci. 69*, 37-46.

Lucas, A. D., Chadwick, N., Warren, B. F., Jewell, D. P., Gordon, S., Powrie, F., and Greaves, D. R. (2001). The transmembrane form of the CX3CL1 chemokine fractalkine is expressed predominantly by epithelial cells in vivo. *Am. J. Pathol. 158*, 855-866.

Ma, M., Geiger, J. D., and Nath, A. (1994). Characterization of a novel binding site for the human immunodeficiency virus type 1 envelope protein gp120 on human fetal astrocytes. *J. Virol. 68*, 6824-6828.

Ma, Q., Jones, D., Borghesani, P. R., Segal, R. A., Nagasawa, T., Kishimoto, T., Bronson, R. T., and Springer, T. A. (1998). Impaired B -lymphopoiesis, myelopoiesis, and derailed cerebellar neuron migration in CXCR4 and SDF 1 deficient mice. *Proc. Natl. Acad. Sci. 95*, 9448-9453.

McArthur, J. C. (1987). Neurologic manifestations of AIDS. *Medicine (Baltimore) 66*, 407-437.

McGeer, P. L., and McGeer, E. G. (1995). The inflammatory response system of brain:implication for therapy of Alzheimer and other neurodegenerative diseases. *Brain Res. Review. 21*, 195-218.

Meltzer, M. S., Skillman, D. R., Gomatos, P. J., Kalter, D. C., and Gendelman, H. E. (1990). Role of mononuclear phagocytes in the pathogenesis of human immunodeficiency virus infection. *Annu. Rev. Immunol. 8*, 169-194.

Merrill, J. E., and Chen, I. S. (1991). HIV-1, macrophages, glial cells, and cytokines in AIDS nervous system disease. *Faseb. J. 5*, 2391-2397.

Messam, C. A., and Major, E. O. (2000). Stages of restricted HIV-1 infection in astrocyte cultures derived from human fetal brain tissue. *J. Neurovirol. 6 Suppl. 1*, S90-94.

Meucci, O., Fatatis, A., Simen, A. A., Bushell, T. J., Gray, P. W., and Miller, R. J. (1998). Chemokines regulate hippocampal neuronal signaling and gp120 neurotoxicity. *Proc. Natl. Acad. Sci. 95*, 14500-14505.

Meucci, O., Fatatis, A., Simen, A. A., and Miller, R. J. (2000). Expression of CX3CR1 chemokine receptors on neurons and their role in neuronal survival. *Proc. Natl. Acad. Sci. U S A. 97*, 8075-8080.

Meucci, O., and Miller, R. (1996). gp120-induced neurotoxicity in hippocampal pyramidal neuron cultures: protective action of TGF-beta1. *J. Neurosci. 16*, 4080-4088.

Michael, N. L. (2002). Host genetics and HIV--removing the mask. *Nat. Med. 8*, 783-785.

Miller, R. J., and Meucci, O. (1999). AIDS and the brain: is there a chemokine connection? *Trends Neurosci. 22*, 471-479.

Miura, Y., Koyanagi, Y., and Mizusawa, H. (2003a). TNF-related apoptosis-inducing ligand (TRAIL) induces neuronal apoptosis in HIV-encephalopathy. *J. Med. Dent. Sci. 50*, 17-25.

Miura, Y., Misawa, N., Kawano, Y., Okada, H., Inagaki, Y., Yamamoto, N., Ito, M., Yagita, H., Okumura, K., Mizusawa, H., and Koyanagi, Y. (2003b). Tumor necrosis factor-related apoptosis-inducing ligand induces neuronal death in a murine model of HIV central nervous system infection. *Proc. Natl. Acad. Sci. U S A. 100*, 2777-2782.

Mizoue, L. S., Bazan, J. F., Johnson, E. C., and Handel, T. M. (1999). Solution structure and dynamics of the CX3C chemokine domain of fractalkine and its interaction with an N-terminal fragment of CX3CR1. *Biochemistry 38*, 1402-1414.

Mizoue, L. S., Sullivan, S. K., King, D. S., Kledal, T. N., Schwartz, T. W., Bacon, K. B., and Handel, T. M. (2001). Molecular determinants of receptor binding and signaling by the CX3C chemokine fractalkine. *J. Biol. Chem. 276*, 33906-33914.

Moser, B., and Loetscher, P. (2001). Lymphocyte traffic control by chemokines. *Nat. Immunol. 2*, 123-128.

Mrak, R. E., Sheng, J. G., and Griffin, W. S. T. (1995). Glial Cytokines in Alzheimer's Disease: Review and Pathogenic Implications. *Human Pathology. 26*, 816-823.

Murphy, P. M. (2001). Viral exploitation and subversion of the immune system through chemokine mimicry. *Nat. Immunol. 2*, 116-122.

Nakajima, K., Honda, S., Tohyama, Y., Imai, Y., Kohsaka, S., and Kurihara, T. (2001). Neurotrophin secretion from cultured microglia. *J. Neurosci. Res. 65*, 322-331.

Navia, B. A., Jordan, B. D., and Price, R. W. (1986). The AIDS dementia complex: I. Clinical features. *Annals of Neurology. 19*, 517-524.

Nishida, K., Markey, S. P., Kustova, Y., Morse, H. C., 3rd, Skolnick, P., Basile, A. S., and Sei, Y. (1996). Increased brain levels of platelet-activating factor in a murine acquired immune deficiency syndrome are NMDA receptor-mediated. *J. Neurochem. 66*, 433-435.

Nottet, H. S., Jett, M., Flanagan, C. R., Zhai, Q. H., Persidsky, Y., Rizzino, A., Bernton, E. W., Genis, P., Baldwin, T., Schwartz, J. H., et al. (1995). A regulatory role for astrocytes in HIV-1 encephalitis. An overexpression of eicosanoids, platelet-activating factor, and tumor necrosis factor-alpha by activated HIV-1-infected monocytes is attenuated by primary human astrocytes. *J. Immunol. 154*, 3567-3581.

Ohagen, A., Ghosh, S., He, J., Huang, K., Chen, Y., Yuan, M., Osathanondh, R., Gartner, S., Shi, B., Shaw, G., and Gabuzda, D. (1999). Apoptosis induced by infection of primary brain cultures with diverse human immunodeficiency virus type 1 isolates: evidence for a role of the envelope. *J. Virol. 73*, 897-906.

Park, D. S., Morris, E. J., Stefanis, L., Troy, C. M., Shelanski, M. L., Geller, H. M., and Greene, L. A. (1998). Multiple pathways of neuronal death induced by DNA-damaging agents, NGF deprivation, and oxidative stress. *J. Neurosci. 18*, 830-840.

Peng, H., Huang, Y., Rose, J., Erichsen, D., Herek, S., Fujii, N., Tamamura, H., and Zheng, J. (2004). Stromal cell-derived factor 1 mediated CXCR4 signaling in rat and human cortical neural progenitor cells. *Journal of Neuroscience Research 76*, 35-50.

Perno, C. F., Cooney, D. A., Currens, M. J., Rocchi, G., Johns, D. G., Broder, S., and Yarchoan, R. (1990). Ability of anti-HIV agents to inhibit HIV replication in monocyte/macrophages or U937 monocytoid cells under conditions of enhancement by GM-CSF or anti-HIV antibody. *AIDS Res. Hum. Retroviruses. 6*, 1051-1055.

Perrella, O., Carreiri, P. B., Perrella, A., Sbreglia, C., Gorga, F., Guarnaccia, D., and Tarantino, G. (2001). Transforming growth factor beta-1 and interferon-alpha in the AIDS dementia complex (ADC): possible relationship with cerebral viral load? *Eur. Cytokine Netw. 12*, 51-55.

Perrella, O., Carrievi, P., Guarnaccia, D., and Soscia, M. (1992a). Cerebrospinal fluid cytokines in AIDS dementia. *J. Neurol. 239*, 387-388.

Perrella, O., Finelli, L., and Carrieri, P. B. (1992b). The role of cytokines in AIDS-dementia complex. *Acta Neurol. (Napoli) 14*, 342-344.

Perry, S. W., Hamilton, J. A., Tjoelker, L. W., Dbaibo, G., Dzenko, K. A., Epstein, L. G., Hannun, Y., Whittaker, J. S., Dewhurst, S., and Gelbard, H. A. (1998). Platelet-activating factor receptor activation. An initiator step in HIV-1 neuropathogenesis. *J. Biol. Chem. 273*, 17660-17664.

Pestka, S., Krause, C. D., Sarkar, D., Walter, M. R., Shi, Y., and Fisher, P. B. (2004). Interleukin-10 and related cytokines and receptors. *Annu. Rev. Immunol. 22*, 929-979.

Petito, C. K., Vecchio, D., and Chen, Y. T. (1994). HIV antigen and DNA in AIDS spinal cords correlate with macrophage infiltration but not with vacuolar myelopathy. *J. Neuropathol. Exp. Neurol. 53*, 86-94.

Poluektova, L., Gorantla, S., Faraci, J., Birusingh, K., Dou, H., and Gendelman, H. E. (2004). Neuroregulatory events follow adaptive immune-mediated elimination of HIV-1-infected macrophages: studies in a murine model of viral encephalitis. *J. Immunol. 172*, 7610-7617.

Prehn, J. H., Bindokas, V. P., Marcuccilli, C. J., Krajewski, S., Reed, J. C., and Miller, R. J. (1994). Regulation of neuronal Bcl2 protein expression and calcium homeostasis by transforming growth factor type beta confers wide-ranging protection on rat hippocampal neurons. *Proc. Natl. Acad. Sci. U S A. 91*, 12599-12603.

Prehn, J. H., and Miller, R. J. (1996). Opposite effects of TGF-beta 1 on rapidly- and slowly-triggered excitotoxic injury. *Neuropharmacology. 35*, 249-256.

Renauld, J. C. (2003). Class II cytokine receptors and their ligands: key antiviral and inflammatory modulators. *Nat. Rev. Immunol. 3*, 667-676.

Rizzardi, G. P., Lazzarin, A., and Pantaleo, G. (2002). Potential role of immune modulation in the effective long-term control of HIV-1 infection. *J. Biol. Regul. Homeost. Agents. 16*, 83-90.

Rossi, D., and Zlotnik, A. (2000). The biology of chemokines and their receptors. *Annu. Rev. Immunol. 18*, 217-242.

Rostasy, K., Egles, C., Chauhan, A., Kneissl, M., Bahrani, P., Yiannoutsos, C., Hunter, D. D., Nath, A., Hedreen, J. C., and Navia, B. A. (2003). SDF-1alpha is expressed in astrocytes and neurons in the AIDS dementia complex: an in vivo and in vitro study. *J. Neuropathol. Exp. Neurol. 62*, 617-626.

Rottman, J. B., Ganley, K. P., Williams, K., Wu, L., Mackay, C. R., and Ringler, D. J. (1997). Cellular localization of the chemokine receptor CCR5. Correlation to cellular targets of HIV-1 infection. *Am. J. Pathol. 151*, 1341-1351.

Ryan, L. A., Cotter, R. L., Zink, W. E., Gendelman, H. E., and Zheng, J. (2002). Macrophages, Chemokines and Neuronal Injury in HIV-1 Associated Dementia. *Cellualr and Molecular Biology. 48*, 125-138.

Ryan, L. A., Peng, H., Erichsen, D. A., Huang, Y., Persidsky, Y., Zhou, Y., Gendelman, H. E., and Zheng, J. (2004). TNF-Related Apoptosis-Inducing Ligand Mediates Human Neuronal Apoptosis: Links to HIV-1 Associated Dementia. *J. Neuroimmunol. 148*, 127-139.

Sacktor, N., Lyles, R. H., Skolasky, R., Kleeberger, C., Selnes, O. A., Miller, E. N., Becker, J. T., Cohen, B., and McArthur, J. C. (2001). HIV-associated neurologic disease incidence changes: Multicenter AIDS Cohort Study, 1990-1998. *Neurology 56*, 257-260.

Saha, R. N., and Pahan, K. (2003). Tumor necrosis factor-alpha at the crossroads of neuronal life and death during HIV-associated dementia. *J. Neurochem. 86*, 1057-1071.

Sanders, V. J., Mehta, A. P., White, M. G., and Achim, C. L. (1998). A murine model of HIV encephalitis: xenotransplantation of HIV-infected human neuroglia into SCID mouse brain. *Neuropathol. Appl. Neurobiol. 24*, 461-467.

Sattentau, Q. J., and Weiss, R. A. (1988). The CD4 antigen: physiological ligand and HIV receptor. *Cell 52*, 631-633.

Scorziello, A., Florio, T., Bajetto, A., Thellung, S., and Schettini, G. (1997). TGF-beta1 prevents gp120-induced impairment of Ca2+ homeostasis and rescues cortical neurons from apoptotic death. *J. Neurosci. Res. 49*, 600-607.

Shaheen, F., and Collman, R. G. (2004). Co-receptor antagonists as HIV-1 entry inhibitors. *Curr. Opin. Infect. Dis. 17*, 7-16.

Shapshak, P., Duncan, R., Minagar, A., Rodriguez de la Vega, P., Stewart, R. V., and Goodkin, K. (2004). Elevated expression of IFN-gamma in the HIV-1 infected brain. *Front. Biosci. 9*, 1073-1081.

Shi, B., Rainha, J., Lorenzo, A., Busciglio, J., and Gabuzda, D. (1998). Neuronal Apoptosis Induced by HIV-1 Tat Protein and TNF-a: Potentiation of Neurotoxicity Mediated by Oxidative Stress and Implications for HIV-1 Dementia. *J. Neurovirol. 4*, 281-290.

Shiraishi, K., Fukuda, S., Mori, T., Matsuda, K., Yamaguchi, T., Tanikawa, C., Ogawa, M., Nakamura, Y., and Arakawa, H. (2000). Identification of fractalkine, a CX3C-type chemokine, as a direct target of p53. *Cancer Res. 60*, 3722-3726.

Sippy, B. D., Hofman, F. M., Wallach, D., and Hinton, D. R. (1995). Increased expression of tumor necrosis factor-alpha receptors in the brains of patients with AIDS. *J. Acquir. Immune Defic. Syndr. Hum. Retrovirol. 10*, 511-521.

Song, L., and Pachter, J. S. (2004). Monocyte chemoattractant protein-1 alters expression of tight junction-associated proteins in brain microvascular endothelial cells. *Microvasc. Res. 67*, 78-89.

Soontornniyomkij, V., Wang, G., Pittman, C. A., Wiley, C. A., and Achim, C. L. (1998). Expression of brain-derived neurotrophic factor protein in activated microglia of human immunodeficiency virus type 1 encephalitis. *Neuropathol. Appl. Neurobiol. 24*, 453-460.

Srinivasan, D., Yen, J. H., Joseph, D. J., and Friedman, W. (2004). Cell type-specific interleukin-1beta signaling in the CNS. *J. Neurosci. 24*, 6482-6488.

Strieter, R. M., Polverini, P. J., Kunkel, S. L., Arenberg, D. A., Burdick, M. D., Kasper, J., Dzuiba, J., Van Damme, J., Walz, A., Marriott, D., and et al. (1995). The functional role of the ELR motif in CXC chemokine-mediated angiogenesis. *J. Biol. Chem. 270*, 27348-27357.

Stumm, R. K., Zhou, C., Ara, T., Lazarini, F., Dubois-Dalcq, M., Nagasawa, T., Hollt, V., and Schulz, S. (2003). CXCR4 regulates interneuron migration in the developing neocortex. *J. Neurosci. 23*, 5123-5130.

Tang, J., and Kaslow, R. A. (2003). The impact of host genetics on HIV infection and disease progression in the era of highly active antiretroviral therapy. *Aids 17 Suppl. 4*, S51-60.

Tong, N., Perry, S. W., Zhang, Q., James, H. J., Guo, H., Brooks, A., Bal, H., Kinnear, S. A., Fine, S., Epstein, L. G., et al. (2000). Neuronal fractalkine expression in HIV-1 encephalitis: roles for macrophage recruitment and neuroprotection in the central nervous system. *J. Immunol. 164*, 1333-1339.

Tran, P. B., and Miller, R. J. (2003). Chemokine receptors: signposts to brain development and disease. *Nat. Rev. Neurosci. 4*, 444-455.

Tyor, W. R., Glass, J. D., Griffin, J. W., Becker, P. S., McArthur, J. C., Bezman, L., and Griffin, D. E. (1992). Cytokine expression in the brain during acquired immune deficiency syndrome. *Ann. Neurol. 31*, 349-360.

Vallat, A.-V., Girolami, U. D., He, J., Mhashikar, A., Marasco, W., Shi, B., Gray, F., Bell, J., Keohane, C., Smith, T. W., and Gabuzda, D. (1998). Localization of HIV-1 co-receptors CCR5 and CXCR4 in the brain of children with AIDS. *Am. J. Path. 152*, 167-178.

van der Meer, P., Ulrich, A. M., Gonzalez-Scarano, F., and Lavi, E. (2000). Immunohistochemical analysis of CCR2, CCR3, CCR5, and CXCR4 in the human brain: potential mechanisms for HIV dementia. *Exp. Mol. Pathol. 69*, 192-201.

van Marle, G., Henry, S., Todoruk, T., Sullivan, A., Silva, C., Rourke, S. B., Holden, J., McArthur, J. C., Gill, M. J., and Power, C. (2004). Human immunodeficiency virus type 1 Nef protein mediates neural cell death: a neurotoxic role for IP-10. *Virology. 329*, 302-318.

Walz, A., Peveri, P., Aschauer, H., and Baggiolini, M. (1987). Purification and amino acid sequencing of NAF, a novel neutrophil-activating factor produced by monocytes. *Biochem. Biophys. Res. Commun. 149*, 755-761.

Wang, X. (2001). The expanding role of mitochondria in apoptosis. *Genes Dev.* 15, 2922-2933.

Wesselingh, S. L., Power, C., Glass, J. D., and et al (1993). Intracerebral cytokine messenger RNA expression in acquired immunedeficiency syndrome dementia. *Ann. Neurol. 33*, 576-582.

Westmoreland, S. V., Rottman, J. B., Williams, K. C., Lackner, A. A., and Sasseville, V. G. (1998). Chemokine receptor expression on resident and inflammatory cells in the brain of macaques with simian immunodeficiency virus encephalitis. *Am. J. Pathol. 152*, 659-665.

Wiley, C. A., Schrier, R. D., Nelson, J. A., Lampert, P. W., and Oldstone, M. B. A. (1986). Cellular localization of human immunodeficiency virus infection within the brains of acquired immune deficiency syndrome patients. *Proc. Natl. Acad. Sci. USA 83*, 7089-7093.

Williams, K., Schwartz, A., Corey, S., Orandle, M., Kennedy, W., Thompson, B., Alvarez, X., Brown, C., Gartner, S., and Lackner, A. (2002). Proliferating cellular nuclear antigen expression as a marker of perivascular macrophages in simian immunodeficiency virus encephalitis. *Am. J. Pathol. 161*, 575-585.

Wright, J. L., and Merchant, R. E. (1992). Histopathological effects of intracerebral injections of human recombinant tumor necrosis factor-alpha in the rat. *Acta Neuropathol. (Berl) 85*, 93-100.

Wu, D. T., Woodman, S. E., Weiss, J. M., McManus, C. M., D'Aversa, T. G., Hesselgesser, J., Major, E. O., Nath, A., and Berman, J. W. (2000). Mechanisms of leukocyte trafficking into the CNS. *J. Neurovirol. 6 Suppl. 1*, S82-85.

Wyss-Coray, T., Masliah, E., Toggas, S. M., Rockenstein, E. M., Brooker, M. J., Lee, H. S., and Mucke, L. (1996). Dysregulation of signal transduction pathways as a potential mechanism of nervous system alterations in HIV-1 gp120 transgenic mice and humans with HIV-1 encephalitis. *J. Clin. Invest. 97*, 789-798.

Xiao, B. G., and Link, H. (1998). Immune regulation within the central nervous system. *J. Neurol. Sci. 157*, 1-12.

Yoshimura, T., Matsushima, K., Oppenheim, J. J., and Leonard, E. J. (1987). Neutrophil chemotactic factor produced by lipopolysaccharide (LPS)-stimulated human blood mononuclear leukocytes: partial characterization and separation from interleukin 1 (IL 1). *J. Immunol. 139*, 788-793.

Zhang, K., McQuibban, G. A., Silva, C., Butler, G. S., Johnston, J. B., Holden, J., Clark-Lewis, I., Overall, C. M., and Power, C. (2003). HIV-induced metalloproteinase processing of the chemokine stromal cell derived factor-1 causes neurodegeneration. *Nat. Neurosci. 6*, 1064-1071.

Zhang, L., He, T., Talal, A., Wang, G., Frankel, S. S., and Ho, D. D. (1998). In vivo distribution of the human immunodeficiency virus/simian immunodeficiency virus coreceptors: CXCR4, CCR3, and CCR5. *J. Virol. 72*, 5035-5045.

Zhao, M. L., Kim, M. O., Morgello, S., and Lee, S. C. (2001). Expression of inducible nitric oxide synthase, interleukin-1 and caspase-1 in HIV-1 encephalitis. *J. Neuroimmunol. 115*, 182-191.

Zheng, J., Bauer, M., Cotter, R. L., Ryan, L. A., Lopez, A., Williams, C., Ghorpade, A., and Gendelman, H. E. (2000a). Fractalkine mediated macrophage activation by neuronal injury: relevance for HIV-1 associated dementia. Paper presented at: 30th Annual meeting of society for neuroscience (New Orleans, Society for Neuroscience).

Zheng, J., Ghorpade, A., Niemann, D., Cotter, R. L., Thylin, M. R., Epstein, L., Swartz, J. M., Shepard, R. B., Liu, X., Nukuna, A., and Gendelman, H. E. (1999a). Lymphotropic virions affect chemokine receptor-mediated neural signaling and apoptosis: implications for human immunodeficiency virus type 1-associated dementia. *J. Virol. 73*, 8256-8267.

Zheng, J., Niemann, D., Bauer, M., Leisman, G. B., Cotter, R. L., Ryan, L. A., Lopez, A., Williams, C., Ghorpade, A., and Gendelman, H. E. (2000b). a-Chemokines and their Receptors in the Neuronal Signaling: Relevance for HIV-1-associated Dementia. Paper presented at: 7th Conference on Retroviruses and Opportunistic Infections (San Francisco, Foundation for Retrovirology and Human Health).

Zheng, J., Niemann, D., Bauer, M., Williams, C., Lopez, A., Erichsen, D., Ryan, L. A., Cotter, R. L., Ghorpade, A., Swindells, S., and Gendelman, H. E. (2001). HIV-1 glia interactions in interleukin-8 and growth-related oncogene a secretion, neuronal signaling and demise: relevance for HIV-1-associated dementia. Paper presented at: 8th conference on retroviruses and opportunistic infections (Chicago, Foundation for retrovirology and human health).

Zheng, J., Thylin, M., Ghorpade, A., Xiong, H., Persidsky, Y., Cotter, R., Niemann, D., Che, M., Zeng, Y., Gelbard, H., et al. (1999b). Intracellular CXCR4 signaling, neuronal apoptosis and neuropathogenic mechanisms of HIV-1-associated dementia. *J. Neuroimmunol. 98*, 185-200.

Zhou, N., Fang, J., Mukhtar, M., Acheampong, E., and Pomerantz, R. J. (2004). Inhibition of HIV-1 fusion with small interfering RNAs targeting the chemokine coreceptor CXCR4. *Gene Ther. 11*, 1703-1712.

Zink, M. C., Coleman, G. D., Mankowski, J. L., Adams, R. J., Tarwater, P. M., Fox, K., and Clements, J. E. (2001). Increased macrophage chemoattractant protein-1 in cerebrospinal fluid precedes and predicts simian immunodeficiency virus encephalitis. *J. Infect. Dis. 184*, 1015-1021.

Zou, Y. R., Kottmann, A. H., Kuroda, M., Taniuchi, I., and Littman, D. R. (1998). Function of the chemokine receptor CXCR4 in haematopoiesis and in cerebellar development. *Nature 393*, 595-599.

Zujovic, V., Benavides, J., Vige, X., Carter, C., and Taupin, V. (2000). Fractalkine modulates TNF-alpha secretion and neurotoxicity induced by microglial activation [In Process Citation]. *Glia 29*, 305-315.

In: Neuro-AIDS
Editors: A. Minagar and P. Shapshak, pp. 81-100

ISBN:1-59454-610-X
© 2006 Nova Science Publishers, Inc.

Chapter IV

Drug Abuse and Neuro-AIDS

Avindra Nath[1,2,], Kurt F. Hauser[3],*
Mark Prendergast[4] and Joseph Berger[5]
Departments of [1]Neurology, [2]Neuroscience,
Johns Hopkins University, Baltimore, Maryland, USA;
[3]Departments of Anatomy and Neurobiology, [4]Psychology,
[5]Neurology and Internal Medicine, University of Kentucky,
Lexington, Kentucky, USA.

Abstract

In certain populations around the world, the HIV pandemic is driven by drug abuse. Mounting evidence suggests that these patient populations may have accelerated and more severe neurocognitive dysfunction as compared to non-drug abusing HIV infected populations. Many drugs of abuse are CNS stimulants, hence it stands to reason that these drugs may synergize with neurotoxic substances released during the course of HIV infection. Clinical and laboratory evidence suggest that the dopaminergic systems are most vulnerable to such combined neurotoxicity although multiple regions of the brain may be involved. Identifying common mechanisms of neuronal injury is critical to developing therapeutic strategies for drug abusing HIV-infected populations. This chapter reviews 1) the current evidence for neurodegeneration in the setting of combined HIV infection and use of methamphetamine, cocaine, heroin or alcohol, 2) the proposed underlying mechanisms involved in this combined neurotoxicity, and 3) future directions for research. This manuscript also suggests therapeutic approaches based on our current understanding of the neuropathogenesis of dementia due to HIV infection and drugs of abuse.

Keywords: HIV, dementia, methamphetamine, cocaine, alcohol, opiates, heroin

---

[*] Correspondence concerning this article should be addressed to Avindra Nath MD, Department of Neurology, 600 N. Wolfe St, Pathology 509, Baltimore, MD 21287. Tele: 443-287-4656; e-mail: anath1@jhmi.edu.

Introduction

Drug abuse and HIV are truly interlinked epidemics. Nearly two and one half million Americans use heroin and as many as 30 % of injecting drug users are HIV seropositive. Drug abuse also accounts for nearly half of the HIV infections in women in United States, however, the effect of drug abuse on incidence, rate of progression, or severity of HIV dementia is not entirely clear. However, studying the combined effects of drug abuse and HIV on the brain has been challenging. These patients are often poly-drug abusers. Moreover, the amounts and frequency of drug use vary widely amongst patient groups and within single individuals and these patients are often co-infected with hepatitis C (Murrill et al, 2002) making it difficult to determine the degree to which the drugs may alter brain function. Nonetheless, several patient based studies have been performed and many are currently underway. In this chapter, we review the clinical, pathological and pathophysiological studies which when taken together clearly show that drug abuse in conjunction with HIV infection has synergistic effects on brain function.

Epidemiology and Clinical Manifestations

Unlike HIV-seronegative older adults whose rates of drug abuse and mood disorders decline substantially compared with younger adults, this decline is not observed for older HIV seropositive adults (Rabkin et al, 2004). Although the number of studies addressing both the cognitive dysfunction in HIV seropositive individuals and the role of drugs of abuse in their genesis remain limited, the weight of evidence suggests a synergistic effect between HIV and drug abuse on cognitive embarrassment. An early study found no major differences in cognitive functioning amongst asymptomatic HIV-infected persons with or without a history of drug abuse (Concha et al, 1997). However, a later study showed that a history of injection drug use and presentation with prominent psychomotor slowing were associated with more rapid neurologic progression (Bouwman et al, 1998). Furthermore, in some HIV infected drug abusers an accelerated form of HIV dementia may be observed (Nath et al, 2001).

Long-term methamphetamine use has also been associated with neuronal damage as determined by case reports (Bartzokis et al, 1999b; Pascual-Leone and Dhuna, 1990; Pascual-Leone et al, 1990; Weiner et al, 2001), animal models , pathological materials (Wilson et al, 1996a; Wilson et al, 1996b), and magnetic resonance spectroscopy brain imaging (Ernst et al, 2000). Autopsy studies confirm injury to dopaminergic neurons in methamphetamine as well as cocaine abusers (Wilson et al, 1996a; Wilson et al, 1996b). Although infrequent, cocaine use has been associated with persistent dyskinesias including choreoathetoid movements and tics (Bartzokis et al, 1999b; Pascual-Leone and Dhuna, 1990; Weiner et al, 2001) and seizures (Pascual-Leone et al, 1990). Interestingly, some investigators have proposed the use of psychostimulants in the treatment of HIV dementia (Brown, 1995); however, the effects of these drugs on cerebral function in the setting of HIV infection has not been well studied.

Since common drugs of abuse including cocaine, amphetamines, and opiates, all have dopaminergic activation properties, this suggests that these drugs may accelerate the loss of an already compromised dopaminergic system in patients with HIV infection. We recently reported a patient with HIV dementia and a history of cocaine and methamphetamine use who developed a progressive resting tremor, dystonia and athetoid movements (Nath et al, 2001). Furthermore, preliminary studies suggest that intravenous drug abusers with HIV infection had more severe neuronal loss and shrunken neuronal cells in the substantia nigra, compared to patients who died of AIDS without a history of drug abuse (Reyes et al, 1991).

Many features of AIDS dementia mirror symptoms observed in the setting of dopamine deficient states, e.g., Parkinson's disease. Evidence for involvement of the dopaminergic systems in HIV dementia includes the clinical features of the illness, the neuronal loss of deep nuclear structures as determined by magnetic resonance spectroscopy and pathological materials, the shared neurochemistry of the disorders (Berger and Arendt, 2000). Furthermore, patients with AIDS, when treated with even mild dopaminergic blocking drugs, such as prochlorperazine, perpherazine, trifluperazine, low dose haloperidol, thiothixine, chlorpromazine, or metoclopramide, can develop severe parkinsonism (Edelstein and Knight, 1987; Hollander et al, 1985; Hriso et al, 1991; Kieburtz et al, 1991; Mirsattari et al, 1999; Mirsattari et al, 1998). In one study, a comparison was made with psychotic patients without HIV infection receiving neuroleptics (Hriso et al, 1991). The likelihood of developing parkinsonian symptoms was 2-4 times higher in patients with AIDS when controlled for mean drug dose and body weight. Such symptoms developed in 50% of AIDS patients who received less than 4 mg/kg of chlorpromazine equivalents per day and 78% of those who received more than 4 mg/kg per day (Hriso et al, 1991). These observations suggest an already compromised dopaminergic system in HIV-infected individuals receiving these drugs.

The principal source of dopamine and its metabolites in the cerebrospinal fluid is from the dopaminergic system in the brain; dopamine levels in the CSF are thus good reflection of the integrity of dopaminergic neurons. CSF neurotransmitter levels provide a sensitive indicator of neuronal dysfunction and abnormalities can be detected in the asymptomatic phases of neurological disease (Hornykiewicz, 1998). Similarly, CSF homovanillic acid levels are diminished in patients with AIDS and more severely so in patients with AIDS dementia (Berger et al, 1994; Larsson et al, 1991). A study of monoamine metabolites in CSF of asymptomatic SIV infected rhesus macaques showed increased levels of 3,4-dihydroxyphenylacetic acid in the CSF suggesting increased dopamine turnover in early stages of infection (Koutsilieri et al, 1997b).

Alcohol abuse and/or dependence is frequently observed in HIV-infected individuals and likely represents a significant risk factor for HIV infection (Weinhardt et al, 2001). Individuals who abuse alcohol often engage in high-risk sexual behavior (Baldwin et al, 2000) and have significant compromise of immune function, resulting from direct immunotoxicity and nutritional deficiency (Dingle and Oei, 1997; Watzl and Watson, 1992). This latter point, in particular, may suggest that HIV-positive individuals who abuse alcohol are at increased risk for both the development of AIDS and other HIV-related symptoms, such as HIV-associated dementia complex (Pillai et al, 1991; Tabakoff, 1994; Tyor and Middaugh, 1999).

Studies exploring possible interactions between alcohol abuse and development of HIV-1 related symptoms are, to date, inconclusive. A small number of studies have examined cognitive function in alcoholics infected with HIV and find no evidence of a link between greater neuropsychological impairment and HIV-1 positive status (Bornstein et al, 1993; Heaton et al, 1995). However, as Basso and Bornstein (Basso and Bornstein, 2000) correctly point out, these studies and related neuroimaging studies (McArthur et al, 1990; Meyerhoff et al, 1995) did not conduct the critical comparisons between neuropsychological function in alcoholic and non-alcoholic HIV-1 seropositive individuals. Comparisons in these studies were typically conducted between seropositive and seronegative patients. Further, these studies did not account for individual differences in the patients' history of alcohol detoxification, a factor that can dramatically affect neuropsychological functioning (Craig and Mosier, 1978). It is unclear, then, if the presence of alcoholism worsens the neuropathological and behavioral effects of HIV-1 infection in seropositive individuals. Recent studies suggest that opiate use may be associated with the development of asymptomatic peripheral neuropathies in HIV infected patients (Morgello et al, 2004), but this area has not been well studied.

Neuropathology in HIV Infected Drug Abusers

Neuropathological studies, in general, have shown significant differences in the brains of HIV seropositive drug abusers when compared to a control HIV-seropositive population. However, these differences were not consistently demonstrated; perhaps reflective of differences in the study populations and techniques employed. Bell and colleagues demonstrated a marked severity of HIV encephalitis (HIVE) in drug abusers (Bell et al, 1998). A particularly striking involvement of dopaminergic neurons has been reported (Reyes et al, 1991). Drug users with HIVE tend to have more activated microglia than non-drug-using comparison groups, particularly in the thalamus (Arango et al, 2004; Tomlinson et al, 1999). In another study, the same group of investigators found that GFAP-reactive astrocytes in both grey and white matter were significantly more numerous in drug using patients with HIVE when compared to HIV negative drug users or HIV seropositive drug users without HIVE. They were numerous in only one subject who was treatment-naïve suggesting that in this population, HIV infected astrocytes may serve as a reservoir for the virus (Anderson et al, 2003). Drug abuse has no significant effect on B cell infiltrates into the brain of HIV infected patients (Anthony et al, 2004). The above studies have been reported from a cohort in Edinburgh where the population is predominantly an opiate abusing cohort. In a methamphetamine abusing cohort from San Diego, similarly a severe microglial reaction was found in patients with drug abuse and HIVE when compared to patients with HIVE who were non-methamphetamine users. However, in contrast they found that the methamphetamine-using patients with HIVE showed significantly lower gp41 scores suggesting less numbers of HIV infected macrophages/microglia and less severe forms of encephalitis but a higher frequency of ischemic events, and a more pronounced loss of synaptophysin and calbindin immunoreactivity, suggesting damage to non-pyramidal neurons (Langford et al, 2003).

Effect of Drug Abuse on HIV Replication

The "opiate cofactor hypothesis" has been proposed as a mechanism in the pathogenesis of AIDS (Donahoe and Vlahov, 1998), and is based on experimental findings that opioids can modulate HIV propagation in immune cells and suppress immune function. By contrast, the effects of opiates disease progression in non-human primate models of HIV have been less straightforward (Donahoe, 2004), although in recent, carefully controlled studies, chronic, morphine has been shown to markedly increase viral loads in plasma and CSF (Kumar et al, 2004). Opioid drugs and HIV proteins act synergistically to destabilize immune function by affecting monocytes and lymphocytes. Subsets of leukocytes express mu, delta, and kappa opioid receptors, as well as endogenous opioid peptides such as enkephalins, and opioids can modulate neuroimmune function through complex (direct and indirect) actions that involve both peripheral and central neural and non-neural mechanisms (Bidlack, 2000; Chang et al, 1998; McCarthy et al, 2001; Mellon and Bayer, 1998). Although the effects of opioids on immune function have been previously reviewed (Adler et al, 1993; Peterson et al, 2001; Sharp et al, 1998), an emerging concept is that the opioid system can have dichotomous (positive and negative) effects on HIV infection and/or replication in immunocytes. For example, mu receptor stimulation increases HIV expression in monocytic cells (Peterson et al, 1999; Peterson et al, 1993), while kappa receptor activation can have the opposite, inhibitory effect on HIV expression in monocytic and lymphocytic cells (Chao et al, 1996; Chao et al, 2001; Peterson et al, 2001). Mu and kappa receptors have been noted to mediate opposing actions in other systems (Bohn et al, 2000). Interestingly, mu-opioid receptor activation can increase the expression of cytokine receptors, that serve as co-receptors for HIV in susceptible cells including CCR3, CCR5, and CXCR4, while kappa-opioid receptor stimulation can increase CCR2, while decreasing CCR5, expression (Rogers and Peterson, 2003). To add to this complexity, there is evidence for bi-directional heterologous interactions between opioid and chemokine receptors (Rogers et al, 2000) (Rogers and Peterson, 2003). Thus, although opioids can be pro- or anti-inflammatory depending on the particular opioid receptor and cell type that are affected, the typical/net consequence of mu-opioid receptor activation is to suppress immune function thereby promoting disease progression.

Effect of HIV and Drugs of Abuse
on Neuronal Function

In vitro studies show that when neuronal cell lines are exposed to either dopamine, cocaine, or morphine along with supernatants from HIV infected cells, significant neuronal cell death and oxidative stress occurs (Koutsilieri et al, 1997a). An acute exposure to methamphetamine and cocaine may be sufficient to cause neurotoxicity (Turchan et al, 2001). The mechanism by which these substances synergize remains elusive. As demonstrated in these studies, at least in part the mechanism involves mitochondrial dysfunction. Since both gp120 and Tat have been shown to cause toxicity to dopaminergic cells and similarly methamphetamine and cocaine also cause toxicity to dopaminergic systems, we characterized the dopaminergic neurons and receptors in our culture system. We found that only a small proportion of these cells underwent cell death when exposed to HIV proteins and these drugs of abuse (Turchan et al, 2001). This suggests that there must be additional factors, which need to be identified, that cause some neurons in drug abusing individuals to be vulnerable to HIV.

Cocaine

One possible mechanism for cocaine-HIV protein synergy is oxidative stress. Mitochondria have been proposed as critical cellular targets for cocaine toxicity, and prior studies have found that cocaine can decrease mitochondrial respiration and increase the production of reactive oxygen species in animals (Boess et al, 2000). We have found that Tat may produce oxidative damage in vivo (Askenov et al, 2001). Increased oxidative modifications of proteins occurs soon following the injection of Tat into the rat striatum and may be an important mechanism for Tat neurotoxicity. Thus, both cocaine and Tat target the mitochondria, producing oxidative stress, suggesting the possibility for synergistic interactions in producing mitochondrial dysfunction and ultimately cell death. This provides a basis for searching for antioxidant compounds that may decrease or prevent oxidative damage produced by cocaine and HIV interactions.

Methamphetamine

Methamphetamine synergizes with Tat in vivo. Methamphetamine-treated animals demonstrated a 7% decline in striatal dopamine levels while Tat-treated animals showed an 8% reduction. Exposure to both methamphetamine + Tat caused an almost 65% reduction in striatal dopamine. This same treatment caused a 56% reduction in the binding capacity to the dopamine transporter. It should be pointed out that the dose of methamphetamine used in this study did not induce hyperthermia, thus increasing the relevance of this animal model with respect to human disease (Maragos et al, 2002). Microdialysis studies in this animal model show that the synergistic response is accompanied by marked decreases in dopamine release in the striatum (Cass et al, 2003).

The combined effects of methamphetamine and HIV proteins may affect a number of regions within the brain and there maybe some differences in the underlying mechanisms in the different regions. For example, administration of Tat or METH resulted in stimulation of cellular oxidative stress and activation of redox-regulated transcription factors in the cortical, striatal, and hippocampal regions of the mouse brain. In addition, DNA-binding activities of NF-kappaB, AP-1, and CREB in the frontal cortex and hippocampus were more pronounced in mice injected with Tat plus METH compared to the effects of Tat or METH alone. Intercellular adhesion molecule-1 gene expression also was upregulated in a synergistic manner in cortical, striatal, and hippocampal regions in mice which received injections of Tat combined with METH compared to the effects of these agents alone. Moreover, synergistic effects of Tat plus METH on the tumor necrosis factor-alpha and interleukin-1beta mRNA levels were observed in the striatal region (Flora et al, 2003).

Opiates

In the CNS, heroin acts largely via its conversion to morphine, making morphine the most commonly used drug of choice to study opiate effects in vivo and in vitro. Besides their immunomodulatory actions, opioids may directly modulate the response of neurons and macroglia to HIV infection. Interestingly, depending on the target tissue, particular opioid receptor type involved, and pharmacodynamics of receptor activation, opioids can have paradoxical neuroprotective or neurodegenerative effects. The divergent actions likely result from the fact that opioid receptors are highly promiscuous in their interactions with particular intracellular signaling pathways, and opioid receptor-effector coupling differs greatly among cell types (Hauser et al, 1998). In some experimental systems, opioids can be protective (Hauser et al, 1999; Meriney et al, 1991; Polakiewicz et al, 1998). For example, selective a mu opioid receptor agonist stimulates anti-apoptotic effectors downstream to the phosphoinositide 3-kinase (PI-3-K)-dependent signaling cascade in CHO cells stably transfected with mu opioid receptors (Polakiewicz et al, 1998). Morphine may exaggerate HIV-envelope protein gp120-induced early proliferative increases in kidney fibroblasts (Singhal et al, 1998a), and opioids can protect against the detrimental effects of gp120 (Stefano, 1999). More often, however, opioids exaggerate the effects of preexisting, non-opioid proapoptotic or proinflammatory signals, respectively; thereby either reducing cell viability directly (Goswami et al, 1998; Yin et al, 1997), or indirectly through the release of cytotoxic inflammatory intermediaries from immune cells. Mu opioid drugs with abuse liability, such as heroin, morphine, and fentanyl, respectively, can induce toxicity in cerebellar Purkinje cells in vitro (Hauser et al, 1994) and in the limbic system of rats at high dosages (Kofke et al, 1996). Fentanyl has been shown to exacerbate the effects of ischemia-induced damage to the basal ganglia (Kofke et al, 1999). Morphine can induce apoptosis through a caspase-3-dependent pathway in primary human microglia and neurons in vitro (Hu S., et al., 2002). Typically, however, opioids are not intrinsically toxic and morphine alone is rarely toxic to most neuronal types (Gurwell et al, 2001; Hauser et al, 2000). By contrast, there is burgeoning data suggesting that nontoxic concentrations of opioids can significantly exacerbate cell losses if combined with pro-apoptotic agents (Nair et al, 1997; Singhal et al, 1999; Singhal et al, 1997; Singhal et al, 1998b; Yin et al, 1999). Mu agonists enhance staurosporine or wortmannin-induced apoptosis in embryonic chick neurons or neuronal cell lines (Goswami et al, 1998).

Alternatively, opioids may lower the threshold of susceptibility of dopaminergic neurons to viral damage by affecting dopamine turnover. Endogenous opioids, and/or opiate drugs such as morphine or heroin, can activate dopaminergic neurons through several different mechanisms of action (review, Kreek, 2001). Opioids can decrease dopamine levels though the disinhibition of interneurons that synapse on dopaminergic neurons, such as in the ventral tegmental area. Opioids may also modulate the cellular response to dopamine. For example, opioid receptor activation reportedly increases D2, but not D1, dopamine receptor binding sites in the rat striatum (Rooney et al, 1991), which may have considerable functional consequences (De Vries et al, 1999; Vanderschuren et al, 1999). Conversely, in another study, repeated intermittent exposure to morphine increases dopamine D1-receptor-induced adenylyl cyclase activity in rat striatal neurons *in vitro* (Schoffelmeer et al, 1997). Another highly significant issue related to HIV susceptibility is the disruption in dopaminergic function that occurs with the development of tolerance and dependence, or during withdrawal (Koob, 2000). Chronic opiate drug exposure is typically accompanied by disruption of second messenger cascades, altered patterns of gene activation, and increased oxidative stress (Hauser et al, 1998; Koob, 2000; Kreek and Koob, 1998), which may further enhance the vulnerability of neurons to HIV infection.

Several investigators have provided evidence that opioids and HIV-1 Tat protein are synergistically toxic to neurons through a direct action on neural cell targets. Importantly, we have observed synergistic Tat-opioid drug toxicity in human and mouse neural cells, using distinct, yet complementary, experimental approaches (Gurwell et al, 2001); (Turchan et al., unpublished observations). Importantly, the enhanced toxicity is mediated through specific opioid receptors, since the neurodegenerative effects of morphine are concentration-dependent and can be reversed by opioid receptor antagonists (Gurwell et al, 2001). Recent studies from our laboratories demonstrate that the coordinate effects are caused by mitochondrial toxicity through actions involving Akt/PKB, PI-3 kinase, and caspases 1, 3 and 7 activation in human neurons (Turchan et al., unpublished observations). A majority of the neurons in our cultures possess mu, delta, and/or kappa receptor immunoreactivity suggesting that opioids and Tat are acting directly. Alternatively, because a small number of contaminating glia may be present, we cannot be certain that some aspects of the neurotoxicity seen result from opiate-HIV actions via glial intermediaries. Subpopulations of striatal astrocytes (Stiene-Martin et al, 1998), and microglia (Chao et al, 1996) can express opioid receptors. Lastly, opioid drugs with abuse liability act by mimicking endogenous opioid peptides. Thus, besides directly modify the neural response to HIV, opiate drugs may act by affecting endogenous opioid peptide levels, which may further modify the response of the CNS to HIV.

Alcohol

Several deleterious effects of chronic ethanol intake occur that are directly neurotoxic and may render the CNS susceptible to other forms of injury, such as that seen in HIVE. For example, chronic ethanol intake can stimulate the production of reactive oxygen species (Brooks, 1997), inhibition of neuronal growth factors (Walker et al, 1993), and reduced local cerebral glucose utilization (Johnson-Greene et al, 1997). Not surprisingly, long-term ethanol abuse in humans is often associated with the development of mild-moderate neurological abnormalities, including impairment of executive function, even in the absence of Korsakoff's syndrome (Diamond and Messing, 1994).

There is reason to postulate that chronic alcoholism may alter neuronal function and sensitize some glutamatergic receptor systems (eg. *N*-methyl-D-aspartate (NMDA)) to the neurotoxic effects of Tat, gp120, or other HIV-1 proteins. *In vitro* studies of Tat and gp120 indicate that over activity of NMDA-type glutamate receptors, in addition to that of α-amino-3-hydroxy-5-methyl-4-isoxazole propionate-type receptors, likely contributes to the neurotoxic effects of these HIV-1 proteins [see (Epstein and Gelbard, 1999; Lipton, 1998; Nath and Geiger, 1998; Tyor and Middaugh, 1999). Thus, the presence of pharmacological factors that can produce a heightened sensitivity of glutamatergic receptor systems may promote HIV-1 related neurotoxicity.

It is clear that adaptive neuronal changes occur during long-term ethanol exposure that appears to sensitize the brain to excitatory amino acid neurotransmission during withdrawal from ethanol intake (review; Littleton and Little, 1994). An extensive literature has demonstrated that chronic ethanol exposure to animals or primary neuronal cell cultures produces compensatory increases in the density and sensitivity of NMDA-type glutamate receptors in cortical and hippocampal regions (Devaud and Morrow, 1999; Prendergast et al, 2000; Rudolph et al, 1998). This has been reported to result in NMDA receptor-mediated elevations in $[Ca^{2+}]$ during ethanol withdrawal (Hu and Ticku, 1995). The potentiation of NMDA receptor-mediated neuronal death during ethanol withdrawal can readily be blocked by NMDA receptor channel blockers (Ahern et al, 1994; Chandler et al, 1993; Prendergast et al, 2000) indicating that chronic ethanol exposure may sensitize the CNS to the neurotoxic effects of HIV-1 proteins that directly or indirectly stimulate function of this excitatory amino acid receptor system, particularly during periods of reduced ethanol intake.

Effect of HIV and Drugs of Abuse on Glial Cell Function

Opioid receptors are widely expressed by macroglia and macroglial precursors. Sustained exposure to morphine and Tat viral protein induces the preferential death of glial precursors and a small but significant proportion of astrocytes. The increased cell death is mediated by mu-opioid receptors and accompanied by the activation of caspase-3 (Khurdayan et al, 2004). Recent findings suggest that a major consequence of opiate-HIV interactions is to disrupt astroglial function and implicate astroglia as catalysts triggering early destabilizing and proinflammatory effects of opiates in HIV-infected individuals. Combined opiate and Tat exposure synergistically destabilize intracellular calcium and increase oxyradical production (El-Hage et al, 2005; El-Hage, Nath, Hauser, unpublished) in cultured striatal astroglia, while causing massive coordinate increases in the release of proinflammatory chemokines. This includes monocyte chemoattractant protein-1 (MCP-1) and RANTES. MCP-1, in particular, when released by CNS-resident astrocytes triggers an influx of monocyte/macrophages and microglial activation. Assuming the recruitment of macrophages/microglia to infected CNS loci is exacerbated in opiate-abusers; this would likely exaggerate losses in neuronal function and neurotoxicity, synaptic losses, and may eventually culminate in synaptic losses and neuronal death. Considering the unremitting and debilitating consequences of HIV by itself, when combined with chronic opiate abuse, this is likely to augment the progression of the disease in the CNS. The combined effects of other drugs of abuse with HIV on glial cell function have yet to be studied.

Effect of HIV and Drugs of Abuse on Blood Brain Barrier Function

The combined effects of HIV and drugs of abuse on the blood brain barrier has not been well studied. However, an in vitro study showed that cocaine can enhance monocyte migration across the blood brain barrier and induce the expression of adhesion molecules on endothelial cells (Fiala et al, 1998). Similarly, it has been shown that there is disruption of the blood brain barrier in HIV infected patients in vivo (Berger and Avison, 2004) which correlates with early inflammatory changes in the CSF particularly increases in monocyte chemoattractant protein −1 levels (Avison et al, 2004). This has been confirmed autopsy studies from HIV infected patients however drug abuse history of these patients was not known (Petito and Cash, 1992; Power et al, 1993). Several in vitro studies also show that HIV derived proteins can alter endothelial cell function or disrupt the blood brain barrier (Andras et al, 2003; Pu et al, 2003; Toborek et al, 2003).

Therapeutic Strategies

Drug abusing HIV infected patients pose unique challenges for the treating physician. Pharmacological interactions may occur between drugs of abuse and antiretroviral therapies (Fabris et al, 2000; Flexner et al, 2001). Treatment of HIV infected patients requires that they take a large number of medications and adhere strictly to complicated dosing schedules to prevent drug resistance. Patients with neurocognitive impairment have greater difficulties meeting such demands, thus it is not difficult to imagine that drug abusing HIV-infected patients with cognitive impairment would be the most challenging of all to treat. Hence, treatment strategies need to include drugs with long half lives, combination medications (where several medications can be combined into a single pill) and use of dietary supplements. Biotechnological approaches that would allow the incorporation of drugs into plants may be one such strategy. Close attention also needs to be given to drug-drug interactions. Lastly, therapeutic vaccines might be an attractive alternative, since immune responses generated may suppress viral replication for several months.

Drug Abuse Intervention

The extent to which drug abstinence would halt or potentially reverse the progression of the resultant HIV-associated encephalopathy in drug abusing individuals is uncertain, but a logical topic for future study. If abstinence cannot be achieved, then interventions that limit drug use, or negate drug effects at the cellular or molecular level (Robinson and Berridge, 2000), might be beneficial. For example, in heroin abusing populations, even though replacing one opiate with another may not be ideal, methadone or buprenorphine treatment programs are likely to be beneficial by limiting and regulating opiate exposure. Some of the detrimental effects of intravenous heroin abuse may be attributable to high, fluctuating opiate levels and a failure to accommodate to changes in opioid signal intensity (Kreek and Koob, 1998; Nestler and Aghajanian, 1997). The accompanying disruption in normal function by these high drug levels may increase the susceptibility of cells to HIV protein toxins (Gurwell et al, 2001), while sustained, chronic exposure to more moderate dosages are likely to have fewer side effects. Studies on the molecular basis of addiction hold promise, because they would identify the basis to develop pharmacological ways to prevent craving for drugs of abuse.

Gonadal Hormones

Recently, much attention has been given to the neuroprotective properties of estrogens for both chronic neurodegenerative diseases and acute insults such as stroke. *In vitro* studies also show that estrogens can protect against a number of neurotoxic compounds (Green and Simpkins, 2000). The mechanisms by which estrogens protect cells can be broadly classified into two categories, receptor mediated and non-receptor-mediated effects. Estrogen receptors are widely expressed in the brain with some regional differences (Gundlah et al, 2000). Estrogen deficiency has been implicated as a risk factor in the development of several neurodegenerative diseases (Manly et al, 2000; Saunders-Pullman et al, 1999; Slooter et al, 1999) and estrogen replacement may result in improvement of cognitive function (Asthana et al, 1999). The mechanisms by which estrogens protect neurons are currently under intense investigation and may involve receptor-mediated mechanisms or non-receptor-mediated, antioxidative effects. For these reasons, we assessed the combined effects of HIV proteins and the drugs of abuse methamphetamine and cocaine, on neuronal function and determined the extent to which estrogen might protect against these neurotoxic substances (Turchan et al, 2001). We observed that 17β-estradiol at concentrations that are achieved physiologically or can easily be obtained pharmacologically protected against the combined insult of HIV proteins and drugs of abuse. Protection was noted against both cell death and mitochondrial impairment. The protection was specific since no protection was noted with 17α-estradiol. In subsequent experiments, we determined if this protection was mediated via estrogen receptors. The estrogen receptor antagonist ICI 182,780 completely, and tamoxifen partially reversed the neuroprotective effects of 17β-estradiol using cell death as an end point. However these compounds were unable to reverse the neuroprotective effects of estrogen on mitochondrial membrane potential, suggesting that the mitochondrial effects of estrogen are non-receptor mediated. Thus, the toxic effects on mitochondria and neuronal cell survival seems to be independently regulated. However, it seems that 17β-estradiol can protect against both these effects by receptor and non-receptor mediated mechanisms (Turchan et al, 2001).

Antioxidants and Neuroprotectants

It is becoming abundantly clear that oxidative stress plays an important role in the neuropathogenesis of HIV infection. As discussed above, HIV proteins and drugs of abuse may synergize to cause mitochondrial toxicity and generate oxidative stress in susceptible neurons. It is thus necessary to determine the degree to which antioxidants can protect HIV infected drug abusing patient populations from developing neurodegeneration. Antioxidants are an attractive approach since they are easily available as dietary supplements and are present is several plants which includes a variety of plant estrogens that do not have feminizing effects. Some novel compounds are also under development that have both anti-retroviral and antioxidant properties (Turchan et al, 2003). A clinical trial is currently underway with L-deprenyl in patients with HIV dementia. This drug has multiple effects on the central nervous system. It is a specific monoamine oxidase B (MAO-B) inhibitor, it has antioxidant effects, reduces the euphoric effects of cocaine and normalizes blood flow in cocaine addicts. In preliminary studies, it has also been shown to slow the progression of HIV dementia and hence might be an ideal candidate for clinical trials in HIV infected drug abusers (Bartzokis et al, 1999a).

Summary

This review has attempted to familiarize the reader with a broad body of knowledge that focuses chiefly on the synergistic effects of HIV and drugs of abuse in the pathogenesis of HIV dementia. This data was drawn from a broad range of studies including clinical assessments, magnetic resonance spectroscopy, CT and MR imaging, and histopathological observations determined at postmortem examination. Clearly, additional research in this important line of investigation is sorely needed.

References

Adler MW, Geller EB, Rogers TJ, Henderson EE, Eisenstein TK (1993). Opioids, receptors, and immunity. *Adv. Exp. Med. Biol. 335*: 13-20.

Ahern KB, Lustig HS, Greenberg DA (1994). Enhancement of NMDA toxicity and calcium responses by chronic exposure of cultured cortical neurons to ethanol. *Neurosci. Lett. 165*: 211-4.

Anderson CE, Tomlinson GS, Pauly B, Brannan FW, Chiswick A, Brack-Werner R, Simmonds P, Bell JE (2003). Relationship of Nef-positive and GFAP-reactive astrocytes to drug use in early and late HIV infection. *Neuropathol. Appl. Neurobiol. 29*: 378-88.

Andras IE, Pu H, Deli MA, Nath A, Hennig B, Toborek M (2003). HIV-1 Tat protein alters tight junction protein expression and distribution in cultured brain endothelial cells. *J. Neurosci. Res. 74*: 255-65.

Anthony IC, Crawford DH, Bell JE (2004). Effects of human immunodeficiency virus encephalitis and drug abuse on the B lymphocyte population of the brain. *J. Neurovirol. 10*: 181-8.

Arango JC, Simmonds P, Brettle RP, Bell JE (2004). Does drug abuse influence the microglial response in AIDS and HIV encephalitis? *Aids 18 Suppl. 1*: S69-74.

Askenov MY, Hasselrot U, Bansal AK, Wu G, Nath A, Anderson C, Mactutus CF, Booze RM (2001). Oxidative damage induced by the injection of HIV-1 Tat protein in the rat striatum. *Neurosci. Letters 305*: 5-8.

Asthana S, Craft S, Baker LD, Raskind MA, Birnbaum RS, Lofgreen CP, Veith RC, Plymate SR (1999). Cognitive and neuroendocrine response to transdermal estrogen in postmenopausal women with Alzheimer's disease: results of a placebo- controlled, double-blind, pilot study. *Psychoneuroendocrinology 24*: 657-77.

Avison MJ, Nath A, Greene-Avison R, Schmitt FA, Bales RA, Ethisham A, Greenberg RN, Berger JR (2004). Inflammatory changes and breakdown of microvascular integrity in early human immunodeficiency virus dementia. *J. Neurovirol. 10*: 223-32.

Baldwin JA, Maxwell CJ, Fenaughty AM, Trotter RT, Stevens SJ (2000). Alcohol as a risk factor for hiv transmission among american indian and alaska native drug users. *Am. Indian Alsk. Native Ment. Health Res. 9*: 1-16.

Bartzokis G, Beckson M, Newton T, Mandelkern M, Mintz J, Foster JA, Ling W, Bridge TP (1999a). Selegiline effects on cocaine-induced changes in medial temporal lobe metabolism and subjective ratings of euphoria. *Neuropsychopharmacology 20*: 582-90.

Bartzokis G, Beckson M, Wirshing DA, Lu PH, Foster JA, Mintz J (1999b). Choreoathetoid movements in cocaine dependence. *Biol. Psychiatry. 45*: 1630-5.

Basso MR, Bornstein RA (2000). Neurobehavioural consequences of substance abuse and HIV infection. *J. Psychopharmacol. 14*: 228-37.

Bell JE, Brettle RP, Chiswick A, Simmonds P (1998). HIV encephalitis, proviral load and dementia in drug users and homosexuals with AIDS. Effect of neocortical involvement. *Brain 121*: 2043-52.

Berger JR, Arendt G (2000). HIV dementia: the role of the basal ganglia and dopaminergic systems. *J. Psychopharmacol. 14*: 214-21.

Berger JR, Avison M (2004). The blood brain barrier in HIV infection. *Front. Biosci. 9*: 2680-5.

Berger JR, Kumar M, Kumar A, Fernandez JB, Levin B (1994). Cerebrospinal fluid dopamine in HIV-1 infection. *AIDS 8*: 67-71.

Bidlack JM (2000). Detection and function of opioid receptors on cells from the immune system. *Clin. Diagn. Lab. Immunol. 7*: 719-23.

Boess F, Ndikum-Moffor FM, Boelsterli UA, Roberts SM (2000). Effects of cocaine and its oxidative metabolites on mitochondrial respiration and generation of reactive oxygen species. *Biochem. Pharmacol. 60*: 615-23.

Bohn LM, Belcheva MM, Coscia CJ (2000). Mu-opioid agonist inhibition of kappa-opioid receptor-stimulated extracellular signal-regulated kinase phosphorylation is dynamin-dependent in C6 glioma cells. *J. Neurochem. 74*: 574-81.

Bornstein RA, Fama R, Rosenberger P, Whitacre CC, Para MF, Nasrallah HA, Fass RJ (1993). Drug and alcohol use and neuropsychological performance in asymptomatic HIV infection. *J. Neuropsychiatry Clin. Neurosci. 5*: 254-9.

Bouwman FH, Skolasky RL, Hes D, Selnes OA, Glass JD, Nance-Sproson TE, Royal W, Dal Pan GJ, McArthur JC (1998). Variable progression of HIV-associated dementia. *Neurology. 50*: 1814-20.

Brooks PJ (1997). DNA damage, DNA repair, and alcohol toxicity--a review. *Alcohol. Clin. Exp. Res. 21*: 1073-82.

Brown GR (1995). The use of methylphenidate for cognitive decline associated with HIV disease. *Int. J. Psychiatry. Med. 25*: 21-37.

Cass WA, Harned ME, Peters LE, Nath A, Maragos WF (2003). HIV-1 protein Tat potentiation of methamphetamine-induced decreases in evoked overflow of dopamine in the striatum of the rat. *Brain Res. 984*: 133-142.

Chandler LJ, Newsom H, Sumners C, Crews F (1993). Chronic ethanol exposure potentiates NMDA excitotoxicity in cerebral cortical neurons. *J. Neurochem. 60*: 1578-81.

Chang SL, Wu GD, Patel NA, Vidal EL, Fiala M (1998). The effects of interaction between morphine and interleukin-1 on the immune response. *Adv. Exp. Med. Biol. 437*: 67-72.

Chao CC, Gekker G, Hu S, Sheng WS, Shark KB, Bu DF, Archer S, Bidlack JM, Peterson PK (1996). kappa opioid receptors in human microglia downregulate human immunodeficiency virus 1 expression. *Proc. Natl. Acad. Sci. U S A. 93*: 8051-6.

Chao CC, Gekker G, Sheng WS, Hu S, Peterson PK (2001). U50488 inhibits HIV-1 expression in acutely infected monocyte-derived macrophages. *Drug Alcohol Depend. 62*: 149-54.

Concha M, Selnes OA, Vlahov D, Nance-Sproson T, Updike M, Royal W, Palenicek J, McArthur JC (1997). Comparison of neuropsychological performance between AIDS-free injecting drug users and homosexual men. *Neuroepidemiology 16*: 78-85.

Craig JR, Mosier WM (1978). Clinical and laboratory findings on admission to an alcohol detoxification service. *Int. J. Addict. 13:* 1207-15.

De Vries TJ, Schoffelmeer AN, Binnekade R, Vanderschuren LJ (1999). Dopaminergic mechanisms mediating the incentive to seek cocaine and heroin following long-term withdrawal of IV drug self-administration. *Psychopharmacology. (Berl) 143*: 254-60.

Devaud LL, Morrow AL (1999). Gender-selective effects of ethanol dependence on NMDA receptor subunit expression in cerebral cortex, hippocampus and hypothalamus. *Eur. J. Pharmacol. 369*: 331-4.

Diamond I, Messing RO (1994). Neurologic effects of alcoholism. *West J Med 161*: 279-87.

Dingle GA, Oei TP (1997). Is alcohol a cofactor of HIV and AIDS? Evidence from immunological and behavioral studies. *Psychol. Bull. 122*: 56-71.

Donahoe RM (2004). Multiple ways that drug abuse might influence AIDS progression: clues from a monkey model. *J. Neuroimmunol. 147*: 28-32.

Donahoe RM, Vlahov D (1998). Opiates as potential cofactors in progression of HIV-1 infections to AIDS. *J. Neuroimmunol. 83*: 77-87.

Edelstein H, Knight RT (1987). Severe parkinsonism in two AIDS patients taking prochlorperazine [letter]. *Lancet 2*: 341-2.

El-Hage N, Gurwell JA, Singh IN, Knapp PE, Nath A, Hauser KF (2005). Synergistic increases in intracellular Ca^{2+}, and the release of MCP-1, RANTES, and IL-6 by astrocytes treated with opiates and HIV-1 Tat. *Glia 50:*91-106.

Epstein LG, Gelbard HA (1999). HIV-1-induced neuronal injury in the developing brain. *J. Leukoc. Biol. 65*: 453-7.

Ernst T, Chang L, Leonido-Yee M, Speck O (2000). Evidence for long-term neurotoxicity associated with methamphetamine abuse: A 1H MRS study. *Neurology 54*: 1344-1349.

Fabris P, Tositti G, Manfrin V, Giordani MT, Vaglia A, Cattelan AM, Carlotto A (2000). Does alcohol intake affect highly active antiretroviral therapy (HAART) response in HIV-positive patients? *J. Acquir. Immune Defic. Syndr. 25*: 92-3.

Fiala M, Gan XH, Zhang L, House SD, Newton T, Graves MC, Shapshak P, Stins M, Kim KS, Witte M, Chang SL (1998). Cocaine enhances monocyte migration across the blood-brain barrier. Cocaine's connection to AIDS dementia and vasculitis? *Adv. Exp. Med. Biol. 437*: 199-205.

Flexner CW, Cargill VA, Sinclair J, Kresina TF, Cheever L (2001). Alcohol use can result in enhanced drug metabolism in HIV pharmacotherapy. *AIDS Patient Care STDS 15*: 57-58.

Flora G, Lee YW, Nath A, Hennig B, Maragos W, Toborek M (2003). Methamphetamine potentiates HIV-1 Tat protein-mediated activation of redox-sensitive pathways in discrete regions of the brain. *Exp. Neurol. 179*: 60-70.

Goswami R, Dawson SA, Dawson G (1998). Cyclic AMP protects against staurosporine and wortmannin-induced apoptosis and opioid-enhanced apoptosis in both embryonic and immortalized (F-11kappa7) neurons. *J. Neurochem. 70*: 1376-82.

Green PS, Simpkins JW (2000). Neuroprotective effects of estrogens: potential mechanisms of action. *Int. J. Dev. Neurosci. 18*: 347-58.

Gundlah C, Kohama SG, Mirkes SJ, Garyfallou VT, Urbanski HF, Bethea CL (2000). Distribution of estrogen receptor beta (ERbeta) mRNA in hypothalamus, midbrain and temporal lobe of spayed macaque: continued expression with hormone replacement. *Brain Res. Mol. Brain Res. 76*: 191-204.

Gurwell JA, Nath A, Sun Q, Zhang J, Martin KM, Chen Y, Hauser KF (2001). Synergistic neurotoxicity of opioids and human immunodeficiency virus-1 Tat protein in striatal neurons in vitro. *Neuroscience 102*: 555-63.

Hauser KF, Foldes JK, Turbek CS (1999). Dynorphin A (1-13) neurotoxicity in vitro: opioid and non-opioid mechanisms in mouse spinal cord neurons. *Exp. Neurol. 160*: 361-75.

Hauser KF, Gurwell JA, Turbek CS (1994). Morphine inhibits Purkinje cell survival and dendritic differentiation in organotypic cultures of the mouse cerebellum. *Exp. Neurol. 130*: 95-105.

Hauser KF, Harris-White ME, Jackson JA, Opanashuk LA, Carney JM (1998). Opioids disrupt Ca2+ homeostasis and induce carbonyl oxyradical production in mouse astrocytes in vitro: transient increases and adaptation to sustained exposure. *Exp. Neurol. 151*: 70-6.

Hauser KF, Houdi AA, Turbek CS, Elde RP, Maxson W, 3rd (2000). Opioids intrinsically inhibit the genesis of mouse cerebellar granule neuron precursors in vitro: differential impact of mu and delta receptor activation on proliferation and neurite elongation. *Eur. J. Neurosci. 12*: 1281-93.

Heaton RK, Grant I, Butters N, White DA, Kirson D, Atkinson JH, McCutchan JA, Taylor MJ, Kelly MD, Ellis RJ, et al. (1995). The HNRC 500--neuropsychology of HIV infection at different disease stages. HIV Neurobehavioral Research Center. *J. Int. Neuropsychol. Soc. 1*: 231-51.

Hollander H, Golden J, Mendelson T, Cortland D (1985). Extrapyramidal symptoms in AIDS patients given low-dose metoclopramide or chlorpromazine [letter]. *Lancet 2*: 1186.

Hornykiewicz O (1998). Biochemical aspects of Parkinson's disease. *Neurology 51*: S2-9.

Hriso E, Kuhn T, Masdeu JC, Grundman M (1991). Extrapyramidal symptoms due to dopamine-blocking agents in patients with AIDS encephalopathy. *Am. J. Psychiatry.* *148*: 1558-61.

Hu S, Sheng WS, Lokensgard JR, Peterson PK (2002). Morphine induces apoptosis of human microglia and neurons. *Neuropharmacology 42:*829-36.

Hu XJ, Ticku MK (1995). Chronic ethanol treatment upregulates the NMDA receptor function and binding in mammalian cortical neurons. *Brain Res. Mol. Brain Res. 30*: 347-56.

Johnson-Greene D, Adams KM, Gilman S, Koeppe RA, Junck L, Kluin KJ, Martorello S, Heumann M (1997). Effects of abstinence and relapse upon neuropsychological function and cerebral glucose metabolism in severe chronic alcoholism. *J. Clin. Exp. Neuropsychol. 19*: 378-85.

Khurdayan VK, Buch S, El-Hage N, Lutz SE, Goebel SM, Singh IN, Knapp PE, Turchan-Cholewo J, Nath A, Hauser KF (2004). Preferential vulnerability of astroglia and glial precursors to combined opioid and HIV-1 Tat exposure in vitro. *Eur. J. Neurosci. 19*: 3171-82.

Kieburtz KD, Epstein LG, Gelbard HA, Greenamyre JT (1991). Excitotoxicity and dopaminergic dysfunction in the acquired immunodeficiency syndrome dementia complex. Therapeutic implications. *Arch. Neurol. 48*: 1281-4.

Kofke WA, Garman RH, Garman R, Rose ME (1999). Opioid neurotoxicity: fentanyl-induced exacerbation of cerebral ischemia in rats. *Brain Res. 818*: 326-34.

Kofke WA, Garman RH, Stiller RL, Rose ME, Garman R (1996). Opioid neurotoxicity: fentanyl dose-response effects in rats. *Anesth. Analg. 83*: 1298-306.

Koob GF (2000). Neurobiology of addiction. Toward the development of new therapies. *Ann. N Y Acad. Sci. 909*: 170-85.

Koutsilieri E, Gotz ME, Sopper S, Sauer U, Demuth M, ter Meulen V, Riederer P (1997a). Regulation of glutathione and cell toxicity following exposure to neurotropic substances and human immunodeficiency virus-1 in vitro. *J. Neurovirol. 3*: 342-9.

Koutsilieri E, Gotz ME, Sopper S, Stahl-Hennig C, Czub M, ter Meulen V, Riederer P (1997b). Monoamine metabolite levels in CSF of SIV-infected rhesus monkeys (Macaca mulatta). *Neuroreport 8*: 3833-6.

Kreek MJ (2001). Drug addictions. Molecular and cellular endpoints. *Ann. N. Y. Acad. Sci. 937*: 27-49.

Kreek MJ, Koob GF (1998). Drug dependence: stress and dysregulation of brain reward pathways. *Drug. Alcohol. Depend. 51*: 23-47.

Kumar R, Torres C, Yamamura Y, Rodriguez I, Martinez M, Staprans S, Donahoe RM, Kraiselburd E, Stephens EB, Kumar A (2004). Modulation by morphine of viral set point in rhesus macaques infected with simian immunodeficiency virus and simian-human immunodeficiency virus. *J. Virol. 78*: 11425-8.

Langford D, Adame A, Grigorian A, Grant I, McCutchan JA, Ellis RJ, Marcotte TD, Masliah E (2003). Patterns of selective neuronal damage in methamphetamine-user AIDS patients. *J. Acquir. Immune Defic. Syndr. 34*: 467-74.

Larsson M, Hagberg L, Forsman A, Norkrans G (1991). Cerebrospinal fluid catecholamine metabolites in HIV-infected patients. *J. Neurosci. Res. 28:* 406-9.

Lipton SA (1998). Neuronal injury associated with HIV-1: approaches to treatment. *Annu. Rev. Pharmacol. Toxicol. 38*: 159-77.

Littleton J, Little H (1994). Current concepts of ethanol dependence. *Addiction 89*: 1397-412.

Manly JJ, Merchant CA, Jacobs DM, Small SA, Bell K, Ferin M, Mayeux R (2000). Endogenous estrogen levels and Alzheimer's disease among postmenopausal women. *Neurology 54*: 833-7.

Maragos WF, Young KL, Turchan JT, Guseva M, Pauly JR, Nath A, Cass WA (2002). Human immunodeficiency virus-1 Tat protein and methamphetamine interact synergistically to impair striatal dopaminergic function. *J. Neurochem. 83*: 955-63.

McArthur JC, Kumar AJ, Johnson DW, Selnes OA, Becker JT, Herman C, Cohen BA, Saah A (1990). Incidental white matter hyperintensities on magnetic resonance imaging in HIV-1 infection. Multicenter AIDS Cohort Study. *J. Acquir. Immune. Defic. Syndr. 3*: 252-9.

McCarthy L, Wetzel M, Sliker JK, Eisenstein TK, Rogers TJ (2001). Opioids, opioid receptors, and the immune response. *Drug Alcohol Depend. 62*: 111-123.

Mellon RD, Bayer BM (1998). Evidence for central opioid receptors in the immunomodulatory effects of morphine: review of potential mechanism(s) of action. *J. Neuroimmunol. 83*: 19-28.

Meriney SD, Ford MJ, Oliva D, Pilar G (1991). Endogenous opioids modulate neuronal survival in the developing avian ciliary ganglion. *J. Neurosci. 11*: 3705-17.

Meyerhoff DJ, MacKay S, Sappey-Marinier D, Deicken R, Calabrese G, Dillon WP, Weiner MW, Fein G (1995). Effects of chronic alcohol abuse and HIV infection on brain phosphorus metabolites. *Alcohol Clin. Exp. Res. 19*: 685-92.

Mirsattari SM, Berry ME, Holden JK, Ni W, Nath A, Power C (1999). Paroxysmal dyskinesias in patients with HIV infection. *Neurology 52*: 109-14.

Mirsattari SM, Power C, Nath A (1998). Parkinsonism with HIV infection. *Mov. Disord. 13*: 684-9.

Morgello S, Estanislao L, Simpson D, Geraci A, DiRocco A, Gerits P, Ryan E, Yakoushina T, Khan S, Mahboob R, Naseer M, Dorfman D, Sharp V (2004). HIV-associated distal sensory polyneuropathy in the era of highly active antiretroviral therapy: the Manhattan HIV Brain Bank. *Arch. Neurol. 61*: 546-51.

Murrill CS, Weeks H, Castrucci BC, Weinstock HS, Bell BP, Spruill C, Gwinn M (2002). Age-specific seroprevalence of HIV, hepatitis B virus, and hepatitis C virus infection among injection drug users admitted to drug treatment in 6 US cities. *Am. J. Public Health. 92*: 385-7.

Nair MP, Schwartz SA, Polasani R, Hou J, Sweet A, Chadha KC (1997). Immunoregulatory effects of morphine on human lymphocytes. *Clin. Diagn. Lab. Immunol. 4*: 127-32.

Nath A, Geiger JD (1998). Neurobiological Aspects of HIV infections: neurotoxic mechanisms. *Prog. Neurobiol. 54*: 19-33.

Nath A, Maragos W, Avison M, Schmitt F, Berger J (2001). Accelerated HIV dementia with methamphetamine and cocaine use. *J. Neurovirol. 7*: 66-71.

Nestler EJ, Aghajanian GK (1997). Molecular and cellular basis of addiction. *Science 278*: 58-63.

Pascual-Leone A, Dhuna A (1990). Cocaine-associated multifocal tics. *Neurology 40*: 999-1000.

Pascual-Leone A, Dhuna A, Altafullah I, Anderson DC (1990). Cocaine-induced seizures. *Neurology 40*: 404-7.

Peterson PK, Gekker G, Hu S, Lokensgard J, Portoghese PS, Chao CC (1999). Endomorphin-1 potentiates HIV-1 expression in human brain cell cultures: implication of an atypical mu-opioid receptor. *Neuropharmacology 38*: 273-8.

Peterson PK, Gekker G, Lokensgard JR, Bidlack JM, Chang A, Fang X, Portoghese PS (2001). kappa-Opioid receptor agonist suppression of HIV-1 expression in CD4(+) lymphocytes. *Biochem. Pharmacol. 61*: 1145-51.

Peterson PK, Gekker G, Schut R, Hu S, Balfour HH, Jr., Chao CC (1993). Enhancement of HIV-1 replication by opiates and cocaine: the cytokine connection. *Adv. Exp. Med. Biol. 335*: 181-8.

Petito CK, Cash KS (1992). Blood-brain barrier abnormalities in AIDS: immunohistochemical localization of serum proteins in postmortem brain. *Ann. Neurol. 32*: 658-666.

Pillai R, Nair BS, Watson RR (1991). AIDS, drugs of abuse and the immune system: a complex immunotoxicological network. *Arch. Toxicol. 65*: 609-17.

Polakiewicz RD, Schieferl SM, Gingras AC, Sonenberg N, Comb MJ (1998). mu-Opioid receptor activates signaling pathways implicated in cell survival and translational control. *J. Biol. Chem. 273*: 23534-41.

Power C, Kong PA, Crawford TO, Wesselingh S, Glass JD, McArthur JC, Trapp BD (1993). Cerebral white matter changes in AIDS dementia: alterations of the blood-brain barrier. *Ann. Neurol. 34*: 339-350.

Prendergast MA, Harris BR, Blanchard JA, 2nd, Mayer S, Gibson DA, Littleton JM (2000). In vitro effects of ethanol withdrawal and spermidine on viability of hippocampus from male and female rat. *Alcohol. Clin. Exp. Res. 24*: 1855-61.

Pu H, Tian J, Flora G, Lee YW, Nath A, Hennig B, Toborek M (2003). HIV-1 Tat protein upregulates inflammatory mediators and induces monocyte invasion into the brain. *Mol. Cell Neurosci. 24*: 224-37.

Rabkin JG, McElhiney MC, Ferrando SJ (2004). Mood and substance use disorders in older adults with HIV/AIDS: methodological issues and preliminary evidence. *Aids 18 Suppl. 1*: S43-8.

Reyes MG, Faraldi F, Senseng CS, Flowers C, Fariello R (1991). Nigral degeneration in acquired immune deficiency syndrome (AIDS). *Acta Neuropathol. 82*: 39-44.

Robinson TE, Berridge KC (2000). The psychology and neurobiology of addiction: an incentive-sensitization view. *Addiction 95 Suppl. 2*: S91-117.

Rogers TJ, Peterson PK (2003). Opioid G protein-coupled receptors: signals at the crossroads of inflammation. *Trends Immunol. 24*: 116-21.

Rogers TJ, Steele AD, Howard OM, Oppenheim JJ (2000). Bidirectional heterologous desensitization of opioid and chemokine receptors. *Ann. N. Y. Acad. Sci. 917*: 19-28.

Rooney KF, Armstrong RA, Sewell RD (1991). Increased dopamine receptor sensitivity in the rat following acute administration of sufentanil, U50,488H and D-Ala2-D-Leu5-enkephalin. *Naunyn. Schmiedebergs. Arch. Pharmacol. 343*: 458-62.

Rudolph JG, Lemasters JJ, Crews FT (1998). Effects of chronic ethanol exposure on oxidation and NMDA-stimulated neuronal death in primary cortical neuronal cultures. *Alcohol. Clin. Exp. Res. 22*: 2080-5.

Saunders-Pullman R, Gordon-Elliott J, Parides M, Fahn S, Saunders HR, Bressman S (1999). The effect of estrogen replacement on early Parkinson's disease. *Neurology 52*: 1417-21.

Schoffelmeer AN, Hogenboom F, Mulder AH (1997). Kappa1- and kappa2-opioid receptors mediating presynaptic inhibition of dopamine and acetylcholine release in rat neostriatum. *Br. J. Pharmacol. 122*: 520-4.

Sharp BM, Roy S, Bidlack JM (1998). Evidence for opioid receptors on cells involved in host defense and the immune system. *J. Neuroimmunol. 83*: 45-56.

Singhal PC, Kapasi AA, Reddy K, Franki N, Gibbons N, Ding G (1999). Morphine promotes apoptosis in Jurkat cells. *J. Leukoc. Biol. 66*: 650-8.

Singhal PC, Reddy K, Franki N, Sanwal V, Gibbons N (1997). Morphine induces splenocyte apoptosis and enhanced mRNA expression of cathepsin-B. *Inflammation 21*: 609-17.

Singhal PC, Sagar S, Reddy K, Sharma P, Ranjan R, Franki N (1998a). HIV-1 gp120 envelope protein and morphine-tubular cell interaction products modulate kidney fibroblast proliferation. *J. Investig. Med. 46*: 243-8.

Singhal PC, Sharma P, Kapasi AA, Reddy K, Franki N, Gibbons N (1998b). Morphine enhances macrophage apoptosis. *J. Immunol. 160*: 1886-93.

Slooter AJ, Bronzova J, Witteman JC, Van Broeckhoven C, Hofman A, van Duijn CM (1999). Estrogen use and early onset Alzheimer's disease: a population-based study. *J. Neurol. Neurosurg. Psychiatry. 67*: 779-81.

Stefano GB (1999). Substance abuse and HIV-gp120: are opiates protective? *Arch. Immunol. Ther. Exp. 47*: 99-106.

Stiene-Martin A, Zhou R, Hauser KF (1998). Regional, developmental, and cell cycle-dependent differences in mu, delta, and kappa-opioid receptor expression among cultured mouse astrocytes. *Glia 22*: 249-59.

Tabakoff B (1994). Alcohol and AIDS--is the relationship all in our heads? *Alcohol. Clin. Exp. Res. 18*: 415-6.

Toborek M, Lee YW, Pu H, Malecki A, Flora G, Garrido R, Hennig B, Bauer HC, Nath A (2003). HIV-Tat protein induces oxidative and inflammatory pathways in brain endothelium. *J. Neurochem. 84*: 169-79.

Tomlinson GS, Simmonds P, Busuttil A, Chiswick A, Bell JE (1999). Upregulation of microglia in drug users with and without pre-symptomatic HIV infection. *Neuropathol. Appl. Neurobiol. 25*: 369-79.

Turchan J, Anderson C, Hauser KF, Sun Q, Zhang J, Liu Y, Wise PM, Kruman I, Maragos W, Mattson MP, Booze R, Nath A (2001). Estrogen protects against the synergistic toxicity by HIV proteins, methamphetamine and cocaine. *BMC Neurosci. 2*: 3.

Turchan J, Pocernich CB, Gairola C, Chauhan A, Schifitto G, Butterfield DA, Buch S, Narayan O, Sinai A, Geiger J, Berger JR, Elford H, Nath A (2003). Oxidative stress in HIV demented patients and protection ex vivo with novel antioxidants. *Neurology 60*: 307-14.

Tyor WR, Middaugh LD (1999). Do alcohol and cocaine abuse alter the course of HIV-associated dementia complex? *J. Leukoc. Biol. 65*: 475-81.

Vanderschuren LJ, Wardeh G, De Vries TJ, Mulder AH, Schoffelmeer AN (1999). Opposing role of dopamine D1 and D2 receptors in modulation of rat nucleus accumbens noradrenaline release. *J. Neurosci. 19*: 4123-31.

Walker DW, Heaton MB, Lee N, King MA, Hunter BE (1993). Effect of chronic ethanol on the septohippocampal system: a role for neurotrophic factors? *Alcohol. Clin. Exp. Res. 17*: 12-8.

Watzl B, Watson RR (1992). Role of alcohol abuse in nutritional immunosuppression. *J. Nutr. 122:* 733-7.

Weiner WJ, Rabinstein A, Levin B, Weiner C, Shulman LM (2001). Cocaine-induced persistent dyskinesias. *Neurology 56*: 964-5.

Weinhardt LS, Carey MP, Carey KB, Maisto SA, Gordon CM (2001). The relation of alcohol use to HIV-risk sexual behavior among adults with a severe and persistent mental illness. *J. Consult. Clin. Psychol. 69*: 77-84.

Wilson JM, Kalasinsky KS, Levey AI, Bergeron C, Reiber G, Anthony RM, Schmunk GA, Shannak K, Haycock JW, Kish SJ (1996a). Striatal dopamine nerve terminal markers in human, chronic methamphetamine users. *Nat. Med. 2*: 699-703.

Wilson JM, Levey AI, Bergeron C, Kalasinsky K, Ang L, Peretti F, Adams VI, Smialek J, Anderson WR, Shannak K, Deck J, Niznik HB, Kish SJ (1996b). Striatal dopamine, dopamine transporter, and vesicular monoamine transporter in chronic cocaine users. *Ann. Neurol. 40*: 428-39.

Yin D, Mufson RA, Wang R, Shi Y (1999). Fas-mediated cell death promoted by opioids. *Nature 397*: 218.

Yin DL, Ren XH, Zheng ZL, Pu L, Jiang LZ, Ma L, Pei G (1997). Etorphine inhibits cell growth and induces apoptosis in SK-N-SH cells: involvement of pertussis toxin-sensitive G proteins. *Neurosci. Res. 29*: 121-7.

In: Neuro-AIDS   ISBN: 1-59454-610-X
Editors: A. Minagar and P. Shapshak, pp. 101-119   © 2006 Nova Science Publishers, Inc.

Chapter V

Viral Load on HIV-1 Associated Dementia: Neuropathology and Drug Efficacy

*Robert K. Fujimura**

Geriatric Research, Education, and Clinical Center,
Veterans Affairs Medical Center, Miami, Florida, USA.

Abstract

HIV-1 associated dementia (HAD) is the most severe and morbid neuronal disorder caused by HIV-1 invasion of the brain. Apparent causative agents are the viral proteins acting as neurotoxins that induce neuronal apoptosis. Part I reviews contributions of viral load determinations on neuropathogenesis of HAD and efficacy tests of AIDS drugs. They serve important roles in elucidation of the mechanisms of pathogenesis and for drug development. Part II goes in detail on polymerase chain reaction (PCR) methods utilized for determination of viral load. These methods include comparative PCR for viral DNA load, competitive reverse transcription PCR for viral structural RNA and regulatory mRNA load, and real-time PCR for viral cDNA load.

Keywords: HIV-1 associated dementia (HAD), viral load, neuropathogenesis, AIDS drugs, polymerase chain reaction (PCR), comparative PCR, multispliced and unspliced viral RNA, real time PCR

---

* Correspondence concerning this article should be addressed to Robert K Fujimura, PhD, GRECC, Veterans Affairs Medical Center, Rm NH 207, 1201 NW, 16th ST, Miami FL, 33125. Email: kanjirob@bellsouth.net

Part I: Neuropathology and Drug Efficacy

Three neurological syndromes are recognized to be caused by HIV-1 infection of the brain: meningoencephalitis, which occurs during the initial acute phase of HIV-1 infection in as much as half of the cases; HIV-1–associated minor cognitive/motor disorder, which occurs in 80% of the cases; and HIV-1–associated dementia (HAD), which is less frequent but the most severe and morbid disorder (Fujimura et al., 1996). The defining symptom of HAD is cognitive dysfunction (lack of attention, abnormalities in visuospatial skills, memory, and learning) accompanied by motor and/or behavioral dysfunction (Fujimura et al., 1996). These abnormalities are accompanied by the loss of cortical neurons, prompting the question: Does the loss of cortical neurons cause the cognitive and motor/behavioral dysfunction, or is the dysfunction caused by changes in other factors occurring before neuron death? Finding the answer to this still-elusive question would greatly facilitate the elucidation of the mechanisms of HAD.

1. Neuropathology of HIV-1–Associated Dementia

Reactive microglia and multinucleated giant cells are the main morphological features of HAD (Budka et al., 1991; Navia et al., 1986). The presence of infected microglial cells correlates with the clinical severity of dementia (Glass et al., 1995).

Clinico-pathological data suggest that the progression of HAD correlates with neuronal loss and brain viral load (Asare et al., 1996; Bell et al., 1998). However, the presence of HIV-1 in neurons has only rarely been observed, suggesting that neuronal loss is due to neurotoxins (Fujimura et al., 1998; Kandanearatchi et al., 2003). Apparently, HIV-1–infected macrophages/microglia produce viral neurotoxins that induce apoptosis of neurons. They include the viral coat protein, gp120 (Kanmogne et al., 2002), and many regulatory proteins, e.g., tat (Fujimura et al, 1998; Kaul and Lipton, 2004).

Pathways to neuronal damage appear to be initiated by the binding of Gp120 of the viral surface to β chemokine receptors CCR5 or CCR3 of macrophages and microglia, but also to α chemokine receptor CXCR4 (Kaul and Lipton, 2004). HIV-1 gp120 proteins and gp160 peptides may be directly involved in blood-brain barrier damage and neuronal cell death (Kanmogne et al., 2002). TNF-α released by infected microglia and macrophages may also causes neuronal injury. The level of TNF-α mRNA correlates with the severity of HAD, but the role of TNF-α in neuronal dysfunction remains unknown (Saha and Pahan, 2003).

The NMDA receptor is an additional receptor leading to neurological dysfunction (Kaul and Lipton, 2004). HIV-1 infection creates excitotoxic conditions, which stimulate the NMDA receptors. Activated NMDA receptors induce neuronal apoptosis, involving Ca+2 overload, activation of p38 mitogen-activated protein kinase (MAPK), caspase activation, free-radical formation, lipid peroxidation, chromatin condensation, and release of cytochrome c from mitochondria (Kaul and Lipton, 2004). These proteins are released or activated by permeabilization of mitochondrial outer membrane, thus inducing apoptosis leading to cell death (Ferri and Kroemer, 2001; Green and Kroemer, 2004).

There is evidence that astrocytes may also produce viral neurotoxins (Ranki et al., 1995; Brack-Werner R, 1999). The severity of HAD correlates with apoptosis of astrocytes (Thompson et al., 2001). Astrocytes have chemokine receptors and are infected, but the infection is abortive and synthesizes multispliced (MS) RNA, which codes for viral regulatory proteins, e.g., Tat, Nef, and Rev (Tornatore et al., 1994; Saito Y et al., 1994; Takahashi et al., 1996; Ranki et al., 1995). Extracellular Tat is reported to cause mitochondria dysfunction in neurons, but Tat-producing astrocytes are protected from cell death (Chauhan et al., 2003).

Chemokine receptors are also present on neurons, and the Nef sequence was found more frequently than the gag sequence in neurons from CA1 and CA3 of the hippocampus (Torres-Munoz et al., 2001), suggesting abortive infection also occurs in some neurons.

The elucidation of pathogenesis would be furthered by determining the viral load in these cell types – microglia, multinucleated giant cells, astrocytes, and neurons; these cells could be isolated by microdissection of tissue sections (Rekhter and Chen, 2001; Mikulowska-Mennis et al., 2002). Unspliced (US) and MS viral RNA infected and abortive infected cells could be differentiated (Fujimura et al., 2004). In this manner, abortive infected astrosytes and neurons could be identified in the brain tissues from patients with varying severity of HAD and their significance could be ascertained. For example, production of regulatory proteins, neurotoxins, could be determined (Ranki et al., 1995).

2. Efficacy Test of AIDS Drugs

With highly active antiretroviral drug therapy (HAART), the viral load in plasma and cerebrospinal fluid (CSF) can be kept at an undetectable level (Eggers et al., 2003; Bestetti et al., 2004). However, the penetration of the brain by the drugs is inefficient, and the brain may act as a reservoir of HIV-1 (Schrager and D'Souza, 1998), where a small amount of HIV-1 is continuously replicated and mutated (Cunningham et al., 2000). For example, the concentration of zidovudine in the CSF is reported to be less than 10% of that observed in the plasma (Burger et al., 1993). Recently developed reverse transcriptase and protease inhibitors penetrate the brain better, but the brain is still suspected to be a reservoir of the virus (Cunningham et al., 2000; Kandanearatchi et al., 2003). When HAART therapy is discontinued, virus from a reservoir invades the rest of the body through the blood stream, infecting T-lymphocytes and macrophages and causes an immediate rise in viral load, which may have mutated to drug-resistant forms (Bestetti et al., 2004); thus the HAART combination may not be as effective as once thought.

Therapeutic drugs target essential viral coded enzymes – reverse transcriptase, protease, and integrase (Jonckheere et al., 2000; Esposito, 1999; Asante-Applah, 1999). Nucleoside and nonnucleoside inhibitors to reverse transcriptase were the first therapeutic drugs developed, followed by protease inhibitors. These three types are the therapeutic components of HAART. Effective therapy depends on the continuous development of new drugs to take the place of the older drugs as they lose effectiveness because of viral resistance (Cashion et al., 1999). The integrase inhibitor is one of the new drugs under development (Tarrago-Litvak et al., 2002; Hazuda et al., 2004). This inhibitor may be effective in preventing establishment of abortive infected cells; presumably the integration of viral sequences is essential for expression of regulatory proteins even in these cells.

The viral load in cerebral spinal fluid (CSF) may be an effective gauge of the virus in the brain. Elevated viral CSF RNA levels in cognitively impaired patients were decreased by HAART therapy to undetectable levels and improved cognitive impairment (Ellis et al., 1997; McArthur et al., 1997; Robertson et al., 1998; Tashima, 1998; Tozzi et al., 1999; Cohen RA et al., 2001; McCoig et al., 2002; Husstedt et al., 2002; Letendre et al., 2004).

Viral RNA levels were determined generally by a commercial kit, which measures US RNA.

Astrocytes are detectable in CSF, and they were shown to increase in later stages of HAD (Pemberton and Brew, 2001). MS RNA differentially determined in these astrocytes as the ratio of MS to US RNA could be used as a gauge for the levels of abortive infection. The method developed by us to determine this ratio could be used for this purpose (Fujimura et al., 2004).

Kandanearatchi and associates (2003) used a human brain aggregate system consisting of neurons, astrocytes, microglia, and oligodendrocytes in a composition similar to that in the human cortex to study the efficacy of various drug combinations for suppressing viral replication and preventing neuronal loss. They concluded that more investigation is needed to determine the most effective combination for reducing HAD. In their system, MS RNA could also be determined, and changes in the ratio of MS to US RNA may detect the presence of abortive infection. In addition, quantification of the HIV-1 DNA load would determine the extent of the viral sequence integrated in host cellular chromosomes (Fujimura et al., 1997a) and hence the existence of cells acting as reservoir of the virus.

As discussed above, the quantification of HIV-1 provirus and MS and US viral RNA, would facilitate our understanding of HAD pathogenesis as well as differentiating the efficacy of therapeutic drugs to abortive and normal infections. The development of commercial kits has facilitated the viral RNA load determination and has been applied to testing the efficacy of therapeutic drugs. However, for studies on pathogenesis, the US RNA load determination is not sufficient; the MS RNA load, as well as viral DNA load, needs to be determined in order to obtain the over-all view of viral activities. For these studies, real-time PCR methods would be more applicable as is discussed in Part II.

Part II: Quantification of Viral DNA and RNA Using Polymerase Chain Reactions

Polymerase chain reactions (PCR) have become the methods of choice for quantifying minute amounts of nucleic acids in tissue, blood, cerebral spinal fluid, and body fluid to study gene expression and mutations, to determine viral loads, and to test the efficacy of therapeutic drugs. PCR methods are rapid, sensitive, specific, and reproducible; these advantages are further enhanced by the real-time PCR methodology.

1. Basic Principles of Polymerase Chain Reactions

In essence, polymerase chain reactions involve the rapid replication of a DNA template *in vitro* through many cycles utilizing nucleoside triphosphates as precursors and temperature-stable DNA polymerase as the catalyst to elongate primers, which are specific and unique for the sequence of interest. All of the reagents are available commercially and guaranteed to be pure and stable within the stated expiration date. Only DNA and RNA samples prepared in an investigator's laboratory may be of uncertain quality and/or quantity. The basic conditions for these reactions are essentially the same and provided by manufacturer's protocols, requiring only optimization for $MgCl_2$, primer concentrations, and annealing temperature of primers to a template for each system under study.

The reaction is initiated at a high temperature (denaturation) to separate double-stranded DNA into single-stranded templates; the temperature is lowered to anneal the primers, which are elongated rapidly and progressively along the templates. The products, double-stranded DNA, are denatured for the next round of synthesis. The temperature is rapidly altered to the temperature required at each step of the reaction using a reliable commercial thermal cycler (e.g., Perkin-Elmer, GeneAmp PCR System 9600). The reactions are repeated through many cycles, and data from the log phase of amplification are used for analysis.

The amplification is expressed by the equation:

$$N_n = (E)^n N_o \tag{1}$$

where N_o is the number of the DNA sequence initially present, N_n is the number of molecules amplified after the cycle number n, and E is the efficiency of amplification. In the ideal case, $E = 2$, and when amplification is not ideal, which is the usual case, E is less than 2 and separated into $(1+E)$, where the final number of a product is assumed to be greater than the initial number of the sequence prior to amplification.

The equation shows that the number of the product depends on the initial number of the sequence and the efficiency of amplification. Therefore, to determine the initial number of the target sequence from the number of amplified product, E needs be determined and should be constant from the first cycle to the cycle n. For the determination of relative ratio between two specimens, the E needs not be determined, but required to be constant.

Methods for viral DNA load and viral RNA load (both MS and US) are described in detail below.

2. Viral DNA Load Determination (Fujimura and Bockstahler, 1995; Fujimura et al., 1997a)

A viral DNA load determination method is described for DNA extracted from cryopreserved tissues, which are flash frozen in liquid nitrogen at the time of autopsy and stored at −80°C until extraction. The method can be applied to tissues preserved by other methods with slight modifications. The life cycle of HIV-1 suggests that most of the viral DNA (provirus) is integrated in host cell chromosomes.

Extraction and Purification of DNA

DNA is extracted from brain tissues following the safety precautions described for a P2 laboratory using P3 procedures.

Frozen tissue is immediately placed on a pre-cooled (at least to $-20°C$) agate motor and immersed in guanidium isothiocyanate solution (e.g., TRIzol reagent, Invitrogen), and thawed at room temperature. The tissue is crushed and ground with an agate pestle as soon as possible, transferred to a centrifuge tube, and homogenized by gentle mixing in a vortex mixer. DNA is extracted according to the manufacturer's procedure.

Standard DNA

The standard DNA should be structurally similar to that of the DNA targeted for analysis. Therefore, it should be linear double-stranded DNA in the presence of a large excess of cellular DNA. For the present example, a single copy of HIV-1 DNA present per cellular genome was used (for example, TH4-7-5 cells, Brack-Werner et al., 1992). A copy of HIV-1 DNA in such a cell was shown to amplify with efficiency equal to that of the β-actin gene (Fujimura and Bockstahler, 1995).

Standards used in most of the published data are plasmid DNAs containing the HIV DNA sequence under study. Plasmids replicate more efficiently than linear chromosomal DNA fragments. Consequently when the HIV-1 DNA sequence in chromosomal fragments is used as the standard, the viral DNA load is 5- to 20-fold higher than when one in plasmid is the standard. Most of the HIV-1 DNA in a tissue is integrated in a chromosomal DNA, and the standard integrated in a chromosome is more appropriate.

Primers

A gag sequence of HIV-1 was identified with primer pairs known as SK 38 (positive strand) and SK 39 (negative strand), which encloses a conserved 115bp sequence of the *gag* region (Ou et al., 1988). The number of copies of cellular genome was determined relative to a segment of β-actin gene (420bp) known to be present one copy per genome (Ng et al., 1985; Fujimura and Bockstahler, 1995). The primers were labeled at the 5' end with T4 polynucleotide kinase and γ-^{32}P ATP. Specific activity was adjusted with unlabeled primers to a convenient specific activity (e.g., 5×10^5 cpm per 0.16 pmol) corrected for decay at the date of use.

Comparative Quantitative PCR

The limiting factor for the determination is the available amount of a target specimen; the amount should be sufficient for at least duplicate, independent experiments. A maximum number of specimens at the minimum of three different concentrations (e.g., 2, 6, 20 ng) of each were run concomitantly in a thermal cycler unit, with the standard DNA and occasionally with DNA from an uninfected subject, each at a minimum of three different concentrations. PCR was carried out in a thermal cycler with the reaction conditions optimized for each pair of primers. The products were labeled at the last cycle of PCR by diluting 1/10 of the product into a fresh reaction mixture containing ^{32}P primers of known specific activity.

In this manner, the number of copies of each product was calculated after the products were separated by gel electrophoresis. The gels were partially dried on a filter paper used as a support, and radioactivity of the product was determined by a phosphorimager unit. Southern hybridization using a probe, SK19, for the region amplified by SK 38/39 yielded results consistent with the direct analysis with the labeled probe as described.

Data Analysis

Each set of an experiment included a standard sample — a reconstituted mixture of three different amounts of TH4-7-5 DNA in the excess but fixed amount of cellular DNA from the HIV-1 negative brain. On the log-log plot, the ratios of amplified products of HIV-1 *gag* to β-actin on the y-axis, and the number of copies of HIV-1 DNA per cellular genome for the standard DNA on the x-axis resulted in a straight line. The ratio can be compared only when the lines for the samples being compared are displaced in parallel in the plot. The parallel lines suggest that the efficiency of amplification between these samples were the same as was shown by Raeymaekers (1993).

The number of copies of HIV-1 DNA in a specimen can be calculated by the equation:

$$(\text{HIV/celluar genome})_s = (\text{SK})_s/b_{sk} \tag{2}$$

where SK_s is the amount (in phosphorimager unit) of the SK 38/39 sequence amplified for the specimen s; b_{sk} is the slope of the concentration dependence curve for the SK 38/39 sequence amplification of the standard DNA. The slope was determined for the standard, included in the experiment with the specimen, from the best-fit straight-line equation of the amount amplified in a phosphor imager unit vs. the amount of HIV-1 DNA in the standard. The standard deviation was calculated among the repeats. The data can be plotted and analyzed by using mathematical software (e.g., PSI-Plot, Poly Software International, Salt Lake City, UT).

Results of a Study

Fujimura and associates (1997b) used the method as described to compare the viral DNA load in three to four regions of the brain from nine cases, seven of which were diagnosed postmortem with HAD. They found that the HIV-1 DNA load in the medial temporal lobe region (including the hippocampus) is larger than the frontal lobe, and the load is greater in HAD cases than in the one case without dementia. Other investigators have usually analyzed only the frontal lobe and on that basis have concluded that there is no clear association of HIV-1 DNA load and HIV-1–associated dementia (e.g.Johnson et al., 1996). The results of Fujimura and associates (1997b) suggested that the viral DNA load in the medial temporal lobe is better related to HAD.

3. HIV-1 Genomic Viral RNA (Unspliced RNA) Load Determination

The most convenient way to determine HIV-1 viral RNA (US RNA) load is to use a commercial kit developed for determining viral RNA load in human plasma. The results with the kits are highly reproducible and may be used for other systems. As an example, the Amplicor HIV-1 Monitor Test Kit (Roche) was applied to RNA extracted from brain tissues (Fujimura et al., 2004) and described herein.

RNA was extracted from HIV-1 infected brain tissue or from the infected cultured cells using guanidium isothiocyanate solution (e.g., TRIzol reagent, Invitrogen). The kit is provided with micro-well plates; each well of the first row performs the reverse transcription of viral RNA to cDNA and amplifies cDNA in the presence of a quantitation standard (QS) RNA using HIV-1 specific *gag* primers, which are biotinylated for detection. The QS is a noninfectious RNA with the same primer binding sequence as the target viral RNA and a unique probe binding sequence that allows QS to be distinguished from the target viral RNA. The products were denatured after PCR amplification. Each sample was serially 5-fold diluted into one column of 5 rows of the wells coated with the HIV-1 *gag* specific probe and two rows of wells coated with QS specific probe. The reaction was stopped with a weak acid and absorbance read at 450 nm using an automated microwell plate reader. The detailed protocol accompanies the kit.

The permissible range of the kit is from 400 to 750,000 copies of HIV-1 RNA. For the copy number to fall into that range, several concentrations were used. For infected H9 cells, 2 to 200 pg of a RNA preparation were used, and for an infected brain tissue, 50 to 100 ng of RNA were used. For RNA from H9 cells, 100 μl of human HIV-1 negative plasma provided with the kit or 2 μg of RNA from a brain tissue of a HIV-1 sera-negative case was added as a carrier. Addition of a large excess of brain RNA did not alter the resulting copy number.

4. Determination of the Ratio of Multispliced to Unspliced HIV-1 RNA Load

The MS RNA codes for regulatory proteins synthesized at early stages of HIV-1 replication cycle, and the full-length US RNA codes for *gag* and reverse transcriptase (Pavlakis et al., 1991). Inside infected brain tissues, the full-length US RNA is synthesized in microglia and multinucleated giant cells and exists mainly in virus particles; the MS RNA exists during active viral replication in these cells but may also be preferentially synthesized in astrocytes by abortive infection (Tornatore et al., 1994; Saito Y et al., 1994; Ranki et al., 1995).

Differentiation of Unspliced and Multispliced RNA (Furtado et al.1995)

By proper choice of primers, US and MS RNAs can be categorized into two sizes. The primer pair selected for the US RNA flanks the major splice donor site just upstream of the *gag* start-codon, which is utilized by all of the MS and SS (single spliced) transcripts. The size of the derived cDNA product is 315 bp, which is exclusively from the US RNA species that is the complete genomic RNA. The primer pair selected for the MS RNA utilizes the sequence in the first exon of *tat/rev* as the upstream primer and the sequence in the second exon as the downstream primer. This primer pair yields a slightly larger PCR product from the regulatory mRNA sequence and thus differentiates from the US RNA by gel electrophoresis.

Preparation of Standard Competitive RNA

The copy numbers of US and MS RNAs are determined with the respective standard competitive RNA constructed for each type of RNAs. Both standard RNAs have the same sequence as the respective target RNAs except for the deletion, so that both the target RNA and its standard recognize the same primer pair and compete for it equally. However, because the molecular sizes of both standard RNAs are distinctly smaller than the respective target RNA, the target and its standard can be differentiated by gel electrophoresis.

To generate the standard for US RNA, pBH10R3 (Brack-Werner, 1992) was PCR amplified with the MF687and MF1001D primer pair. [The primers labeled MF were designed by Furtado and associates, 1995.] The MF1001D primer has additional sequences added to the 3' terminal of 1001 in order to induce a deletion 70 nucleotides in length. For the MS RNA standard, cDNA synthesized from an HIV-1–infected brain tissue was PCR amplified with the MF6022 and MF8707D primer pair. The MF 8707D primer has additional sequences on the 3' terminal of MF 8707 designed to induce a deletion 85 nucleotides long. Both products were inserted into Phagemids pBluescript II SK+ (Stratagene, La Jolla, CA) using the XbaI site created in the upstream primers and the XhoI site created in the downstream primers. The plasmids with the respective deletions were transfected into XL1-Blue Subcloning-Grade Competent Cells (Stratagene, La Jolla, CA), selected, grown, and stored at –20°C in growth media with 50% glycerol. Each respective plasmid preparation, when digested with XhoI and XbaI simultaneously, contained the insert of expected size — 250 bp for US cDNA and 280 bp for MS cDNA. To prepare the US or MS cRNA standard, the appropriate culture was grown from a single colony, and plasmid was extracted, cut with XhoI, purified, and transcribed by T3 RNA polymerase. The product RNA was checked with gel electrophoresis to make certain that it had the anticipated size. [The sequence of the product may also be checked.] The RNA concentration of each preparation was determined from the UV absorbency at 260 nm. Each preparation was diluted in lysis buffer containing RNAse inhibitor, divided into a convenient volume, and stored at –85°C.

Preliminary, HIV-1 gag (US) RNA Load Determination

The competitive RT PCR method is most accurate when the competitor and the test RNA exist in about equal number. Therefore, prior to competitive RT-PCR, the viral RNA load for a specimen was determined using the Amplicor HIV-1 Monitor kit (Roche Diagnostics, Soverville, NJ) as described in section 3.

Competitive RT-PCR

A competitive RT-PCR method (Furtado et al.1995) was modified for one-tube RT-PCR with a commercially available kit (e.g., Titan One Tube RT-PCR kit, Roche).

The reaction mixture was made according to the manufacturer's protocol, adjusted to the optimal $MgCl_2$ concentration. Reaction tubes were made with a constant amount of a target RNA. For US RNA, the amount used for the first determination was based on the copy number determined by the Amplicor HIV-1 Monitor kit, and it was mixed with varying amounts of its standard RNA. For MS RNA, the amount was assumed to be the same as for the US RNA for the initial determination. The reverse transcription step was immediately followed by PCR, adjusting the temperature for each step with a thermo cycler (e.g., Perkin-

Elmer GeneAmp PCR system 9600). As described for the viral DNA load, the products were labeled with one additional cycle with 5' end-labeled primer pair of a known specific activity and quantified with a phosphorimager. The image quantification program of Molecular Dynamics (Sunnyvale, CA) was used to quantify in each lane US or MS viral RNA and the respective standard RNA.

In the first assay with each specimen, the RNA preparation was also subjected to PCR alone to exclude DNA contamination. Detected DNA was removed with RNAse-free DNAse. The specificity of the products of each specimen obtained in the first determination was also tested by Southern blot hybridization with the respective probes for MS and US RNAs.

Ratio of MS to US RNA in RNA from Tissues across the Brain (Fujimura et al., 2004)

The number of copies of US or MS viral RNA in each lane was the ratio of the fraction of each type of viral RNA to the fraction of respective standard RNA multiplied by the number of copies of the standard RNA initially added to each reaction mixture. The number of copies was determined near the equivalence point between US or MS RNA and the respective standard and corrected to 1 μg of cellular or tissue RNA. The value for the equivalence point becomes closer to the target RNA with each repeat and is used for the next repeat. This is especially the case for the MS RNA, the copy number of which was a guess for the first determination. The ratio of MS to US RNA was determined in each specimen from respective copy number.

Statistical Analysis

All statistical analysis was performed with SAS; models were fitted using the PROC GLM function (SAS Institute Inc., Cary, NC, 1985). Univariate one-way repeated measures analyses of variance (RANOVA's) was used to account the reproducibility of determination and differences among brain regions as factors in these analytical models.

Statistical analysis showed that assays repeated on different dates for each RNA preparation were not significantly different. However, significant differences were detected between specimens obtained from different regions of the brain. Further analysis using post hoc LSMEANS showed that the ratios could be compared between neuroanatomical regions and between different cases and was greatest in the frontal lobe in the case studied, and the difference was statistically different from that of the basal ganglia, medial temporal and temporal lobe.

5. Viral Load Determination by Real Time PCR

Introduction

With the advent of real time PCR, it is feasible to compare viral nucleic acids from a larger number of specimens simultaneously (e.g., for the Roche Light Cycler, 32 samples; for the PE Biosystem GeneAmp 5700, 96 samples), more accurately, reproducibly, and rapidly than previously possible. The method described herein is applicable for determination of the ratio of copy number of cDNA made from US or MS RNA (target) with respect to a housekeeping gene (reference). The primer pairs used in the previous section for cDNA for respective RNA could be used for real-time PCR, although one that amplifies a shorter segment (100 to 200bp) is optimal. Large numbers of specimens with clinical data are available from the National NeuroAIDS Tissue Consortium, and the maximum number accommodated by the instrument could be analyzed. The real-time PCR procedures herein are described for Roche LightCycler. The instrument shows real-time the increase in cDNA copy number as the increase in fluorescence at each cycle of PCR amplification, and its software determines the threshold point of the rise in the fluorescence for each sample.

Detection of Real-Time PCR Products

The LightCycler has three channels for fluorescence detection – channel F1 (530 nm) for Fluorescein and SYBR Green I; channel F2 (640 nm) for LC Red 640; and channel F3 (710 nm) for LC Red 705. This unit can detect the product in three different ways:

Hydrolysis (TaqMan) Probe: The target-specific fluorescent probe is labeled with a reporter dye fluorescein phosphoramidite (FAM) at the 5'end and a quencher dye 5-carboxy-tetramethly-rhodamine (TAMRA) at the ninth nucleotide of the probe sequence. As DNA polymerase extends the primers, the probe is hydrolyzed by the 5' exonuclease activity associated with the polymerase, thus removing the quencher and increasing the fluorescence. This activity is detected at channel F1.

SYBR Green 1: The dye binds to the minor groove of double-stranded DNA. At the beginning of each amplification cycle, DNA is denatured and fluorescence is minimal. At the annealing step, the primers hybridize to the target sequence, resulting in binding of some SYBR Green 1. Then, at the end of each elongation step, DNA templates are double stranded and binding of the dye reaches a maximum. Thus, during the logarithmic phase of synthesis, fluorescence increases logarithmically. This activity is also detected in channel F1.

Hybridization (FRET) probes: Two sequence-specific oligonucleotide probes labeled with two different dyes are designed to hybridize to the target sequences on the amplified DNA fragments in tandem, head to tail. The head hybridization probe (#1) is labeled with fluorescein, the donor dye, at the 3' end. The tail hybridization probe (#2) is labeled with red 640, the acceptor dye, at the 5' end. During the annealing phase, the probes hybridize to the amplified DNA fragments in head-to-tail arrangement, bringing the two dyes into close proximity. Fluorescein (#1) is excited by the light from the LightCycler's light-emitting diode (LED), and the energy emitted from the excited fluorescein excites red 640 on probe #2, which emits red fluorescent light. This energy transfer occurs by fluorescence resonance energy transfer (FRET), which is detected by channel F2. At the end of the annealing step of each cycle, red 640 fluorescence is at a maximum. For the elongation step, the temperature is slightly raised and the probes are displaced, quenching the fluorescence. In this procedure, two different sequences could be labeled in the same reaction – the first one with #2 probe and the second one with #3 probe labeled with red 705, which is detected by channel F3 by the same mechanism. Therefore, the copy numbers of both the target and the reference could be determined simultaneously in the same reaction tube.

Among these three methods, SYB green is the most sensitive and easy to use, requiring no probe. It detects all the double-stranded products — e.g., primer-primer and other unwanted products — and therefore easily detects the presence of unwanted byproducts.

When an experimental system is optimized and only the wanted products are formed in sufficient amounts, then FRET probes can be used. SYB green method is generally applicable and described herein.

Experimental Procedure

To improve reproducibility when running many samples from an RNA preparation, cDNA is synthesized from the RNA sample in a large quantity to eliminate the variations caused by reverse transcription. Therefore, the reverse transcription step is separate from the real-time PCR step. RNA is reverse transcribed to cDNA in a sufficient amount to perform all the experiments planned, using a cDNA synthesis kit (e.g., Roche, 1st strand DNA synthesis kit for RT-PCR) and random primers.

For real-time PCR of a cDNA preparation, a kit (e.g., Roche, Light Cycler DNA Master SYBR Green 1) is used to prepare reaction mixtures according to the manufacturer's protocol. Briefly, the instrument is set up for quantification using its software so that PCR reaction started from denaturation of DNA, followed by amplification cycles generally set for 45 cycles, detection of fluorescence at F1 channel for SYBR green; each amplification cycle consists of denaturation, annealing, elongation, and detection at "single." The detection at each cycle is done at a temperature higher than the melting point (Mp) of the product of primer dimers but lower than that of the target or reference product. The program includes the melting curve determination at the end of the PCR reactions, consisting of one cycle of denaturation, slow annealing followed by a quick rise in temperature to 95° C, and then cooling at the slowest rate, 0.1° C/sec, with "continuous" detection. At the end, temperature is lowered to at least 35° C. The product size in each tube is determined by gel electrophoresis in the presence of a marker column as reference. At the optimized conditions, the Mp profile shows one peak and gel electrophoresis shows one product of the expected size.

Data Analysis

For the quantification phase of the program, the LightCycler yields a real time PCR profile (a sigmoid curve) for each sample in a capillary tube with the value for crossing point, (Cp), a cycle number at the threshold of the detection of the fluorescence. Two methods are available in the LightCycler program to determine Cp – "fit point" and "second derivative maximum." By the fit point method, Cp of the threshold point is determined manually as the number of cycle at the rise of the fluorescence curve appreciably above the background, which is chosen at the crossing point between the straight line drawn through the back ground and the line drawn through the straight line region of the rise, which depends on the investigator's judgment. By the second derivative maximum method, the Cp of the threshold points is determined by the software of the instrument from the initial region of the rise in the sigmoid curve, and the Cp given is the maximum point of the second derivative of the region.

The copy number of cDNA amplified and its efficiency of amplification are calculated from equation 1 given previously. The LightCycler provides the software to determine both the absolute and relative quantification, and the procedure for its use is given in its website: www.roche-applied-science.com/lightcycler-online. It gives the list of technical notes available (LightCycler technical note). These technical notes are given in detail for both absolute and relative quantification. For determination of the ratio of the genes expressed or cDNA amounts, relative quantification is appropriate and the software is provided for the data analysis (LightCycler technical note No. LC 13/2001). More complete information on all aspects of real time PCR for any instrument is given at www.gene-quantification.de/

Here three methods for the ratio determination are described (I) Linear Regression (Ramakers et al., 2003); (II) Relative Quantification (Pfaffl, 2001); (III) Delta-Delta Cp (Livak and Schmittgen, 2001), in the order of increasing requirements for assumptions.

Linear Regression analysis of logarithmic form of the basic equation for amplification (equation 1 at the beginning section) is used for (I) linear regression method, which is:

$$\text{Log } N_n = \log N_o + n \text{Log E} \tag{3}$$

when $\text{Log } N_n$ is plotted vs n, the intercept is $\log N_o$ and Log E is the slope to n, where n is the number of cycles around the threshold point of the sigmoid curve. By this approach, N_o and E is obtained from each sigmoid curve, where N_n is in the fluorescence unit. E, the efficiency of amplification, is the antilog of the slope. N_o is the starting copy number of cDNA, from which the number of its mRNA present in the initial RNA preparation is calculated. Thus the absolute number of each amplified cDNA is calculated by this method and the ratio is obtained between N_o of the target and reference in each preparation. This does not require the assumption that PCR efficiencies of all the samples compared are the same. However, the N_o is an apparent number and greatly affected by the variation in E. N_o of the target and the reference genes for comparison between specimens should be done at the same E for each gene. The linear logarithmic region used for the calculation should include the minimum of three integral cycle numbers including the cycle number at threshold point obtained by the second derivative method (RKF prefers to use four or more from the linear region). The mathematical program is available from Ramakers and associates (2003) on request, but any mathematical software can be used such as PSI-Plot used in the previous section.

For (II) the relative quantification method, the efficiency, E, is calculated from the slope of the plot of the cycle number vs. log cDNA at several concentrations. Therefore, each cDNA preparation needs to be subjected to real time PCR at several dilutions (minimum of three) for both the target and reference genes. Equation 1 is used to express the number of cDNA of target and reference genes and solving for the initial ratio of N_{oT} to N_{oR}, the expression for the ratio becomes:

$$N_{oT} / N_{oR} = (E_R)^{Cp\,R}/(E_T)^{Cp\,T} \tag{4}$$

when this ratio is compared between two different specimens such as MS RNA from CSF of a patient treated with HAART to CSF prior to the treatment, the expression of the ratio becomes:

$$\text{Ratio} = [(E_R)^{Cp\,R}/(E_T)^{Cp\,T}]_{s1}/ (E_R)^{Cp\,R}/(E_T)^{Cp\,T}]_{s2} \tag{5a}$$

$$= (E_T)^{\Delta CpT(s2-s1)}/(E_R)^{\Delta CpR(s2-s1)} \tag{5b}$$

where s1 is the specimen after the treatment and s2 is the specimen before the treatment.

Here E is calculated by the equation: $E = 10^{[-1/slope]}$ (RKF prefers to determine E for each curve from the slope of equation 3). Cp is the cycle number at which the fluorescence rises appreciably above the background fluorescence. It is earlier than the threshold point determined by the second derivative maximum method, and Pfaffl prefers to determine manually by the fit point method (Pfaffl, 2001). Pfaffl and associates (2002) have a software called REST, which analyzes the data and obtains the ratio according to equation 5b. When the Cp of the reference gene is the same in s1 and s2, the $\Delta Cp = 0$, and $(E_R)^0 = 1$, and equation 5b simplifies to equation 6:

$$\text{ratio} = (E_T)^{\Delta CpT(s2-s1)} \tag{6}$$

When the amplification efficiencies for the target and the reference are the same for two specimens, then the equation for the ratio of target to reference between two specimens becomes that of method (III), the delta-delta method, as derived by Livak and Schmittgen (2001):

$$\text{ratio} = 2^{-\Delta\Delta Cp} \tag{7}$$

where the efficiency is the same and assumed to be 2. Therefore, this is for the ideal case, and probably would not be applicable to RNA extracted from the brain tissue nor CSF.

For the comparison of the ratio of the initial amount of cDNA of a target gene to a reference gene, the minimal requirement is the amplification efficiency for the gene under comparison between the two specimens to be the same, as shown for the target gene (T) and the reference gene (R) in equation 5b. This was tested for RNA extracted from cryopreserved specimens from seven different human hippocampal tissues, six of which had histological abnormalities and one was an age matched control (obtained from Dr. Dennis Dickson, Mayo Clinic, Jacksonville FL). CDNA was prepared and tested for the ribosomal elongation factor 1a (EF), a housekeeping gene (R). The same amount of RNA was reverse transcribed from the seven specimens and 20ng of each cDNA was subjected to real-time PCR with the EF primer pair. The data were transformed into the logarithmic form (equation 3) and log E and its standard deviation (SD) were obtained from the linear region of the curve using PSI Plot. The regression analysis of the plot of the log fluorescence vs. cycle number yielded the correlation of 0.9992 to 0.9999 for seven specimens. The standard deviation of log E for each specimen showed that each value was within 95% of the normal distribution of the others. Therefore, the efficiency of amplification for cDNA of EF for all seven specimens was considered the same, and the target genes normalized to EF could be compared among seven specimens using equation 5b, if their efficiencies of amplification are shown to be the same by the same method of analysis.

RKF concluded that this method of data analysis could be used to determine changes in viral RNA (US or MS) load affected by HAART treatment, or its relationship with the severity of neurological abnormalities among HAD cases, or across neuroanatomical regions. For the Light Cycler, 15 specimens and a control could be run with a target and reference genes, simultaneously.

Acknowledgements

RKF, the author, thanks the editorial assistant of Mrs. Virginia Roos at the office of Geriatric Research, Education, Clinical Center (GRECC), Veteran Affairs Medical Center, Miami, FL. The research on HIV-1 viral load was initiated at Dr. Larry Bockstahler's laboratory while RKF was a senior fellow of the National Research Council at Center for Devices and Radiological Health, US Food and Drug Administration, Rockville MD. All the subsequent experiments were performed at Dr. Paul Shapshak's laboratory at Department of Psychiatry and Behavioral Sciences, University of Miami School of Medicine, Miami, FL, with active collaboration of Dr. Paul Shapshak and Dr. Karl Goodkin. RKF was supported by DA04787S2, NIDA. Research at Dr. Paul Shapshak's laboratory was supported in part by NIH grants DA04787, DA 07909, DA 12580, DA 14533, and AG 19952. This manuscript was written and the studies on real time PCR were done at GRECC, Department of Veterans Affairs Medical Center, Miami,FL; supported in part by the South Florida VA Foundation for Research and Education." The tissue specimens used to test the methods of analysis of data from real time PCR were obtained from Dr. Dennis Dickson, Mayo Clinic, Jacksonville, FL.

References

Asante–Appiah E, Skalka AM (1999) HIV-1 integrase: structural organization, conformational changes, and catalysis. *Adv. Virus Res. 52*:351-369.

Asare E, Dunn G, Glass J et al. (1996) Neuronal pattern correlates with the severity of HIV-associated dementia complex: usefulness of spatial pattern analysis in clinico-pathological studies. *Am. J. Pathol. 148*:31-38.

Bell JE, Brettle RP, Chiswick A, Simmonds P (1998) HIV encephalitis, provial load and dementia in drug users and homosexuals with AIDS effect of neocortical involvement. *Brain 121*:2043-2052.

Bestetti A, Presi S, Pierotti C et al. (2004). Long-term virological effect of highly active antiretroviral therapy on cerebrospinal fluid and relationship with genotypic resistance. *J. Neurovirol. 10 Suppl. 1*: 52-57.

Brack-Werner R, Kleinschmidt A, Ludvigsen A et al. (1992) Infection of human brain cells by HIV-1: restricted virus production in chronically infected human glial cell lines. *AIDS 6*: 273-285.

Brack-Werner R (1999) Astrocytes:HIV cellular reservoirs and important participants in neuropathogenesis. *AIDS 13*:1-22.

Budka, H. Wiley CA, Kleihues P et al. (1991). HIV-Associated disease of the Nervous System: Review of Nomenclature and proposal for Neuropathology-Based Terminology. *Brain Pathology. 1*:143-152.

Burger DM, Kraaijeveld CL, Meenhorst PL et al.(1993) Penetration of zidovudine into the cerebrospinal fluid of patients infected with HIV. *AIDS 7*:1581-1587.

Cashion MF, Banks WA, Bost KL, Kastin AJ (1999) Transmission routes of HIV-1 gp120 from blood to lymphoid tissues. *Brain Res. 822*: 26-33.

Chauhan A, Turchan J, Pocernich C et al. (2003). Intracellular Human Immunodeficiency Virus Tat Expression in Astrocytes Promotes Astrocyte Survival but Induces Potent Neurotoxicityat Distant Sites via Axonal Transport. *J. Biol. Chem. 278*: 13512-13519.

Cohen RA, Boland R, Paul R et al., (2001) Neurocognitive performance enhanced by highly active antiretroviral therapy in HIV infected women. *AIDS 15*:341-345.

Cunningham PH, Smith DG, Satchell C et al. (2000) Evidence for independent development of resistance to HIV-1 reverse transcriptase inhibitors in the cerebrospinal fluid. *AIDS 14*:1949-1954.

Eggers C, Hertogs K, Sturenburg HJ et al. (2003). Delayed central nervous system virus suppression during highly active antiretroviral therapy is associated with HIV encephalopathy, but not with viral drug resistance or poor central nervous system drug penetration. *AIDS 17*: 1897-1906.

Ellis RJ, Hsia K, Spector SA (1997) Cerebrospinal fluid human immunodeficiency virus type 1 RNA levels are elevated in neurocognitively impaired individuals with acquired immunodeficiency syndrome. HIV Neurobehavioral Research Center Group. *Ann. Neurol. 42*:679-688.

Esposito D, Craigie R(1999) HIV integrase structure and function. *Adv. Virus Res. 52*:319-333.

Ferri KF and Kroemer G (2001) Mitochondria – the suicide organelles. *BioEssays. 23*:111-115.

Fujimura RK and Bockstahler LE (1995) Polymerase chain reaction method for determining ratios of human immunodeficiency virus proviral DNA to cellular genomic DNA in brain tissues of HIV-infected patients. *J. Virol. Methods. 55*: 309-325.

Fujimura RK, Bockstahler LE, Goodkin K, et al. Neuropathology and Virology of HIV Associated Dementia. (1996) *Rev. in Med. Virol. 6*: 141-150.

Fujimura RK, Shapshak P, Feaster D (1997a) A rapid method for comparativequantitative polymerase chain reaction of HIV-1 proviral DNA extracted from cryopreserved brain tissues.

Fujimura RK, Goodkin K, Petito CK, et al. (1997b) HIV-1 proviral DNA load across neuroanatomical regions of individuals with evidence for HIV-1 associated dementia. *JAIDS HR;16*:146-152.

Fujimura RK, Shapshak P, Segal DM et al. (1998) Viral and Host Determinants of Neurovirulence of HIV-1 Infection. *Adv. in Exp. Med. and Biol. 437*: 241-253.

Fujimura RK, Khamis I, Shapshak P, Goodkin K (2004) Regional quantitative comparison of Multispliced to Unspliced ratios of HIV-1 RNA copy number in infected human brain. *J. Neuro-AIDS 2 (4)*: 45-60.

Furtado MR, Kingsley LA, and Wolinsky SM (1995) Changes in the viral mRNA expression pattern correlate with a rapid rate of CD4+ T-cell number decline in HumanImmunodeficiency Virus type 1-infected individuals. *J. Virol. 69*: 2092-2100.

Glass, J.D., Fedor, H., Wesselingh, S.L., McArthur, J.C. (1995) Immunocytochemcical Quantitation of Human Immunodeficiency Virus in the Brain: Correlations with Dementia. *Ann. Neurol. 38*:755-762.

Green DR and Kroemer G (2004) The Pathophysiology of Mitochondrial Cell Death. *Science 305*:626-629.

Hazuda DJ, Young SD, Guare JP et al. (2004) Integrase Inhibitors and Cellular Immunity Suppress Retroviral Replication in Rhesus Macaques. *Science 305*:528-532.

Husstedt I, Frohne L, Bockenholt S et al. (2002) Impact of highly active antiretroviral therapy on cognitive processing in HIV infection: Cross-sectional and longitudinal studies of event-related potentials. *AIDS Res. Hum. Retrovir. 18*:485-490.

Johnson RT, Glass JD, McArthur D, Chesebro BW (1996) Quantitation of human immunodeficiency virus in brains of demented and non-demented patients with acquired immunodeficiency syndrome. *Ann. Neurol. 39*:392-395.

Jonckheere H, Anne J, De Clercq E (2000) The HIV-1 reverse transcription (RT) process as target for RT inhibitors. *Med. Res. Rev. 20*: 129-154.

Kandanearatchi A, Williams B, Everall IP (2003) Assessing the efficacy of highly active antiretroviral therapy in the brain. *Brain Pathol. 13*:104-110.

Kanmogne GD, Kennedy RC, Grammas P. (2002). HIV-1 gp120 proteins and gp160 peptides are toxic to brain endothelial cells and neurons. *J. Neuropathol. Exp. Neurol. 61*:992-1000.

Kaul M and Lipton SA (2004) Signaling pathways to neuronal damage and apoptosis in human immunodeficiency virus type 1-associated dementia: Chemokine receptors, excitotoxicity, and beyond. *J. NeuroVirol. 10(Suppl.1)*:97-101.

Letendre SL, McCutchan JA, Childers ME et al. (2004) Enhancing antiretroviral therapy for human immunodeficiency virus cognitive disorders. *Ann. Neurol. 56*:416-423.

Livak KJ, Schmittgen TD (2001) Analysis of Relative Gene Expression Data Using Real-Time Quantitative PCR and the 2-Δ ΔCT Method. *Methods 25*:402-408.

McArthur JC, McClernon DR, Cronin MF (1997) Relationship between human immunodeficiency virus-associated dementia and viral load in cerebrospinal fluid and brain. *Ann. Neurol. 42*:689-698.

McCoig C, Castrjon MM, Castano E. et al., (2002). Effect of combination antiretroviral therapy on cerebrospinal fluid HIV RNA, HIV resistance, and clinical manifestations of encephalopathy. *J. Pediatr. 141*:36-44.

Mikulowska-Mennis A, Taylor TB, Vishnu P (2002) High-quality RNA from cells isolated by laser capture microdissection. *Biotechniques 33*:176-179.

Navia BA, Cho E-S, Petito CD, Price RW. (1986) The AIDS Dementia Complex: II. Neuropathology. *Ann. Neurol. 19*:525-535.

Ng SY, Gunning P, Eddy R et al. (1985) Evolution of the functional human β-actin gene and its multi-pseudogene family: conservation of noncoding regions and chromosomal dispersion of pseudogenes. *Mol. Cell Biol. 5*: 2720-2732.

Ou CY, Kwok S, Mitchell SW et al. (1988) DNA amplification for direct detection of HIV-1 in DNA of peripheral blood mononuclear cells. *Science 239*: 295-297.

Pavlakis GN, Schwartz S, D'Agostino DM, Felber BK (1991) Structure, splicing, and regulation of expression of HIV-1: A model for the general organization of lentiviruses and other complex retroviruses. In: *Annual Review of AIDS Research*. Kennedy R, Wong-Staal F, and Koff WC (Eds) Marcel Dekker, New York, pp41-63.

Pemberton LA, Brew BJ. (2001). Cerebrospinal fluid S-100beta and its relationship with AIDS dementia complex. *J. Clin. Virol. 22*:249-253.

Pfaffl MW. (2001) A new mathematical model for relative quantification in real-time RT-PCR. *Nucleic Acids Res. 29*: 2002-2007.

Pfaffl MW, Horgan GW, Dempfle L. (2002) Relative expression software tool (REST©) for group-wise comparison and statistical analysis of relative expression results in real-time PCR. *Nucleic Acids Res. 30*, No.9 e36.

PSI-Plot, version 4 (1995). Poly Software International. Salt Lake City, UT.

Ranki A, Nyberg M, Ovod V (1995) Abundant expression of HIV Nef and Rev proteins in brain astrocytes in vivo is associated with dementia. *AIDS 9*:1001-1008.

Raeymaekers L (1993) Quantitative PCR: theoretical considerations with practical implications. *Anal. Biochem. 214*: 582-585.

Ranmakers C, Ruijter JM, Deprez RH, Moorman AF. (2003). Assumption-free analysis of quantitative real-time polymerase chain reaction (PCR) data. *Neurosci. Lett.* 339: 62-66.

Rekhter MD, Chen J (2001) Molecular analysis of complex tissues is facilitated by laser capture microdissection: critical role of upstream tissue processing. *Cell Biochem. Biophys. 35*:103-113.

Robertson K, Fiscus S, Kapoor C et al. (1998). CSF, plasma viral load and HIV associated dementia. *J. Neurovirol. 4*:90-94.

Saha RN, Pahan K. (2003). Tumor necrosis factor-alpha at the crossroads of neuronal life and death during HIV-associated dementia. *J. Neurochem. 86*:1056-1071.

Saito Y, Sharer LR, Epstein LG et al. (1994) Overexpression of nef as a marker for restricted HIV-1 infection of astrocytes in postmortem pediatric central nervjous tissues. *Neurology RR*: 474-481.

SAS, User Guide: Statistics 5th Edition. (1985) SAS Institute Inc. Cary, North Carolina

Schrager LK, D'Souza MP (1998) Cellular and anatomical reservoirs of HIV-1 in patients receiving potent antiretroviral combination therapy.

Stordeur P, Poulin LF, Craciun L et al. (2002) Cytokine mRNA quantification by real-time PCR. *J. Immunol. Methods. 259*:55-64.

Takahashi K, Wesselingh SL, Griffin DE et al.(1996) Localization of HIV-1 in Human Brain Using Polymerase Chain reaction, in situ hybridization and immunocytochemistry. *Ann. Neurol. 39*:705-711.

Tarrago-Litvak L, Andreola ML, Fournier M et al. (2002) Inhibitors of HIV-1 reverse transcriptase and integrase: classic and emerging therapeutical approaches. *Curr. Pharm. Des. 8*:595-614.

Tashima KT, (1998) Cerebrospinal fluid levels of antiretroviral medications. *JAMA 280*:879-880.

Thompson KA, McArthur JC, Wesselingh SL. (2001). Correlation between neurological progression and astrocyte apoptosis in HIV-associated dementia. *Ann. Neurol. 49*:745-752.

Tornatore C, Meyers K, Atwood W et al.(1994) Temporal Patterns of Human Immunodeficiency Virus Type 1 Transcripts in Human Fetal Astrocytes. *J. Virol. 68*:93-102.

Torres-Mufioz J, Stockton P Tacoronte N (2001) Detection of HIV-1 gene sequences in hippocampal neurons isolated from post-mortem AIDS brains by laser capture microdissection. *J. Neuropathol. Exp. Neurol. 60*: 885-892.

Tozzi V, Balestra P, Galgani S (1999) Positive and sustained effects of highly active antiretroviral therapy on HIV-1 associated neurocognitive impairment. *AIDS 13*:1889-1897.

In: Neuro-AIDS
Editors: A. Minagar and P. Shapshak, pp. 121-165

ISBN: 1-59454-610-X
© 2006 Nova Science Publishers, Inc.

Chapter VI

Allostasis in HIV Infection and AIDS

Francesco Chiappelli[1-3]*, Paolo Prolo[1-4], Milan Fiala[3,4], Olivia Cajulis[5], Javier Iribarren[4], Alberto Panerai[6], Negoita Neagos[2,3], Fariba Younai[1] and George Bernard[1,4]

[1]Division of Oral Biology and Medicine, UCLA School of Dentistry;
[2]Psychoneuroimmunology Group, Inc; [3]West-Los Angeles Veterans
Administration Medical Center; [4]UCLA Semel Institute Center for Community Health;
[5]Dental Group of Sherman Oaks, Inc.[6]Department of Pharmacology,
University of Milan, Italy.

Abstract

Allostasis is the set of intertwined psycho-social and physico-physiological responses that regulate the psychobiological adaptation to change in homeostasis. Homeostatic change is consequential to stimuli, which can include chronic immunological challenges such as infection with human immune deficiency virus (HIV), and the associated pathologies, which signify progression to the acquired immune deficiency syndrome (AIDS). This chapter examines salient aspects of the current state of knowledge of the psychoneuroendocrino-pathology in HIV/AIDS, and it proposes potential avenues for research and clinical breakthrough in the next decade.

Keywords: Psychoneuroendocrinology, Psychoneuroimmunology, Allostasis, Evidence-based medicine.

* Correspondence concerning this article should be addressed to Francesco Chiappelli, CHS 63-090, UCLA School of Dentistry, Los Angeles, CA 90095-1668. Chiappelli@dent.ucla.edu.

1. Introduction

Current statistics indicate that, in the twenty-five years since its outbreak, the human immunodeficiency virus (HIV) has infected more than 60 million people. The acquired immune deficiency syndrome (AIDS) that results from the progression of HIV disease has led to the deaths of over 20 million people. The HIV/AIDS pandemic shatters lives and families across the industrialized and the Third worlds. In excess of 14 million children have been orphaned by HIV/AIDS, a number that is expected to more than triple by 2010.

It is estimated that the number of individuals afflicted with HIV/AIDS now exceeds 40 million worldwide, and that 95% of these patients live and die in countries of the developing world. In the Third world, HIV/AIDS blunts and reverses industrial development because it kills men and women in their prime and most productive years. It erodes the very fabric of society, and of the family. The HIV/AIDS pandemic is tragic all the more because a generation of young people today – millions of sexually active, adolescent young men and women around the world - have never known an HIV/AIDS-free world. Many people afflicted by HIV/AIDS are so debilitated that they cannot hold steady employment, or do household chores. Other people with AIDS experience phases of intense life-threatening illness followed by phases in which they function normally. To face the gargantuan proportion of this world-encompassing pandemic, health care resources in both rich and poor countries are insufficient, and lack the means to battle HIV/AIDS through education, prevention, awareness and treatment programs.

Between 850,000 and 950,000 Americans live today with HIV infection, and suffer from the devastating effects on health, performance, and overall quality of life. As new therapies extend life expectancy of HIV-seropositive patients, long term adverse impacts on the quality of life become increasingly important. From the clinical perspective, highly active antiretroviral therapy (HAART), which effectively arrests individuals in the asymptomatic stages of HIV/AIDS, does not eradicate HIV from the body and does not diminish the clinical signs of HIV dementia. Rather, HAART has changed the problem from one that strikes with severity and quickly leads to death to a process of slow, chronic cognitive decline. Whereas the incidence of NeuroAIDS has dropped, its prevalence among asymptomatic HIV-seropositive patients has increased (Kandanearatchi et al, 2003; McArthur et al, 2003)

As we discuss below (*vide infra*), sleep disturbance and fatigue are prevalent and disabling symptoms in a majority of individuals with HIV/AIDS. Sleep complaints are among the first symptoms of HIV infection (Sciolla, 1995). Decreasing CD4+ lymphocyte counts in asymptomatic HIV-seropositive patients correlate with symptoms of the sickness behavior (*vide infra*), including fatigue, increased napping, diminished alertness, difficulty falling asleep, and frequent awakening during sleep. The onset of disturbances in sleep architecture (e.g., rapid eye movement, REM) occurs early in the course of HIV disease and appears to be a characteristic of the long clinical latency preceding the progression to AIDS development of AIDS (Sciolla, 1995). Sleep disturbance and fatigue in HIV/AIDS could interfere with daily activities, diminish quality of life, and contribute to a greater risk of unemployment.

A recent survey in the US has established that African Americans name HIV/AIDS the most urgent health problem, while Latinos consider it the second most urgent behind cancer, as does the overall US public. A majority of African Americans (56%), and two thirds of young African Americans (age 18-29) say, in the Spring of 2004, that the US is losing ground when it comes to the problem of HIV/AIDS – a significant increase since the Fall of 2003. By contrast, 30% of Latinos and one third of the whites surveyed asserted that the US is losing ground in the war on HIV/AIDS. The same survey reveals that 80% of African Americans, 49% of whites, 45% of Latinos and 64% of people under the age of thirty across ethnicities say that the Federal government spends too little money fighting the HIV/AIDS epidemic in the US. It is the general belief (57% of the respondents) that spending more money on HIV/AIDS prevention in the US will lead to meaningful progress in slowing the epidemic nationally and world-wide (Kaiser Family Foundation, national survey, Spring 2004).

Here and abroad, the public is fairly well informed about the HIV/AIDS pandemic: most realize that there is no cure for AIDS, and those drugs, when available and when administered promptly, can lengthen the lives of those with HIV. Many individuals in the US (30%), and many more in Third World countries, which are HIV seropositive do not know they are infected with HIV. This is critically serious in view of the fact that people in general, and in developing countries in particular are unaware of key prevention issues. A large majority of the public (71%) say that most of what they know about HIV/AIDS comes from the media. Less than 10% of respondents state to have received information about HIV/AIDS from a doctor, health professional, health agencies, or educator in the US (Kaiser Family Foundation, National survey, Spring 2004). The dearth of information in developing countries is even more appalling.

Case in point the Philippines, where official reports both by the Department of Health and by the United Nations office for AIDS (UNAIDS) indicate that the prevalence of HIV/AIDS is low. Compared to its neighbors in South-East Asia, where HIV/AIDS is rampant and spreading rapidly, the Philippines reports a total of 1,921 cases since 1984, of whom, published statistics indicate, 255 have died of AIDS (Philippines National Epidemiology Center statistics). What is indeed remarkable is that (putative) containment of the HIV/AIDS epidemic in the Philippines is obtained despite an overwhelming drug abuse and sexually transmitted infections. Both the Philippines Department of Health and the UN office for drug abuse (UN-ODCCP) concur in estimating that about 10% of Filipinos use and abuse Shabu, the local term for amphetamine. The drug, which was transported illegally to the Philippines predominantly from China and other sources until recently, is now manufactured locally and is accessible at relatively low cost. Moreover, a 2003 survey by the Philippines Department of Health established that Filipinos are at high risk of contracting sexually transmitted infections and HIV in as high as one third of the contacts with sex workers. The rise in at-risk behavior reflects the reported rise in sexual promiscuity among Filipinos, with more young adults engaging in pre-marital sex and having multiple partners.

The incongruent data between global trends in the inter-relationship among HIV/AIDS, drug abuse, and sexually transmitted diseases, and the statistics reported by Department of Health and UN offices about the Philippines causes grave concern. An abrupt rise in the prevalence of HIV/AIDS among Filipinos in the next decade is feared, with catastrophic social and economic consequences in Asia and worldwide. This danger threatens the large numbers of Filipino emigrants to the Americas, Europe, Asia and Australia, who return home regularly for visits during holidays. It is a real possibility that the epidemic of HIV/AIDS is about to explode in the Philippines, and this scenario is appalling for global health, and is a tragic prospect for the Philippines.

Most people do not have symptoms when they first become infected with HIV. Some people have flu-like symptoms within a month or two after exposure to the virus, including fever, headache, tiredness, nausea, and enlarged lymph nodes. During the initial period, people are very infectious, and HIV is present in large quantities in genital and other body fluids (e.g., serum). Symptoms later disappear, and subjects may remain asymptomatic HIV-seropositive for up to ten years, during which time the virus continues to be actively multiplying, infecting, and killing cells of the immune system that express the cluster of differentiation #4 (CD4), which acts as a primary ligand for HIV. The most obvious consequence of HIV infection is a decline in the number of CD4+ T lymphocytes. The Center for Disease Control (CDC) has established the onset of AIDS to correspond to the point in the course of HIV disease when the number of CD4+ T cells drops from about $1000/\text{mm}^3$ to 200 and below. Our data confirm these trends (cf., Figures 3 and 4, *vide infra*). Because CD4+ cells play a critical role in immune regulation, HIV infection leads to progressive weakening of cell-mediated immune surveillance, which precipitates a plethora of cancers, bacterial, fungal and parasitic infections systemically as well as locally (e.g., oral cavity, *vide infra*). Lymph nodes, where immune responses take place, enlarge and become sensitive to palpation, and a spectrum of additional symptoms associated with AIDS ensue. This symptomatology includes weakness and lethargy, cachexia and weight loss, skin rashes, and yeast infections, memory loss and other signs of AIDS-related dementia (e.g., seizures, lack of coordination, confusion and forgetfulness, depression, coma), altered sleep and neuroendocrine rhythmicity, viral infection, and a variety of other opportunistic infections, and tumors (e.g., Kaposi's sarcoma, cervical cancer, lymphomas). This chapter examines current and future areas of psycho-social/psycho-pathological research in HIV and AIDS, from the fundamental perspective of mind-body interaction (i.e., psychoneuroimmunology), depicted in Scheme 1.

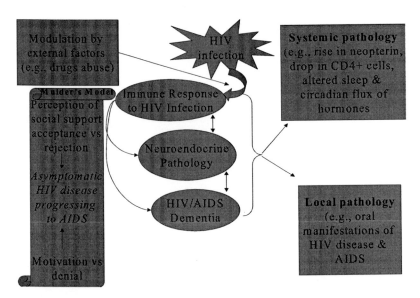

Scheme 1. Mind-Body Interaction Model in HIV/AIDS.

2. Psycho-Social Domain

Social support networks have been studied extensively in health psychology. Both the quality and the quantity of social support are beneficial to health and to well being. Certain coping styles, such as action-oriented, cognitive, emotional, and avoidance behavior are critical. Good social support promotes psychological well being which in turn promotes good health (Green, 1993). This axiom lies at the core of psychosomatic medicine and psychoneuroimmunology. By contrast, lack of adequate social support may favor the onset of depression, and its associated psychoneuroendocrine pathology. Feelings of isolation, alienation, and loneliness have been linked to a lack of social support. Factor analysis has identified four sources of beneficial social support for HIV/AIDS gay men, which can be summarized as acceptance and support provided by friends, relatives, partner, and organization (i.e., religious or lay). Blame and fear lead to rejection, and constitute barriers in providing social support (Schwarzer et al, 1994).

Faith, prayer, support and acceptance offered by religious organizations or affiliations are important aspects of intervention, which are gaining increasing scientific support. People are raised around the world in an environment that espouses one religion or another. Religions use different codes to structure people's lives. These codes contribute to the enforcement of societal discipline (Solomon, 1996). Religion and spirituality rest on faith, prayer, as well as support and acceptance by the religious community. Modern medicine often ignores the depth of spirituality, which is often limited to recording the patient's religion. Religion and spirituality are not synonymous, and the latter may encompass religious practices. Patients with chronic illness tend to use faith and prayer as fundamental spiritual coping mechanisms, in addition to support and acceptance from the religious organization (Narayanasamy, 2002). Faith and prayer are an important component of spiritual life across cultures: they sustain people in times of crisis and emotional turmoil, and serve as an effective means of holistic complementary medical intervention (Lo, 2003). Holistic complementary care addresses the physical, psychological, social and spiritual dimensions, while promoting spiritual well-being, which is often undervalued in traditional medicine, and favors the use of faith and prayer in helping the patients find meaning in life and peace in death (Lo, Brown, 1999), with significant improvement in overall physiological health.

In the case of HIV/AIDS, research provides substantial elements to begin to dissect these important psychosocial variables. Faith-based religious institution play a key role in the education of the patients, the caregivers and public, and provide, in so doing, compassionate care to the patients. For example, individual members of the Catholic Church have done much to respond to the HIV/AIDS pandemic over the course of the last two decades. Whereas the Catholic Bishops in the US have sought to reinforce conservative canonical teachings and values with respect to sexual behavior and marital relationships, the community of faithful and church leaders have developed a vision of church-related HIV/AIDS services that extends beyond the mere providing of care and basic social and pastoral activities, such as helping dying people and their families confront the reality of HIV/AIDS (Vitillo, 1993). Similarly, issues of morality, morbidity, mortality, reality, responsibility are central to the Evangelical Church, and blunt its response to this National and global health crisis (Ayers, 1995). The Black Church has been involved in lending support, providing care, and being actively involved in the health and social welfare of its members. It has been sharply criticized for its lukewarm response and involvement in response to the HIV/AIDS pandemic (Baker, 1999), although trends have changed as of late with a greater shift toward addressing the quality of life of African-American church-going HIV/AIDS patients (Sanders, 1997). The Hindu religion is strongly opposed to extramarital and premarital sex, and condemns these behaviors as responsible for HIV/AIDS. But, HIV/AIDS patients find acceptance and solace in the Hindu religion because of its selfless spirit, and its spiritual teaching about the immortality of the soul. The Islam sect of Soofieism condemns AIDS as a self-inflicted disease caused by promiscuity and the breakdown of morals in society (Naidu, 1997).

Until the turn of the Century, most religious organizations in Africa (e.g., Kenya) ignored HIV/AIDS, and described it as the unfortunate outcome of aberrant or immoral behavior. Churches in Kenya recommended that HIV/AIDS be avoided and controlled by banishing the sick, and by avoiding extramarital and premarital sex, but trends are now reversing (Black, 1997). In Papua/New Guinea, the Church recognizes the sacredness of life in every person. It teaches that human dignity needs to be respected, and advocates that people with AIDS should not be condemned, avoided, or rejected. HIV/AIDS awareness education is emphasized in the context of human sexuality, marriage and religious teaching. In addition to medical programs, Church organizations successfully provide psychological, social, and economic support to HIV/AIDS patients and their families (Bouten, 1996). Several Church organizations in the Western hemisphere, including the US and worldwide, increasingly follow this model of humanistic support, acceptance, teaching and counseling (Tesoriero et al, 2000).

Certain religious organizations, which tend to call for tolerance (Somlai et al, 1997), are founded on a universal belief of duty to support all suffering persons, and to help them receive the best possible care and treatment. In that context, religion is seen as a potential help to patients with chronic diseases, such as HIV/AIDS. On the grounds of edict or morality, religion cannot be a non-participant to this world pandemic, to the same extent as medicine cannot ignore the force of religious faith, prayer, support and acceptance (Solomon, 1996).

Charitas International sponsors educational and awareness-raising seminars at the regional, national, and international levels, and supports service programs in Third world countries to insure medical and social service facilities, food and medical supplies, and HIV testing equipment and expertise. The social support endeavor of Charitas International extends itself to the provision of staff training, transportation, home care programs, and support for homeless persons with HIV/AIDS, orphan care programs, and alternative income-generating projects for commercial sex workers.

Franciscans International, another Catholic organization that works on the front lines of HIV/AIDS issues, serves particularly in hospitals, parishes and community centers, and supports a stronger political will, resulting in more serious policies, to bring appropriate resources and attention to the pandemic. Franciscans International has recognized that the fight against HIV/AIDS must be waged globally by integrating social, cultural, traditional, spiritual and medical realities, and it has joined representatives from Brazil, Senegal, Thailand and Uganda, and UNAIDS, to examine policies to combat HIV/AIDS. The consensus statement from this group is at the forefront of addressing the need to combine prevention and protection of the pandemic, including the lack of infrastructures to welcome the HIV/AIDS patient, the lack of doctors and trained personnel, the danger associated with the mobility of the population and the migration process. Franciscan International stresses that the fight against HIV/AIDS must eliminate the discrimination against HIV-seropositive people, and the need to combat the stigmas surrounding HIV/AIDS, to provide for orphaned children and to overcome cultural beliefs, and misbeliefs.

The Ecumenical Advocacy Alliance consists of over 85 churches and church-related organizations, including Franciscans International and others, that implement HIV/AIDS strategy support groups, and speak out on the causes, prevention, treatment and consequences of the pandemic. As a united voice, they call on governments to fund and support the efforts of the World Health Organization to insure that the people living with HIV/AIDS in the world have access to the necessary drugs by 2005. If concerted action is not taken, it is feared that China, for example, will experience a rise of HIV/AIDS cases to 10 million by 2010.

The South Asia Inter-Religious Council on HIV/AIDS includes representatives from the Hindu, Muslim, Christian, Buddhist, Sikh, Jain and Baha'i faiths, and is now formalized to include representatives of Afghanistan, Bangladesh, Bhutan, India, Maldives, Nepal, Pakistan and Sri Lanka. The Council recognizes that *"[S]piritual leaders are uniquely placed to provide comfort and guidance to those affected by the disease ...Their examples can help end the stigma and discrimination that perpetuate HIV/AIDS"*. This inter-faith religious organization endeavors to carry out inter-religious advocacy efforts, counseling, information, teaching about HIV/AIDS and sexual health, and moral support to young people in their communities (*Associated Press*, 7/15/2004).

Data have established that AIDS progresses more rapidly among HIV-seropositive patients who are experiencing or are particularly sensitive to social rejection (Cole et al, 1997). It is clear that a social support system such as that provided by religious organizations and affiliations is critical to the well being of HIV/AIDS individuals. Social support and acceptance, however, does not need to be rigidly structured within the confines of religion. For instance, CHESS (Comprehensive Health Enhancement Support System) is a successful computer-based support system that provides information, referrals, decision support, and social support to the select group of people living with AIDS/HIV who have access to Internet (Gustafson et al, 1994).

In summary, Mulder (1994) has proposed a general "stress-coping-social support" model with the goal of identifying psychosocial risk factors for progression and to develop effective psychosocial interventions. The model establishes social support as a beneficial mediating variable in HIV/AIDS, but underscores that the underlying psychobiological "causal paths" among stress, coping, social support, and disease progression remain to be elucidated. Scheme 1 illustrates the interaction between the psychoneuroendocrine and the immune systems in HIV/AIDS, and presents intertwined relationships, which are described in this Chapter as the putative fundamental physiologic mechanisms of Mulder's model.

3. Psychoneuroendocrine-Immune Interactions and HIV/AIDS

Western philosophical thought established since Antiquity the dichotomy between spirit and matter. To the pre-Socratic notion of ordered nature (=physis), followed Plato's dualism of body and soul, of eternal forms and sensory experience, of the teleological order of the eternal mind (=demiurge, *demiourgós*) and matter (e.g., the balance among four elements of air, water, earth and fire), of the soul (*psuché*) and the body (*húle*). Aristotle's critique placed reality within the sphere of sensible objects (=phenomena), rather than invisible forms only captured by the mind, and maintained this dualistic view. Change of state was viewed to be driven by a cause (*Causa*) (Chiappelli et al, 2004a), which consists of a "formal cause" (i.e., one derived from the object itself), a "material cause" (i.e., that which will persist through the change process), a "moving cause" (i.e., that which induces the process of change), and a "final cause", the goal or purpose of the change. Whereas the Aristotelian celestial realm is perfect and changeless (i.e., the "unmoved mover"), the terrestrial realm in which the psychosocial and physio-pathological reality of human nature is imbedded is imperfect and constantly changing. The agent-movers of this change can be intrinsic to the human reality (i.e., in modern terms, we would say today in the context of HIV/AIDS, the neuroendocrine-immune pathology consequential to HIV infection, for instance), or extrinsic to it (e.g., psycho-social forces such as social support, environmental forces such as alcohol and drug use and abuse, infection with HIV). Following this tradition of Western thought, René Descartes opened, as it were, Modern thought and reductionism with the establishment of the distinct functions of the body (*res extensa*) from those of the mind (*res cogitans*) (Chiappelli et al, 2004a).

The cognitive schism that resulted led to Modernism, the separation between spirituality and scientism, and to the divisions in the health sciences we find in Western medicine today, and which the current area of "systems biology" attempts to co-join. The renowned XIX Century French physiologist, Claude Bernard (1813-1878) first proposed that maintenance of the internal milieu (*le milieu intérieur, 1856*) is a fundamental feature of physiological regulation. The phrase "homeostasis" was coined. Walter Cannon (1871-1945) over five decades later proposed that organisms engage in a dynamic process of adjustment of the physiological balance of the internal milieu in response to changing environmental conditions. Between the 1950's and the mid 1960's, Hans Selye (1907-1982) established the cardinal points of the "Generalized Stress Response", and demonstrated the concerted physiological responses to stressful challenges.

The early 20th Century biologist, Polany, described consciousness and related perceptions of motivation and control as fundamental phenomena processed by the central nervous system (CNS). The interaction between the psyche and physical health - disease continuum, is now firmly established in the domain of psychosomatic medicine: all forms of human disease are related to alterations in the interaction among genetic, endocrine, nervous, immune and psychic (including consciousness), behavioral, cognitive and emotional) factors. These fundamental concepts, first championed by Speransky (cf., "neuro-dystrophic processes") (Speransky, 1943) and Engle (Engle, 1960), were later precisely outlined by (cf., "psychoneuroimmunology") (Solomon and Moos, 1964; Solomon, 1987).

A long and contentious history had existed in Western philosophical thought between idealists and realists, which has impacted science. Those scientists who were idealists, tended to be influenced by Freud, and emphasized that the "primary reality lies in the world of the mind"; hence the formulation that the pathogenesis of (some) diseases could be laid primarily at the door of intrapsychic conflicts and psychoneuroses. Others espoused realism and recognized that humans are social beings who live with others in mutual interaction, and are a product of shifting cultural, historical, evolutionary, economic, and environmental influences, which they interpret, sometimes internalize, and to which certainly they respond. Many natural and experimentally produced conditions can therefore challenge the person's health, and lead to illness and disease (Hinkle, 1967). It was then concluded in a series of monographs that the behavioral (e.g., avoidance behavior, lethargy) and physiological responses (i.e., pattern of hormonal responses) to certain experimental situation (i.e., stressors, stressful challenges) can be conceptualized as adaptive, only when adaptation *de facto* fails, and the responses are inappropriate, excessive, inadequate, or disorganized. In such instances, they lead to pathological consequences (Mason, 1968). This early view was a precursor to our current conceptualization of allostasis (*vide infra*).

Taken together, these principles have come to represent for many the birth of the scientific domain of the ordered integration between the mind and the hormonal system as monitored and regulated by the brain (i.e., psychoneuroendocrinology). Within the same decade, it was demonstrated that conditioned taste aversion with saccharin (as the conditioned stimulus) produced a significant suppression of hemoagglutinating antibody titers in rats (Ader and Cohen, 1975), which lend substance to the proposition that the central nervous and immune systems are in fact not separate entities, but inter-communicating and cross-regulating physiological systems, whose intertwined nature was mediated by neural and neuroendocrine responses.

Scientific data were *de facto* confirming that *res extensa* and *res cogitans* could not distinct from each other in the living organism. Bernard's homeostasis of the *milieu interieur* was increasingly recognized as a homogeneous and finely regulated set of mechanisms that interact among each other, regulate each other, and modulate each other in a constant process of adaptation to changes brought about by internal (i.e., emotions, perceptions of support vs. alienation), physical (i.e., pain, physical load), and external stimuli (i.e., environment, immune challenge) (Lutgendorf and Costanzo, 2003). It is this set of psychobiological events that are involved in the process of adaptation to change that are now collectively termed allostasis. Currently, by extension, the term also describes the events that involve mind-body systemic regulation to recover from stress, rather than local feedback. Allostatic regulation is the recovery and the maintenance of internal balance and viability amidst changing circumstances consequential to challenges (e.g., stressors, stimuli), and encompasses a range of behavioral and physiological functions that direct the adaptive function of regulating homeostatic systems. Heterostasis describes the situation where the demands upon the organism exceed its inherent physiological limiting capacity (Sterling and Eyer, 1988; McEwen and Wingfield, 2003; Chiappelli and Cajulis, 2004).

The cumulative load of the allostatic process, the allostatic load, produces the pathological side effects of failed adaptation, which are commonly observed in a variety of diseased states. These outcomes lead to and engender mental as well as physical unwellness and sickness, which pertain to the domain of psychosomatic medicine. In most situations, subjects position themselves along a spectrum of allostatic regulation, somewhere between allostasis (=toward regaining physiological balance), and the allostatic overload (=toward physiological collapse, and associated potential onset of varied pathologies).

Case in point in dentistry: the perception of chronic dental pain can be a significantly stressful challenge. The perception of pain in dentistry requires a careful assessment because pain can be a sign of pathology (e.g., dental fracture or fissure, pulpitis, temporomandibular disorder), or it may be secondary to stress-associated tooth grinding. Stressed subjects tend to grind their teeth, which transpires as alterations in dental anatomy, as strain and pain to the periodontal fibroblasts, and, over prolonged periods of time, as increased vertical distance of occlusion and altered angle of Spee (Gesh et al, 2004; Wright et al, 2004). In an ongoing study of the relationship among dental pain, dental anxiety, and the perception of wellness, we have noted that dental patients can be distinguished based on their reports of perceived pain intensity (high pain mean $\pm$SD: 5.5 ± 1.00, vs. low pain: 2.96 ± 0.96, t test, $p=0.0037$). Contrary to expectation, these groups do not differ in terms of reported dental anxiety (1.67 ± 0.58 vs. 1.67 ± 1.15, Wilcoxon $p=0.5$), but perception of pain was found to impact negatively, as hypothesized, upon dental patients overall perception of wellness (2.33 ± 0.58 vs. 3.33 ± 0.58, t $p=0.051$; Pearson $r=-0.52$) (Chiappelli, Cajulis, Prolo, Neagos and Iribarren, in preparation).

In brief, allostasis represents a set of intertwined psycho-social and physico-physiological processes that monitor and mediate the psychobiological regulatory responses to all possible challenge, including challenges to the immune system (e.g., viral infection). It is rests on the complex interaction of variable set points, which are characterized by individual differences, themselves associated with anticipatory behavioral and physiological responses, and vulnerable to physiological overload and to the breakdown of regulatory capacities (McEwen and Wingfield, 2003; Schulkin, 2003; Chiappelli and Cajulis, 2004; Iribarren et al, in press). The allostatic response can be effectively tested experimentally (*vide infra*), including in patients with HIV/AIDS.

Type 1 allostatic load utilizes the psychobiological responses to the challenge as a mean of self-preservation by means of developing and establishing temporary or permanent adaptation skills. The organism aims at surviving the perturbation in the best condition possible, and at normalizing the normal life cycle. In Type 2 allostatic load, the challenge is excessive, sustained, or continued, and drives allostasis chronically. An escape response cannot be found (Iribarren et al, in press). Type I vs. type II allostatic loads are reminiscent of Myers early observations of soldiers during the Civil War who were diagnosed with Di Costa syndrome, a precursor to today's post-traumatic stress disorder (PTSD). The symptomatology was reported to include effort fatigue, dyspnea, a sighing respiration, palpitation, sweating, tremor, an aching sensation in the left pericardium, utter fatigue, an exaggeration of symptoms upon efforts, and occasionally complete syncope. Myers described the syndrome as resembling more closely an abandonment to emotion and fear, rather than the "effort" that normal subjects engage to overcome challenges (Myers, 1870). In current psychological theory, we recognize this behavior as a form of learned helplessness (Seligman, 1972).

The allostatic response consists of a set of psychobiological process, whose relevance to the health-disease continuum is long lasting. Research in the next decade will characterize the fundamental mechanisms of allostasis by defining its underlying psycho-neuroendocrine-immune (i.,e., psychoneuroimmune) pathways. Psychoneuroimmunology was defined as "... *the complex bidirectional interactions between the CNS (mediating both psychic and biologic processes) and the immune system (not only responsible for resistance to infectious diseases and cancer but also serving newly recognized bioregulatory functions)....the field reinforces that view that all disease is multifactorial and biopsychosocial in onset and course – the result of interrelationships among specific etiologic (e.g., bacteria, viruses, carcinogens), genetic, endocrine, nervous, immune, emotional, and behavioral factors...*" (Solomon, 1987).

This view evidently pertains to today's system biology view on HIV/AIDS (Solomon et al, 2000; Antoni, 2003). It was noted that "...*relaxation skills, cognitive coping strategies and social support may mediate ...mood effects ...that these mood changes may mediate adrenal hormone regulation indicated by reductions in 24-h urinary cortisol (with reduced depressed mood) and norepinephrine (with reduced anxiety) and increases in serum DHEA-S and testosterone levels (with reduced depressed mood)... (that these) changes in production of these hormones may explain, in part, ... short-term changes in IgG antibody titers to herpesviruses (with increased DHEA-S-to-cortisol ratio), and longer-term changes in lymphocyte subpopulations such as CD8 suppressor/cytotoxic cells (with reductions in urinary noradrenaline output) and transitional naive CD4 cells (with reductions in urinary cortisol output)...(and that) alterations in mood, neuroendocrine functioning and immunologic status that may have health implications for HIV infection ...*" (Antoni, 2003).

The exquisite nature of the psychoneuroimmune interactive system derives from the degree of overlay of the complexity of the psyche with the short and long feedback loops that directly and indirectly regulate neuroendocrine responses, and the modulation of cellular and humoral, innate and antigen-dependent immunity. Immune surveillance against HIV and AIDS-related opportunistic infections is, in effect, a consequence of behaviors and emotions generated and controlled by the brain in response to intrinsic (e.g., depression, anger, volitional control) and extrinsic forces (e.g., acceptance, social support, environmental triggers). The bridge between the mind and the immune system is the neuroendocrine system in HIV/AIDS, as it is in health (Solomon et al, 2000; Antoni, 2003; Chiappelli et al, 2004a).

Maladaptation of the person to the environment can cause psychological turmoil, with serious psychosomatic *sequelae*. Certain environmental factors have been identified since the time of Hippocrates as putative causative factors in the pathogenesis and in the exacerbation of a wide variety of diseases, from cardiovascular disease to psychiatric disorders. Immune surveillance processes, specifically the production of pro-inflammatory cytokines, can be directly stimulated by negative emotions and stressful experiences and indirectly stimulated by chronic or recurring infections. Accordingly, distress-related immune deregulation may be among the mechanisms behind a diverse set of health risks associated with negative emotions (Kiecolt-Glaser et al, 2002). Most immune outcomes are generally related to the general expression of a certain affect (e.g., happiness, sadness, anger, anxiety), rather than the specific quality of any given mood state (e.g., clinical depression) (Futterman et al, 1994). Autonomic neural activity (e.g., palmar skin conductance, brachial artery systolic blood pressure, electrocradiogram, inter-beat duration between R spikes, finger photoplethysmograph pulse peak amplitude, and peripheral finger photoplethysmograph peak during the final 60 seconds of a 15-min resting period, expressed as the SD of each indicator about its mean under each assessment condition) also play a significant role in mediating the relationship between psychological factors (e.g., introversion, social inhibition) and HIV/AIDS pathogenesis (Cole et al, 2003).

Immune tissues, including primary and secondary lymphoid organs, receive sympathetic and para-sympathetic innervation, which enter the parenchyma of the tissue in association with the vasculature (arterial, venous, lymphatic), and which projects into the parenchyma to form synapse-like junctions with lymphoid and myeloid cells. This innervation is functional, changes immune responsiveness, follows pharmacological manipulation of noradrenergic sympathetic or peptidergic nerves, and directs immune cell migration properties systemically and locally (e.g., the dental pulp; Patel et al, 2003) (Chiappelli et al, 2004a).

Fibers expressing dopamine-β-hydroxylase and/or tyrosine hydroxylase, and other neural markers, are confirmed by immunohisto- and immunocyto-chemical protocols and electron microscopy (Chiappelli et al, 2004a). The case of tyrosine and tryptophan hydroxylase-containing nerve fibers is interesting in the context of neuroimmune interactions because the essential co-factor of these enzymes, tetrahydrobiopterin is intimately related to the product of interferon γ-mediated monocyte/macrophage activation, neopterin (Chiappelli, 1991). The significant rise in serum neopterin observed in HIV-seropositive patients as they progress to AIDS (*vide infra*) may suggest new hypotheses about impaired sympathetic modulation of immunity in HIV/AIDS.

Classic receptor binding studies demonstrate a wide variety of target cells with β-adrenoceptors and receptors for neuropeptides and for a variety of hormones on cells of the immune system. We tested the function of β-adrenergic receptors in perpheral blood mononuclear cells from patients with fibromyalgia, a condition of chronic pain. Activation of G-protein coupled to these receptors leads to an increase in the intracellular level of cAMP. Basal cAMP levels are elevated, albeit not significantly ($p=0.124$) in-patients with fibromyalgia (3.02 ± 0.44 pmol/10^6 cells), compared to control subjects (2.26 ± 0.39 pmol/10^6 cells), and stimulation with millimolar concentrations of isoproterenol leads to a significant rise in intracellular cAMP in both groups. Isoproterenol at 10^{-5}M fails to produce this outcome in the patient group ($p=0.74$), while a significant stimulation of cAMP is obtained in the control group ($p=0.012$), suggesting that circulating lymphocytes in patients with fibromyalgia have fewer functional β-adrenoceptors (Maekawa et al, 2003).

Vasoactive-intestinal peptide innervation also plays a significant role in neuroendocrine-immune regulation, and the polypeptide itself appears to be of particular relevance to the HIV/AIDS problem since an inner five-amino-acid (TDNYT) sequence of the peptide proximal to the N-terminal shares homology with the proposed attachment sequences of the HIV viral envelope (gp120) unto CD4+ cells (Sacerdote et al, 1987, 1988).

Synaptic terminals are subjected to high levels of oxidative and metabolic stress and calcium influx and are therefore sites where neurodegenerative cascades likely begin in many different disorders, including HIV/AIDS-associated dementia. HIV viral proteins, such as Tat, elicit Ca2+-dependent acetyl-choline release by species-specific intra-terminal mechanisms by binding via discrete amino acid sequences to different receptive sites on cholinergic terminals of human and animal model systems (i.e., rat) (Feligioni et al, 2003). Collectively, the data suggest that HIV-derived proteins promote synaptic dysfunction and degeneration, which contribute to the observed deficits in cognitive and motor functions in AIDS patients.

HIV infection selectively targets the basal ganglia resulting in loss of dopaminergic neurons, decreased dopamine levels in the cerebrospinal fluid and increasing susceptibility to Parkinsonism (Mirsattari et al, 1998). HIV proteins gp120 and Tat when injected into the basal ganglia of experimental animals cause selective neuronal loss and gliosis (Jones et al, 1998). Gp120 produces a greater gliotic reaction, compared to Tat, but Tat leads to increased loss of nigro-striatal fibers. Both peptides cause synergistic neurotoxicity when adminstered together at subtoxic dosages, and synergize with other neurotoxic compounds such as glutamate to cause neurotoxicity (Nath et al, 2000). Common drugs of abuse such as methamphetamine and cocaine, which also cause dopaminergic dysfunction, synergize with gp120 and Tat to induce neurotoxicity, in a manner that can be blocked by estrogen. Tat and morphine cause synergistic neurotoxicity in striatal neurons, which can be blocked by naloxone (Nath et al, 2004).

Opioid innervation of lymphoid organs is variable, but little is known of what directs the innervation to specific compartments within the lymphoid tissues (Chiappelli et al, 2004a). The endogenous opioid, β-endorphin (βE) is a 31 aminoacids opioid peptide known in the last thirty years for its activity in the central nervous system (CNS). In the CNS, βE is mostly synthesized in the arcuate nucleus from which it projects in several brain areas. In the periphery βE is synthesized in the intermediate pituitary or its vestigia, and in cells of the immune system, including splenocytes, peripheral blood lymphocytes, and monocytes (Sacerdote et al, 1991a).

The levels of βE in peripheral blood mononuclear cells (PBMC) are independent of those in plasma, and they respond to physiological stimuli, e.g. stress, increase several folds its concentrations (Manfredi et al, 1995). Both βE concentrations and release from PBMC steeply increase after middle age (> 40 years of age), and remain unchanged into advanced aging (> 100 years of age), in a pattern that precedes and then parallels immnosenescence. The PBMC-βE age pattern parallels both the age related increase of memory immune cells (CD45RO+), and the increase of plasma interleukin(IL)-6 concentrations. Pharmacologial studies show that both CNS and PBMC βE are under dopaminergic and GABAergic inhibitory tonic control, as well as serotoninergic tonic stimulatory input. The observation that steroids do not have a direct role in the modulation of PBMC βE (Sacerdote et al, 1991b) is also critical in the context of allostasis and in situations of psychophysiological stress, when βE produced by the CNS and the pituitary, but not that produced by immune cells, is down regulated by the increased steroids (Sacerdote et al 1994a). In HIV/AIDS, the observed decreased CNS dopaminergic tone and content (Mirsattari et al, 1998) could contribute to the parallel increase of the opioid (*vide infra*), whereas the reduction of the opioid inhibitory tone could be beneficial to patients with HIV/AIDS.

Immune cells constitutively produce βE, express receptors for βE, and can produce and release the opioid (Manfredi et al, 1995). βE exerts a physiological inhibitory tone on immune function, since the administration of the opiate receptor antagonists naloxone or naltrexone induces an increase of NK activity and mitogen induced PBMC and splenocyte proliferation (Manfredi et al, 1993). Immune cells utilize for βE the same receptors that are shared by morphine and the other μ opiate receptor agonists. Despite extensive work by our group and others, the role of βE in immune modulation *in vitro* remains mixed and the fundamental mechanisms unclear (Chiappelli et al, 1991, 1992, 2004a).

By contrast, *in vivo* studies have yielded more consistent results, indicating a mainly immunosuppressive role for βE, similarly to what has been observed following the administration morphine and related opiates (Panerai et al, 1995). βE is inhibitory to cellular immunity, and both naloxone and naltrexone exert their effect despite inducing a huge increase of corticosteroids secretion. In addition, the effect of βE on immune responses are preserved in adrenalectomized animals (Taoh et al, 1988, Sacerdote et al, 1994b).

In normal human subjects, PBMC βE concentrations are low in presence of an activated immune system, as it happens in rheumatoid arthritis, Crohn's disease, rejection of organ transplantation and in multiple sclerosis, as well as in PBMC following a stressful challenge, and in pregnancy, and more generally speaking in diseased states with blunted TH1 cytokine patterns (*vide infra*) (Panerai and Sacerdote, 1997). By contrast, βE concentrations are significantly elevated in PBMC from HIV+, and these values rise in parallel with disease progression. βE are also elevated in the mature T cell line (HuT78) chronically infected by the HIV, compared to uninfected cells and to Hut78 cells infected with other viruses (Barcellini et al, 1994). Taken together, these lines of evidence suggest that βE concentrations are elevated when the immune system is depressed, and they are decreased when the immune system is activated, and that the altered cytokine *milieu* could contribute to favor HIV replication (cf., Table 1).

Table 1. Relative βE levels in Response to Stimuli or Pathological States

	Rat/Mouse CNS ß-endorphin	Human PBMC/ mouse splenocytes ß-endorphin	Predominant Cytokine pattern
Stress	↑	↑	Th2
HIV+		↑	Th2
Multiple Sclerosis	↓	↓	Th1
Rheumatoid Arthritis	↓	↓	Th1
Crohn's Disease		↓	Th1
GABA	↓	↓	
Dopamine agonists	↓	↓	
Dopamine antagonists	↑	↑	
Serotonin agonists	↑	↑	
Serotonin antagonists	↓	↓	

In conclusion, the administration of a long lasting opiate receptor antagonist, such as naltrexone, could be effective in decreasing the immunosuppressive effect induced by the augmented production of βE. Dopaminergic drugs (e.g., bromocriptine, pergolide) could inhibit βE synthesis in immune cells, and thus blunt the facilitatory effects of the opioid on virus replication. Taken together, The significance of this line of research to the problem of drug use in HIV/AIDS cannot be overstated.

One among the principal cross-talk between the psychoneuroendocrine and the immune systems involve the hypothalamic-pituitary-adrenal (HPA) axis, and the inter-relationship between adrenal steroids and cytokines (Solomon, 1987; Chrousos and Gold, 1992; Kiecolt-Glaser et al., 2002). Cytokines are a large family of polypeptide mediators classically associated with the regulation of immunity and inflammation. Cytokines modulate hypothalamus-originating responses, such as emotions, appetite, fever, and endocrine regulation. The proinflammatory cytokines, including IL-1β, IL-6 and tumor necrosis factor (TNF)-α regulate the sickness behavior, and the activation of the HPA axis. The HPA response leads to a complex cascade of events that includes sympathetic-adrenal-medullary outcomes (i.e., the locus coeruleus/norepinephrine system), that results in the production of pro-opiomelanocortin (POMC)-derived peptides (i.e., adrenocorticotropic hormone [ACTH]), and cortisol. Feedback regulation dampens hypothalamic and pituitary output (Chiappelli et al, 2004a). The HPA axis involves a network of central and peripheral components, consisting centrally of corticotropin releasing hormone (CRH) and urocortin (a CRH-related peptide), and peripherally of ACTH and cortisol.

The actions of CRH in the brain and in the periphery are mediated through a family of specific receptors, which we have discussed in detail previously (Chiappelli et al, 2004a). In brief, isoforms are encoded by two distinct genes (i.e., CRHR1α and 1β, CRHR2α, 2β and 2γ). The cloning of CRH receptors and their localization in the brain have led to the development of receptor antagonists (e.g., antalarmin, a novel class I CRH receptor antagonist that blunts the effect of CRH on pituitary ACTH with no effect on the adrenal response to stress [Wong et al, 1999]), which may be of potential use in the treatment of certain conditions, perhaps including AIDS-related dementia.

Leptin is increasingly recognized as a stress-related hormone, with multiple role critical to survival. The peptide is a trophic factor for reproductive hormones, which in turn are modulators of cellular immunity. Leptin acts directly at the dorsomedial and the ventromedial nuclei of the hypothalamus, at the pituitary gland, and at the ovary (Prolo et al, 1998). Leptin plays an important role in providing information to the hypothalamus about energy homeostasis by translating the metabolic status of the peripheral adipocyte to the brain. Plasma levels of leptin are pulsatile and present diurnal variations that are inversely correlated with cortisol concentrations (Prolo et al, 1998). Leptin levels are highest between midnight and the early morning hours, and lowest noon to mid-afternoon, and the nocturnal rise in leptin may be associated with the suppression of appetite during sleep. Taken together, these lines of evidence suggest that leptin may be revealed to be not only an important modulator of gonadal hormone-mediated immune surveillance in health and in disease, but an essential messenger in HIV/AIDS-related cachexia. Research to date indicates that there indeed seems to be a significant reduction in leptin secretion with subcutaneous fat loss in HIV-seropositive patients (Pearson correlation of subcutaneous fat with mean leptin secretion: $r = 0.72$, $p < 0.0001$, with leptin pulse amplitude: $r = 0.62$, $p < 0.0001$, with leptin nadir: $r = 0.62$, $p < 0.0001$; regression of subcutaneous fat, but not visceral fat, for leptin secretion $R^2 = 0.57$, $p < 0.0001$) (Koutkia et al, 2004). Conflicting data, however, remain in the literature indicating that leptin will remain at the forefront of the HIV/AIDS research agenda in the next decade (Nowak et al, 1999; van der Merwe et al, 2004).

CRH secreted in the hypophyseal circulation, and urocortin another CRH receptor agonist with ligand properties to both classes of CRH receptors, binds to class I CRH receptors on cells of the anterior pituitary, and elicits the activation of transcription factors for the transcription of POMC mRNA. This gene is translated and spliced into ACTH, β-endorphin, and related peptides. POMC expression is under the regulatory control of arginine-vasopressin (AVP), which is released from the hypothalamus parvocellular division of the paraventricular nucleus, and from the magnocellular neurons of the supraoptic nucleus. Physiological regulation of the HPA axis depends upon the CRH/AVP ratio (Scott and Dinan, 1998; Chiappelli et al, 2004a).

Functional derangement of every endocrine organ has been reported in HIV/AIDS (Bashin et al, 2001). It is possible and even probable that the CRH/AVP ratio is altered during the course of HIV/AIDS, which could shed light on the mixed nature of the data about variations in HPA function in HIV disease. For example, although we have noted no significant changes in cortisol levels in asymptomatic HIV-seropositive individuals vs. AIDS patients (*vide infra*), others have reported significant changes. Early deregulation of the HPA axis can occur following in HIV infection, although the exact physiopathological mechanism is not fully elucidated. Increased CRH production by IL-1β and a role of the HIV envelope glycoprotein (gp 120) have been proposed to explain observed increases in ACTH and cortisol levels in HIV patients (Verges et al, 1989). Significant linear correlations were observed between baseline levels of serum cortisol and both IL-6 ($r = 0.955$; $p = 0.001$) and IL-1β ($r = 0.863$; $p = 0.005$) in HIV-seropositive patients (Biglino et al, 1995). In experimental animals, intracerebroventricular injection of gp120 leads to a marked sickness behavior syndrome, consisting of reduced exploratory behavior, suppressed consumption of food and saccharin solution, and reduced body weight, as well as a significant febrile response, and a significant rise in serum levels of ACTH and corticosterone (Barak et al, 2002). Severe adrenal insufficiency is rare (3%) in HIV-seropositive patients, and appears to be confined to the AIDS group and to be consistently secondary to ACTH deficiency (Catania et al, 1994).

Cortisol and other corticosteroid hormones act via intracellular receptors. The binding of the hormone to the receptor leads to a conformational change and dissociation from its binding protein. Translocation signals induce a dimerization of the receptor complex; the dimer enters the nucleus and binds to glucocorticoid-responsive elements on the chromatin DNA, regulating transcription. Type I corticosteroid receptors preferentially binds to aldosterone, whereas type II receptors preferentially bind to dexamethasone, a synthetic corticosteroid. Corticosterone down-regulates type II receptors and upregulates type I receptors; by contrast, mineralocorticoids down- regulate both types of receptors (Lupien and McEwen 1997; Chiappelli et al, 2004a).

Exposure to an antigenic stimulation activates the production of pro-inflammatory cytokines (i.e., IL-1β, IL-6, TNF-α), which in turn stimulate CRH secretion in the hypothalamus. CRH activates the HPA axis, whose final product, cortisol, suppresses the production of cytokines and of other cytokines engaged in T proliferation and activation (i.e., TH1 cytokines: IL-2, interferon[IFN]-γ). Glucocorticoids not only dampen this specific arm of the immune system, but act as fine and powerful modulators of cellular immunity by specifically dampening pro-inflammatory and TH1 responses, seemigly leaving unaltered TH2-type responses (i.e., antibody production) (Munck and Guyre, 1986). Glucocorticoids enhance and favor the expression of certain cytokine receptors (e.g., IL-1R, IL-2R, IL-4R, IL-6R) at the molecular level by means of glucocorticoid-induced expression of signaling molecules common to several cytokine receptors (e.g., gp130), and increased concentrations of these specific receptors contribute to containing the circulating form of the cytokines that they are in the process of suppressing. That is to say, glucocorticoids act in a specific manner to induce a net cytokine imbalance, a shift in the TH1/TH2 ratio, and a shift in immune surveillance.

Structural and/or functional alterations in adrenal glands, and thuis in glucocorticoids production, have been reported in HIV/AIDS. Most patients with AIDS have elevated basal plasma cortisol levels with abnormal circadian rhythm irrespective of accompanying symptoms of adrenal insufficiency (Bhansali et al, 2000). As noted, only a small subset of HIV-seropositive patients meet criteria for adrenal insufficiency following a short ACTH stimulation test. Baseline and stimulated levels of cortisol generally correlate inversely with ACTH levels in HIV-seropositive patients without symptoms of adrenal insufficiency (Pearson $r = -0.57$, $p<.05$), but this relationship is lost in their cohorts with symptoms of adrenal insufficiency ($r=0.14$). The 24-hour urinary free cortisol levels are similar in both groups, but correlated strongly with baseline and stimulated serum cortisol levels in HIV-seropositive patients with symptoms of adrenal insufficiency (Pearson $r = 0.8$ and $r = 0.9$, respectively, $p < .002$) (Stolarczyk et al, 1998).

Patients with HIV/AIDS who maintain normal cortisol levels, however, such as those in our study (*vide infra*) tend to exhibit an overall clinical symptomatology compatible with glucocorticoid hypersensitivity of the immune system, such as suppression of the innate and the adaptive arms of cellular immunity. The latter could derive from the glucocorticoid-induced inhibition of cytokine networks regulating innate and TH1-driven cellular immunity, as noted above. Indeed, the HIV-1 protein Vpr has glucocorticoid receptor co-activator activity, potently increases the sensitivity of glucocorticoid target tissues to cortisol, and may contribute to the suppression of cellular immune responses in HIV/AIDS. Under experimental conditions, Vpr protein *in vitro* potentiated in a dose-dependent manner glucocorticoid-induced suppression of both mRNA expression and secretion of IL-12 subunit p35 and IL-12 holo-protein, but not IL-12 subunit p40 or IL-10, by normal human monocytes/macrophages stimulated with lipopolysaccharide (LPS) or by heat-killed, formalin-fixed *Staphylococcus aureus* (Cowan strain 1). These outcomes can be blocked by the glucocorticoid antagonist, RU-486 (Mirani et al, 2002).

The neuroendocrine system in general and the HPA axis in particular shows a circadian pattern dependent on the rest-activity/sleep-wake cycle. Immune effectors (e.g., cytokines) appear to be regulated in the same way. These temporal organizations have functional implications for the regulation of psychoneuroendocrine-immune events. The periodicity of ACTH and cortisol levels correlates directly with the active period both in diurnal and in nocturnal animals. Cerebrospinal fluid levels of CRH and pro-inflammatory cytokines present diurnal variations, with higher levels in the evening and lowest levels early in the morning in a pattern opposite to that of plasma cortisol levels (Prolo et al, 2002). Detailed circadian studies are required in the next decade to understand fully human neuroendocrine-immune functions in health and in disease, and more specifically in HIV/AIDS. Multiple evaluation points need to be included in the examination, under rigorous study conditions to establish plasma hormone concentrations, and, through the use of deconvolution methods, to characterize secretion rates, and to assess sequence-dependent patterns. Analyses will produce detailed assessment of parameters such as approximate entropy to quantify the orderliness of sequential measures, such as hormonal and cytokine time series in patients with HIV/AIDS vs. controls (Prolo et al, 2004).

The role of pro-inflammatory cytokines on sleep in health and in HIV/AIDS also remains to be elucidated (Prolo et al, 2004). It has been proposed that subjects with HIV show a sleep behavior similar to that of older subjects, due to their rapid immunosenescence. Aging is associated with 24-h increase of IL-6, with a phase advance of the IL-6 circadian wave (Figure 1) over that of cortisol by 3–5 h, thus suggesting an increasing over-activity of the HPA axis with increasing age, the latter finding being consistent with a previous report in middle-aged patients with early-untreated rheumatoid arthritis (Chrousos et al, 1993). Since higher IL-6 levels are significant correlated with risk of sudden death, this finding may imply that autoimmune diseases may accelerate the senescence process of the immune system (Singh et al, 2002; Luc et al, 2003), as was noted for βE above. The extent to which these observations pertain to the neuroimmunopathology of HIV/AIDS will be fully elucidated in the coming years.

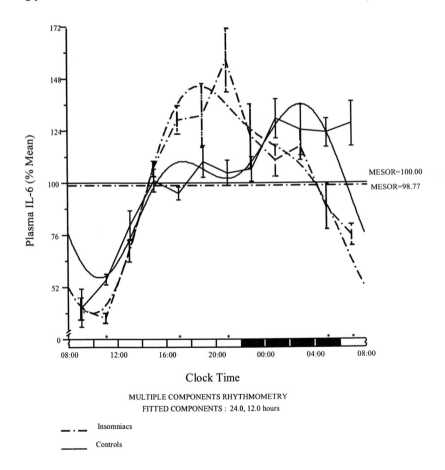

Figure 1. Multiple-component (fitted components: 24 and 12 hours) cosinor analysis of 24-hour plasma IL-6 in insomniacs (dotted line) and controls (solid line) expressed as percent variation from the mean. The thick black line on the abscissa represents the sleep-recording period. MESOR, mid-line estimating statistic of rhythm or rhythm-adjusted mean. *p < .05 (adapted from Fig.2 in Vgontzas et al, 1999).

Despite its somnogenic properties, IL-6 administration or elevation of its endogenous levels result in sleep disturbance when associated with HPA axis activation (Vgontzas et al, 1999). The association of IL-6 and cortisol with wake time is stronger in old adults than in the young subjects. Middle-aged men show increased vulnerability of sleep to stress hormones, compared with the young (Vgontzas et al, 2001, 2003). Changes in sleep physiology associated with aging, including elevations of sleep-disturbing hormones and increased sensitivity of the sleep-controlling target organ to the actions of these hormones, play a significant role in the marked increase of insomnia prevalence with aging. IL-6 peripheral levels correlate negatively with sex steroids levels, positively with the amount of adipose tissue, are decreased after a restful night of sleep, and are elevated in chronic pain/inflammatory syndromes (Irwin, 2002).

Whole saliva collected from normal subjects, with no oral pathology or periodontal disease, every two hours for 24 hours demonstrated for the first time in saliva a circadian pattern for a broad range of cytokines (i.e.e, pro-inflammatory, TH1, TH2, chemochines). The pattern was similar, albeit distinct to that observed in plasma (Figures 2a-2c). At present, we cannot confirm in saliva the observation we made in plasma of a biphasic circadian pattern of IL-6 secretion (Vgontzas et al., 1999).

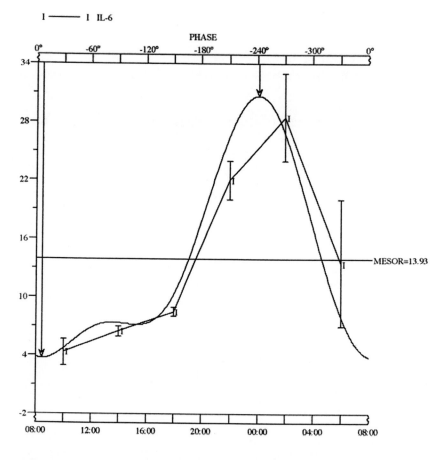

Figure 2a. Whole Saliva Circadian Pattern of IL-6 (representative Normal Health Subjects Healthy 35-years Old Male Subject)

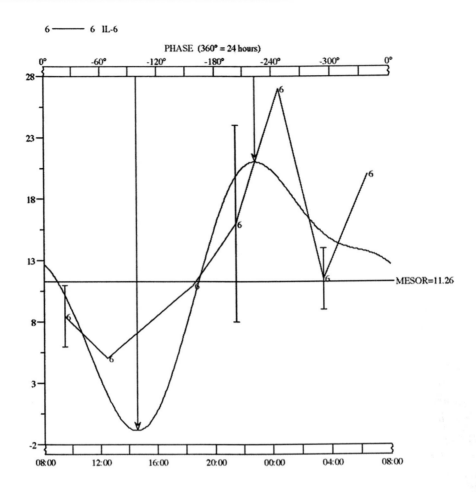

Figure 2b. Whole Saliva Circadian Pattern of IL-6 (representative Normal Health Subjects Healthy 70-years Old Male Subject).

Common complications in HIV/AIDS include peripheral neuropathy, which can be a source of sleep disturbance, as noted above, and exacerbate fatigue symptoms, which in turn could affect long-term survival. For example, certain cytokines (e.g., TNF-α) alter sleep architecture, sleep deprivation alters neuroendocrine and immune responses, immune system activation and neuroendocrine responses alter sleep, and sleep quality appears to affect the course of and susceptibility to HIV/AIDS (Sciolla, 1995). Research needs to confirm these findings, and the observations that psychological distress may impact upon the immune system through its effects on sleep quality (Cruess et al, 2003).

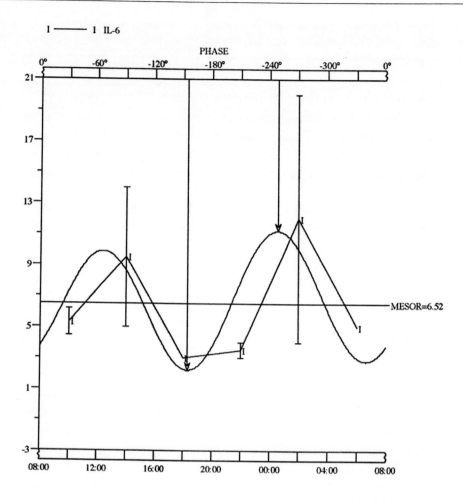

Figure 2c. Whole Saliva Circadian Pattern of IL-6 (representative Normal Health Subjects Healthy 20-years Old Female Subject).

A variety of hormonal and metabolic disturbances arise following HIV infection, the most important of which is the wasting syndrome (i.e., cachexia, a form of hypercatabolic metabolism and depletion of lean body mass attributed to the action of TNFα among other cytokines) associated with progressive HIV infection. Weight loss, and, more specifically, wasting, is a major problem in the care of patients with AIDS, contributing to the morbidity and mortality of the disease. The weight loss associated with HIV infection consists of two components: acute weight loss, resulting primarily from acute secondary opportunistic infections, and chronic weight loss. Wasting has prognostic importance because death generally occurs when patients reach 66% of ideal body weight, similar to the degree of weight loss at which death occurs due to simple starvation. Although fat stores are preferentially depleted during starvation, loss of body cell mass (muscle and viscera) with relatively less fat loss is more common in HIV/AIDS. Anorexia and reduced caloric intake during episodes of opportunistic infection contribute to wasting. Anorexia, in and of it self is a complex disease that is characterized by a variety of neuroendocrine disorders (Chiappelli and Trignani, 1994).

In Anorexia nervosa, dysfunction of the pituitary-thyroid axis is common, but in HIV/AIDS overt clinical or biochemical thyroid dysfunctions are rare. When present, thyroid failure generally results from the destruction of the thyroid gland by opportunistic infections such as *Pneumocystis carinii*, or tumoral processes such as Kaposi sarcoma. Contrary to what is observed in severe non-thyroidal illnesses, the low T3 syndrome and the sick euthyroid syndrome are not marked, and become notable principally in the final stage of AIDS. Hypothyroid-like regulation of the pituitary-thyroid axis, possibly directed to limit hypermetabolism in HIV infection, occurs, suggesting that particular thyroid profiles of clinical importance (e.g., T3, rT3, T3/rT3) may emerge as specific markers and reliable indicators of the progression of HIV infection to AIDS (Lambert, 1994; Koutkia et al, 2002).

Infiltration of endocrine tissue by secondary infectious or malignant processes is not a rare underlying cause of hormonal insufficiency in HIV/AIDS. Case in point is the viral infiltration in the gonads (e.g., testes), and consequential hypothalamic-pituitary-gonadal deregulation. HIV viral DNA is found in 5-20% of spermatogonia and spermatocytes. Testicular infection is reportedly more common with cylomegalovirus, *Mycobacterium avium-intracellulare, Toxoplasma gondii,* or tuberculosis, in association with HIV. Clinical signs of hypogonadism or gonadal pathology, while relatively common in HIV/AIDS, are nonspecific. They are manifested as decreased libido, erectile dysfunction, gynecomastia, and muscle wasting. Low serum testosterone levels, reported in 35-40% of HIV-seropositive asymptomatic patients, tends to rise as the disease progresses to AIDS, where over 50% of the patients typically have serum testosterone and pituitary gonatropin levels below normal (Dobs et al, 1988; Croxson et al, 1989). Decreased serum testosterone may result before substantial loss of lean body mass (e.g., 10% of baseline weight), decreased bone density, psychological changes, and sexual dysfunction occur. Interventions directed at raising serum testosterone levels to supra-physiological doses can increase the perception of quality of life in asymptomatic to HIV-seropositive (Rabkin et al, 1995), but their efficacy and safety remains to be established.

In general terms, endocrine hypofunction in HIV/AIDS is more often than not secondary to the well-known effects of severe illness, which is typically manifested as a significant alterations in the ratio between cortisol and dihydroepiandrosterone (DHEA) (Chiappelli et al, 1994). Changes in cortisol:DHEA ratio and serum IFNγ levels are closely associated with clinical evolution and atherogenic lipid alterations in HIV-associated lipodystrophy (Christeff et al, 2002).

Ongoing analyses reveal that cortisol serum levels between HIV-seropositive (n=85) and HIV-seropositive patients (n=281) are not statistically significantly different (24.85±9.90 μg/dl and 24.51±11.23 μg/dl, respectively). Whereas the serum levels of DHEA drops among HIV-seropositive (median: 39.95 ng/ml), compared to the HIV-seronegative cohorts (median: 50.38 ng/ml), this decrease is not significant. The cortisol/DHEA ratio increases over two-fold, HIV-seropositive, compared to HIV-seronegative individuals (0.77±0.53), a statistically significant rise (Wilcoxon, p=0.015).

Whereas DHEA serum levels significantly correlates with the percent and the number of circulating lymphocytes, and particularly CD4+ T cells (r=0.76, r=0.92, r=0.87, respectively, p<0.05), these relationships are lost among HIV-seropositive patients. The strong positive relationship between DHEA serum levels and the percent and the number of T cells that express the homing receptor for the peripheral lymph node, CD62L, which is statistically significant (r=0.81, r=0.93, respectively, p<0.05) among HIV-seronegative individuals, is all be lost among HIV-seropositive patients (r=-0.20, r=-0.05, respectively). The notable correlation between the cortisol/DHEA ratio and the ratio of CD62L+/CD62L- T cells in HIV-seronegative subjects (r=0.94, p<0.05) disappears among HIV-seropositive patients (r=-0.01).

The percent of CD62L+ T cells drops significantly in the HIV-seropositive patients (18.31$\pm$12.0), compared to their HIV-seronegative cohorts (28.08$\pm$13.04, t test, p<0.0001). By contrast, the 1.13-fold rise in CD62L+/CD62L- ratio among HIV-seropositive patients, compared to HIV-seronegative subjects is not statistically significant. There is a significant drop in naïve helper T cells (CD4+CD45RA+) in HIV-seropositive (9.46+7.89), compared to HIV-seronegative control subjects (13.47+7.81, t test, p<0.0001). The feeble, albeit significant correlation between this cell population and the cortisol/DHEA ratio in HIV-seronegative individuals (r=0.53, p<0.05) is unremarkable among HIV-seropositive patients (r=0.10), as is the correlation between cortisol levels and any cellular immune marker tested in either group (Chiappelli et al, unpubl. obs).

Taken together, these preliminary analyses indicate that a statistically significant relationship exists between the neuroendocrine and the cellular immune system in normal healthy individuals, which vanishes in HIV/AIDS. Research must now be crafted to distinguish the neuroendocrine-immune pathology in asymptomatic HIV disease and in AIDS. One approach might be to stratify the HIV-seropositive sample along the variable of the CD4/CD8 ratio. Neopterin values are found to be within the normal range, albeit rising in HIV-seropositive patients with a CD4/CD8 ratio greater than 0.5 (4.1 mg/ml$\pm$0.67), but rise sharply as CD4/CD8 ratio fall below 0.5 (9.13 mg/ml$\pm$1.6, t test, p=0.007). The overall inverse correlation between the drop in CD4/CD8 ratio and the rise in neopterin serum levels in HIV-seropositive patients is in fact significant (r=-0.81, p<0.05). The association between the drop in CD4/CD8 ratio and the percent of circulating CD4+ cells in that groups is also significant (r=0.88, p<0.05). The drop in %CD4+ cells is usually significantly sharper in patients whose CD4/CD8 ratio is less than 0.5 (35.53$\pm$6.9 vs. 13.68$\pm$9.1, t test, p=0.03), compared to their cohorts whose CD4?CD8 remains steady above 0.5. Cortisol serum levels do not appreciably change during the course of HIV disease, but the cortisol/DHEA ratio drops significantly (p=0.04) when the CD4/CD8 falls below 0.5. The inverse correlation between the cortisol/DHEA ratio and serum neopterin is suggestive, albeit weak (r=-0.70). The percent of T cells endowed with the marker CD62L drops significantly as the CD4/CD8 ratio falls below the 0.5 mark (25.4$\pm$3.1 and 10.7$\pm$5.9, respectively, t test, p=0.02) (Figure 3).

The percent of naïve CD4+ T cells (CD4+CD45RA+) is also significantly decreased as the CD4/CD8 ratio falls below the 0.5 mark (12.9$\pm$1.9 and 5.8$\pm$3.5, respectively, t test, p=0.03). The pattern of disappearance of CD62L+ cells and of CD45RA+ cells strongly overlaps (r=0.996, p<0.05), in a relationship that is best represented by a polynomial equation (Figure 4). The figure confirms that naïve CD4+ T cells largely overlap with T cell endowed with the ability to migrate to the peripheral lymph node, and it is not surprising that the drop in either of these cell populations shows a strong inverse correlation with the rise in serum neopterin (r=-0.985, p<0.05). A somewhat more discrete direct relationship is revealed with the drop in CD4/CD8 ratio, and weak association with the drop in Cortisol/DHEA ratio (r=0.643) (Chiappelli et al, unpub. obs).

Taken together, these data suggest that neither serum cortisol levels, nor the cortisol/DHEA ratio, which are indices of neuroendocrine-immune interaction in HIV-seronegative subjects, retain any association with cellular immune markers during progression of HIV disease to AIDS. This observation, if proven true in subsequent studies and analyses, may point to a critical aspect of HIV/AIDS: that is, the disruption of physiological important interactions and interconnections between the endocrine and the immune systems, specifically between the glucocorticoid regulatory system and T cell-mediated cellular immunity.

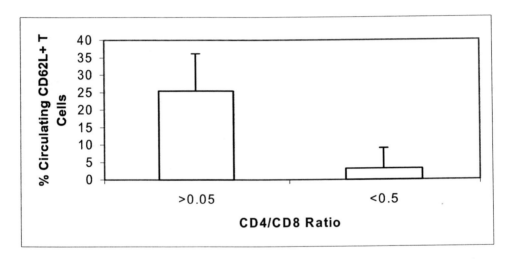

Figure 3. Drop in CD62L+ T Cells as a Function of CD4/CD8 Ration in HIV-Seropositive Subjects.

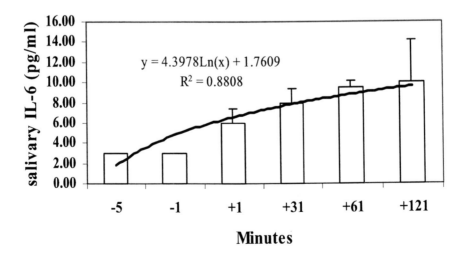

Figure 4. Simultaneous Disappearance of CD62L+ T Cells and Naive T Cells (CD4+CD45RA+) in HIV-seropositive Subjects.

4. Future Directions

The lines of evidence we have presented in this chapter converge to suggest that stress research and HIV/AIDS research are intertwined. Psychobiological manifestations in HIV/AIDS evidently pertain to the same domain of mind-body interactions, which are elucidated in psychoneuroimmunology research. The recent advances in our understanding of the adaptation of the organism to stressful challenges, the allostatic process, presents therefore a new and rich paradigm for research in the psychobiology of HIV/AIDS. Moreover, the dichotomy of Type I and Type II allostatic response provides a theoretical model for the development of novel and improved modes of intervention to treat HIV infection and AIDS.

Three fundamentally distinct challenge stimuli are currently employed in psychobiological research on stress. Psycho-cognitive stimuli include psycho-emotional trauma, which are common in social psychology research but tend to fall in disfavor with medical ethics committees, intellectual challenges (e.g., mental arithmetic, speech delivery), and cognitive dissonance stimuli. The Stoop color-word interference test is an example of the latter that has been used as an effective modality for testing the psychoneuroendocrine-immune response in normal middle-age, non-elderly men and women. This experimental protocol can successfully distinguish two groups of responders based on the salivary and plasma cortisol response to the challenge: 40% of participants are typically high-responders, and the bottom 40% of the respondents are low-responders. The group of low-responders characteristically manifest significantly higher salivary and plasma levels of pro-inflammatory cytokines (e.g., IL-6) in response to the challenge, but lower subjective experience of stress, compared to the high-responders. These observations are suggestive that individual variations exist in the response of the psychoneuroendocrine-immune response (Kunz-Ebrecht et al, 2003). One important *caveat* of the Stroop color-word interference test is that color confusion can be inconsistent in certain subgroups of subjects, especially as subjects advance in age. The Stroop test should not to be used for clinical diagnostic purposes (e.g., diagnosis of HIV/AIDS-related dementia), but rather limited as an experimental tool (Fisher et al, 1990). Cognizant that depression is often part of the psychopathology in HIV/AIDS (*vide supra*), we initiated a study aimed at comparing patients with major depression, as determined by SCID criteria, with age-, sex- and ethnicity-matched control subjects for the response on the Stroop test. Analyses indicate that the median Raw Color-Word score is 20% higher in the control, compared to the depressed subjects (p < 0.05). The median Predicted Interference score based on Color and Word scores is indistinguishable among normal and depressed subjects. However, and confirming the literature (Benoit et al, 1992), our data indicate substantial differences in percentile position of the median T scores: 66% percentile (depressed patients) vs. 42% percentile (normal control subjects) (Iribarren, et al, unpub obs).

A related test, albeit not as widely used in the domain of allostatic research to date is the mirror-tracing challenge, which involves reproducing a pattern by looking at its mirror reflection. Early data indicate attenuated norepinephrine as well as ACTH and cortisol responses to this challenge, as well as to the speech delivery challenge test in asymptomatic HIV-seropositive patients (Kumar et al, 2002).

Physical challenges (e.g., cold pressor test challenge) is another commonly used, simple, rapid and inexpensive, easy-to-perform, and widely recognized experimental stress stimulus in human allostasis studies. The physiological mechanism underlying the response this challenge (i.e., immersion of the non-dominant hand in an ice-bath) involves a response temperature in the form of constriction to blood flow of both superficial and deep tissues of the hand, and consequential strong perception of pain. The cold pressor test is an adequate model to study psychobiological responses to stressful discomfort because cold-induced vasospasms are frequently present in syndromes of chronic pain and chronic stress (Lapossy et al., 1994). The cold pressor test has been used successfully in a variety of experimental models, including elucidating characteristics of endocrine responses in patients with chronic pain. The measure of pain latency (e.g., length of time of hand immersion), is typically significantly shorter in patients with fibromyalgia and secondary concomitant fibromyalgia, for example, compared to healthy control subjects (Carli et al, 2002). One *caveat* of this test lies in the fact that it generates cold-induced vasospasms, which may have adverse effects in subjects with cardio-vascular dysfunctions, a condition that is not uncommon in advanced AIDS. We have demonstrated that HIV induces significant pathology to cardiomyocytes (Gujuluva et al, 2001). Early studies have shown that patients with HIV/AIDS manifest a blunted response in norepinephrine, ACTH and cortisol to the cold-pressor test (Kumar et al, 2002), which may be congruent with the occurrence of autonomic neurophathies observed in HIV/AIDS infection (Freeman et al., 1990).

These observations, taken together with the data cited above on investigations on mirror-star tracing and speech challenges, suggest an alternative interpretation, because they converge by independent mechanisms to support that the neuroendocrine responses are compromised in HIV/AIDS infection. The possibility must also be considered that the attenuated response to the cold pressor challenge may be a consequence of altered pain perception in HIV/AIDS attributable to peripheral neuropathy. The hypothesis has been proposed that these allostatic findings could also be viewed from the perspective that HIV auxiliary protein, vpr, can interact with glucocorticoid receptors (Kino et al., 1999), and that a sequence of pre-gag region in HIV-1 genome has close homology with the sequence in the POMC-promoter region (Licinio et al, 1995). Since HPA axis activity impacts cytokines such as IL-6, and based on our observation that the response to the cold-pressor test includes a significant, time-bound, gender-dependent (response in women significantly higher than in men, $p < 0.05$) 5-7 fold rise in salivary IL-6 levels (Figure 5), these findings appear very important in understanding the CNS pathogenesis in HIV/AIDS.

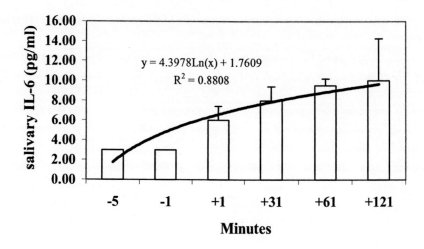

Figure 5. Pattern of Salivary IL-6 Response to the Cold Pressor Challenge in Normal Control Subjects.

This line of research has become all the more significant since recent studies show that highly potent antiretroviral therapies (HAART) may also induce metabolic disorders (Carr et al, 1998), sufficiently powerful to alter the corstisol/DHEA ratio. HAART has changed the problem of HIV/AIDS from one that strikes with severity and quickly leads to death to a process of slow, chronic cognitive decline. Whereas the incidence of NeuroAIDS has dropped, its prevalence among asymptomatic HIV-seropositive patients has increased (Kandanearatchi et al, 2003; McArthur et al, 2003). The clinical manifestations have now evolved from a subacute dementing disease to a more protracted disorder, characterized by decreased resident brain activated myeloid cells (CD14+CD69+), more subtle CNS, neaural and neuroendocrine toxicity associated with changes in neural cell signaling, structural and functional proteins (Kusdra et al, 2002). These effects are likely translated at the level of neural and neuroendocrine modulation of systemic and local immunity since immunological data indicate that HIV infection brings about a sharp drop of peripheral blood CD4+ lymphocytes, which cannot be accounted solely on HIV-mediated CD4+ cell death. The disappearance of CD4+ lymphocytes from the blood compartment in HIV-seropositive patients results from enhanced migration out of the blood, and homing to extravascular tissues, including the brain parenchyma. The increased CD4+ lymphocyte homing rates in HIV-seropositive subjects returns to normal levels, however, following HAART (Chen et al, 2002). Migratory leukocytes can transmit HIV to both T lymphocytes and non-T cells that had previously crossed the endothelial barrier, such as the BBB. Furthermore, these cells can subsequently reverse-migrate out of perivascular reservoirs carrying HIV back across the barrier, thus disseminating HIV (Birdsall et al, 2002). Cytokines are critical to this process: IL-15 stimulates HIV-infected monocytes to produce IL-8, for example, which specifically attract neutrophils and monocytes to inflammation sites and thus favors immune surveillance to pathogens in HIV infection. IL-15 production by peripheral blood mononuclear cells is significantly blunted in HAART-naïve patients. HIV-seropositive patients responsive to HAART showed IL-15 production comparable to that of healthy donors. (D'Ettore et al, 2002). The extent to which HAART alters the circardian pattern of IL-15 and IL-8 has not been elucidated as of yet. HAART also minimizes the oral manifestations of HIV/AIDS, but the effect of HAART on local immunity in the stoma (e.g., salivary cytokines) remains to be examined.

In the initial reports of HIV infection oral candidiasis was described as one of the earliest signs of immunologic dysfunction (Gottilieb et al, 1981; Masur et al, 1981). It was soon recognized that due to progressive immunologic suppression HIV-seropositive patients were at increased risk of developing serious opportunistic infections and neoplasms many of which having their earliest manifestations in the oral cavity. In addition, it was shown that deterioration in the local oral immune responses and changes in the salivary flow rate and composition may facilitate the development of periodontal disease, caries, tooth demineralization and altered sensation all of which leading to compromised masticatory functions and nutrition (EC-Clearinghouse 1993; Navazesh et al, 1993; Younai et al, 2001; Patton et al, 1999). It is important to note that many oral lesions described in association with HIV/AIDS do occur outside of the context of HIV, but many are seen in higher frequency in association with HIV than not and are highly suggestive of HIV infection in undiagnosed in individuals (Shiboski et al, 1994; Ficcara et al, 1994; Feigal et al, 1991).

Oral manifestations can be used for HIV staging and classification (CDC 1993; WHO 1990; Redfield 1986), as predictors of disease progression (Maden et al, 1994, Dodd et al, 1991, Klein et al, 1984), and as indicators of HIV viral load (Younai et al, 2001; Patton et al, 1999; Baqui et al, 1999). After more than two decades since the onset of the HIV pandemic, major disparities in accessing optimal medical care still exist across national standards. In countries where most HIV-positive patients have access to highly active or some form of antiretroviral therapy, the prevalence rates for many types of HIV-related oral manifestations have been reduced (Pinheiro et al, 2004; Nicolatou and Galitis 2004; Patton et al, 2000; Eyeson et al, 2000). By contrast, reports published from countries where access to HIV-specific drugs is not universally available indicate much higher frequencies for oral lesions (Myburgh et al, 2004; Reichart et al, 2003). The variations in the level of HIV care implicate different diagnostic roles for HIV-related oral pathologies depending on the region. In high risk communities, discovering HIV-related oral pathologies may be indicative of undiagnosed and untreated HIV infection while in the presence of appropriate anti-HIV treatments, detection of oral lesions may be indicative of therapeutic failure and immunologic deterioration.

HIV-related oral manifestations are broadly categorized into bacterial, fungal and viral infections, ulcerative conditions and neoplasms:

• Many types of bacterial infections such as *Mycobacterium avium intracellulare, Klebsiella pneumoniae, Enterobacterium cloacae* and Actinomycosis have been described in the oral cavity of HIV infected patients (Greenspan et al, 1990). Periodontal manifestations are considered the most common bacterial infections in this patient population (EC-Clearinghouse 1993). Although conventional gingivitis and periodontitis are common findings among HIV-positive patients, as they are in non-infected patients, HIV-specific periodontal conditions have also been characterized. They range from early gingival manifestations such as Linear Gingival Erythema (LGE, used to be called HIV-G) and Necrotizing Ulcerative Gingivitis (NUG), to more advanced presentations Necrotizing Ulcerative Periodontitis (NUP, used to be called HIV-P) and Necrotizing

Stomatitis (NS). LGE presents as a fiery red band along the margin of gingiva and is most likely related to infections with *Candida* species (Velegraki et al, 1999; Odden et al, 1994; Moore et al, 1993). NUG involves necrosis and destruction of one or more dental papillae, whereas NUP and NS extend beyond the papillae and lead to the exposure of the underlying bone (EC-Clearinghouse 1993).

- Herpes viruses that routinely shed into the oral cavity have increased pathogenic potential in immunosuppressed individuals and are associated with Oral Hairy Leukolpakia (OHL), Kaposi's Sarcoma (KS) and many HIV-associated ulcerations and lymphomas. In addition, human papilloma virus (HPV)-related lesions may be seen in HIV infection. OHL has been described in immunologic deficiency states related to HIV infection (Greenspan et al, 1984), renal and bone marrow transplantation (Greenspan et al, 1989; Epstein et al, 1988), cytotoxic therapy of leukemia (Syrjänen, 1989), and other immunologic dysfunctions (Schiødt et al, 1995). The presence of OHL in an otherwise healthy individual may be attributed to HIV infection or a defect in cell mediated immunity (CDC, 1993). Lesions of OHL appear as asymptomatic, bilateral, corrugated keratotic areas predominantly found on the lateral borders of the tongue; they may present with a flat surface and may also be observed in oral mucosal locations other than the tongue (Kabani et al, 1989). OHL has been reported to resolve with HIV therapies (Phelan et al, 1988). KS is a multifocal vascular neoplasm seen in advanced HIV disease and AIDS. An HHV8-related malignancy, KS is seen as red, blue, or dark purple flat macules in the early stages; lesions become lobulated and ulcerated as the disease progresses (Ficarra et al, 1988). Localized intraoral lesions may be treated with intralesional injections of sclerotic solutions or alpha interferon (American Academy of Oral Medicine, 2001, Sulis et al, 1989). The development of non-Hodgkin's lymphomas (NHL) increases by 60 folds in HIV infection (Beral et al, 1991) and is currently seen in higher frequencies in Africa and Asia compared to the US (reviewed by Patton et al, 2002). Lymphomas seen in association with HIV infection tend to be aggressive and high-grade presenting as a nodular mass enlarging quickly and destroying the underlying bone (Epstein et al, 1992; Piluso et al, 1994). Their medical management requires combination chemotherapy and local radiation therapy with a poor cure rate. Several HPV related lesions have been described in association with HIV infection, Verruca Vulgaris, Condyloma Accuminatum and Focal Epithelaial Hyperplasia (Greenspan et al, 1990). Treatment of these lesions include, surgical excision, laser removal, topical cauterizing agents and interferon injections (American Academy of Oral Medicine, 2001). In the era of effective anti-HIV treatment a significant increase in the prevalence rates of HPV-related lesions have been reported (Greenspan et al, 2001).
- Many deep fungal infections such as Cryptococcosis and Histoplasmosis may have intraoral involvement. Penicilliosis marneffei has recently been reported with dramatically higher frequencies in South-East Asia (for review Patton et al, 2002). Infection with *Candidia albicans* remain the most common HIV-related oral fungal infection that continues to exist even with anti-HIV treatment. Saliva has many antifungal activities that may be altered by HIV infection (for review Younai et al, 2001). They include presence of IgA antibodies (Müller et al, 1991; Sweet et al, 1995) Mucins and Thrombospondin (Bergy et al, 1993; Malamud et al, 1993; Crombie et al, 1998), as

well as several soluble inhibitors such as lysozyme, lactoferrin, defensins (Nakashima et al, 1993; Yamaguchi et al, 1993), and the "secretory leukocyte protease inhibitor (SLPI)" (Mc Neeley et al, 1995). It is possible that qualitative and quantitative alterations in saliva during HIV infection are responsible for alterations in oral defense mechanisms that ordinarily prevent mucosal adherence and colonization by *Candida* species. There are several different clinical variants of oral candidiasis ranging from yellowish pseudomembranous lesions to white plaques to atrophic and erythematous mucosa. The widespread use of antifungal agents for both prevention and treatment of oral candidiasis, especially Fluconazole, has led to the development of fungal resistance complicating the clinical management of this infection.

- Early identification and treatment of oral ulcers in HIV infected patients is crucial to improving quality of life and restoring optimal functions. Other than many viral and bacterial infections and neoplasms that can manifest as an oral ulcer, Aphthous Stomatitis is considered an immune-mediated ulcerative condition seen associated with HIV infection (Phelan et al, 1991). These ulcers are classified based on their appearance, size and clinical course and require treatment only if they interfere with patient's normal functions. Treatment may include palliative care, application of topical antibiotics, corticosteroid compounds, or systemic Thalidomide (American Academy of Oral Medicine, 2001, Rosenstein et al, 1991, Sokol-Anderson et al, 1991;Glick et al, 1992; Youle et al, 1989; Ryan et al, 1992).

- Dry mouth may be a significant finding during the course of HIV infection. The term HIV-related salivary gland disease (HIV-SGD) is used to designate diffuse enlargement of salivary glands and/or xerostomia, both reported to occur in association with HIV infection (Schiødt et al, 1987, 1992). It is estimated that 5% of adult HIV positive patients develop bilateral salivary gland enlargement while 10-30% develop xerostomia (Younai, 2001; Silverman et al, 1986). Recent reports indicate an increase in the prevalence rates of HIV-SGD and xerostomia (Patton et al, 1999) related to HIV infection or medication use (Younai, 2001; Valentine et al, 1992; Dodd et al, 1992). Careful clinical examination is crucial to the diagnosis and management of xerostomia in HIV positive patients.

The third principal mode to test the allostatic response utilizes physiological stimuli (e.g., immune challenge, experimental manipulation of the HPA axis). For example, the dexamethasone-suppression test (DST) is widely used in neuroendocrine and neuroendocrine-immune research to study the functional response of the HPA and of the psychoneuroendocrine-immune response. Administration of 1-5 mg of DEX to normal subjects in the evening (2300 h) results in a flattened cortisol plasma level the following morning and day. The cortisol suppression response is an indication of DEX-sensitivity and normal HPA response. Significant changes in the migratory properties of circulating CD4+ T cells occur in DEX-sensitive control subjects (Chiappelli et al, 1991). The DST challenge can monitor experimentally the allostatic response in a variety of patient populations. In DEX-resistant (i.e., no cortisol suppression following DST) patients with Anorexia nervosa, the migratory properties of circulating CD4+ T cells are not altered (Chiappelli et al, 1991). PTSD has been associated with lower concentrations of cortisol and enhanced suppression of cortisol by DEX following the DST challenge, although discrepancies exist among reports. Neither low basal CORT nor enhanced suppression of CORT are consistent markers of a PTSD diagnosis. This observation is not unique to PTSD: patients with Major Depression and patients with Alzheimer's disease, for example, also stratify along two principal groups: DST suppressors and DST non-suppressors (Iribarren et al, 2004), which prevents the use of the DST as a diagnostic test, but not as an exquisitely useful experimental tool to better understand neuroendocrine-immune interactions in a variety of patient populations (Chiappelli and Trignani, 1994).

Another *caveat* of this protocol is that it provides a static challenge to the HPA axis: it leads to a shut-off, albeit temporarily, of the HPA flux by acting on its feedback system. In that respect it presents a reflection of the regulatory response, rather than of the HPA potential *per se*, as, for example the CRH stimulation test does. Because of the intimate nature of the relationship between neuroendocrine and immune products, it can also be said that the DST challenge is a static challenge of psychoneuroendocrine-immune responses. DST has been used to define and to characterize the fundamental physiological interactions and neuroendocrine-immune pathology in HIV/AIDS (Catania et al, 1990, 1992, 1993). Ovine CRH stimulation of the HPA axis has revealed that about 25% of HIV-seropositive patients with no clinical evidence of AIDS or pituitary or adrenal disease manifest reduced pituitary reserve with high basal ACTH and cortisol, vs. about 25% with reduced adrenal reserve with high basal cortisol and inappropriately normal basal ACTH. The remaining 50% maintain normal HPA axis activity with increased basal cortisol secretion (Azar and Melby, 1993). These observation must be revisited in light of the high- and low-responders characterization of responders to the Stroop test cited above (Kunz-Ebrecht et al, 2003), including consideration of cellular immune changes consequential to these challenges

In conclusion future studies aimed at characterizing the allostatic response in HIV/AIDS will open novel modes of treatment interventions for HIV-seropositive and AIDS patients. Clinical research in HIV/AIDS requires the stringent, rigorous and systematic approach provided by evidence-based medicine. Evidence-based research medicine goes beyond the routine narrative literature review. It systematically evaluates the strength of the available evidence, and generates a consensus statement of the best available evidence in the form of a systematic review of the available research.

The future of clinical and translational research in HIV/AIDS lies in the systematic evaluation of the research evidence in treatment intervention for the patients. This type of "research on research" endeavor requires attentive library search of the published materials (e.g., clinical trials) and informal individual communications with the individual researchers and authors. The collected evidence is then evaluated for research quality along certain standards (e.g., the consolidated standards of randomized trials [CONSORT]), and by means of validated instruments (e.g., Timmer scale, Jadad scale, Wong scale) (Chiappelli et al, 2004b).

The data from separate reports are pooled, when appropriate, for meta-analysis, meta-regression, and Individual Patient Data analyses. The data are analyzed from the perspective of Bayesian modeling in order to interpret data from research in the context of external evidence and judgments (Chiappelli et al, 2004b).

In the context of the treatment of patients with HIV/AIDS and co-morbidities, it is important and timely to generate a systematic review of the clinical research evidence for joint and simultaneous treatment of HIV/AIDS and the co-morbidities, vs. a staggered approach. The summative evaluation of the outcome of such a systematic review will generate a consensus statement that will establish whether or not the problem was framed in a clinically relevant manner (e.g., were the patient population, predictor variables and outcome measures clearly identified, and relevant to the treatment of HIV/AIDS and its co-morbidities within the confines of the research). The statement must discuss the validity of the process of integration (e.g., were the prospective inclusion and exclusion criteria clearly identified, was the search comprehensive and explicitly described, was the validity of the individual studies adequately assessed, was the process of study selection, searching, assessing validity and data abstraction reliable). The statement also produces evidence about the rigor of the process by which information was integrated (e.g., was the individual studies sufficiently similar to warrant their combination in an over-arching hypothesis-driven analysis, are the summary finding representative of the largest and most rigorously performed studies). The quality, presentation, and relevance of the findings must be discussed (e.g., are the key elements of each study clearly displayed, is the magnitude of the findings statistically significant, are the findings homogeneous or heterogeneous, are sensitivity analyses presented and discussed, do the findings suggest and overall net benefit for patients with HIV infection of AIDS). This concerted, systematic and scientific-process driven mode of evaluating current treatment interventions for subjects with HIV/AIDS is timely and urgent to insure that the medical establishment will be prepared to handle the fast-approaching wave of HIV seropositivity and AIDS cases in the next decade.

This method-driven approach to the evaluation of clinical data has the merit that its product, the consensus statement, also generates a cost-effectiveness analysis (i.e., a process of decision analysis that incorporates cost), for example, by a step approach similar as above to assess a) if the problem was framed in a clinically relevant manner, b) the validity of information integrated, c) the rigor of process of integration, and c) the presentation and quality of the findings. The relevant findings in this cost-effectiveness analysis are usually expressed as the incremental cost-effectiveness between joint and simultaneous treatment of HIV/AIDS and its co-morbidities, vs. a staggered approach. The incremental cost-effectiveness ratio, that is the difference in costs between the two strategies divided by the difference in effectiveness between the two strategies are often presented as well.

The consensus statement evaluates each competitive strategy, usually by means of the Markov model-based decision tree. This approach permits to model events that may occur in the future as a direct effect of treatment or as a side effect. The model produces a decision tree that cycles over fixed intervals in time, and incorporates probabilities of occurrence. Even if the difference between the two treatment strategies appears quantitatively small, the Markov model outcome reflects the optimal clinical decision, because it is based on the best possible values for probabilities and utilities incorporated in the tree. The outcome produced of the Markov decision analysis is generally obtained by means of the sensitivity analysis to test the stability over a range probability estimates, and thus reflects the most rational treatment choice.

In the context of psychobiology and allostasis, Rose et al (2003) have established by means of a systematic review of the literature, for instance, that the early optimism about brief early psychological interventions, including debriefing, appear unfounded and not supported by the research evidence. Our current systematic research aimed at comparing self-hypnosis and music therapy, vs. mindful meditation for general anxiety (Lee et al, 2004), by contrast supports the promising observations that a multimodal cognitive-behavioral stress management intervention on anxious mood, perceived stress, 24-hr urinary catecholamine levels, and changes in T-lymphocyte subpopulations over time in asymptomatic HIV-seropositive patients (Antoni et al, 2000).

Considering the present research trends, it is reasonable to predict that future evidence-based research in HIV/AIDS will increasingly examine the domain of the psychobiology and the allostatic response in HIV/AIDS. This should insure the development and testing of novel or improved treatment interventions for HIV-seropositive and AIDS patients based on a holistic, mind-body interaction perspective.

Acknowledgements

This work was supported in part by the Diagnostic Product Co., the Amgen Co., the John D. and Catherine T. MacArthur Foundation, the Kettering Foundation, The Alzheimer's Association, the Harbor-UCLA Research and Education Institute, the UCLA Norman Cousins Program on Psychoneuroimmunology, the UCLA Center for the Interdisciplinary Study of Immunological Diseases, the UCLA School of Dentistry, and the National Institutes of Health (AI 07126; CA16042, DA07683, DA10442), as well as the "AIDS Project" of the Istituto Superiore di Sanita', Italy. The authors thank the students and laboratory assistants who have contributed to the data presented here throughout the years, and in a special manner Drs. PL Meroni and P Sacerdote for their valuable suggestions and help. The authors thank Mr. Greg Dobie for early contributions to a preliminary draft of the manuscript.

References

Ader R, Cohen N. Behaviorally conditioned immunosuppression. *Psychosom. Med.* 1975, 37: 333–40.

American Academy of Oral Medicine, Clinician's Guide to HIV-infected patients 2001.

Antoni MH, Cruess DG, Cruess S, Lutgendorf S, Kumar M, Ironson G, Klimas N, Fletcher MA, Schneiderman N. Cognitive-behavioral stress management intervention effects on anxiety, 24-hr urinary norepinephrine output, and T-cytotoxic/suppressor cells over time among symptomatic HIV-infected gay men. *J. Consult. Clin. Psychol.* 2000 68:31-45.

Antoni MH. Stress management effects on psychological, endocrinological, and immune functioning in men with HIV infection: empirical support for a psychoneuroimmunological model. *Stress.* 2003, ;6:173-88.

Ayers JR. The quagmire of HIV/AIDS related issues which haunt the Church. *J. Pastoral. Care.* 1995 49:201-10.

Azar ST, Melby JC. Hypothalamic-pituitary-adrenal function in non-AIDS patients with advanced HIV infection. *Am. J. Med. Sci.* 1993 305:321-5.

Baker S. HIV/AIDS, nurses, and the black church: a case study. *J. Assoc. Nurses. AIDS Care.* 1999, 10:71-9.

Baqui AAMA, Meiller TF, Habra-Rizk MA et al. Association of HIV viral load with oral diseases. *Oral. Dis.* 1999; 5:294-8.

Barak O, Weidenfeld J, Goshen I, Ben-Hur T, Taylor AN, Yirmiya R. Intracerebral HIV-1 glycoprotein 120 produces sickness behavior and pituitary-adrenal activation in rats: role of prostaglandins. *Brain Behav. Immun.* 2002 6:720-35.

Barcellini W, Sacerdote P, Borghi MO, Rizzardi GP, Fain C, De Giuli Morghen C, Manfredi B, Lazzarin A, Meroni PL, and Panerai AE. Beta-endorphin content in HIV-infected HuT78 cell line and in peripheral lymphocytes from HIV-positive subjects. *Peptides.* 1994 15:769-75.

Bhansali A, Dash RJ, Sud A, Bhadada S, Sehgal S, Sharma BR. A preliminary report on basal and stimulated plasma cortisol in patients with acquired immunodeficiency syndrome. *Indian J. Med. Res.* 2000 112:173-7.

Bhasin S, Singh AB, Javanbakht M. Neuroendocrine abnormalities associated with HIV infection. *Endocrinol. Metab. Clin. North. Am.* 2001 30:749-64,

Benoit G, Fortin L, Lémelin S, Laplante L, Thomas J, EverettJ. L'attention sélective dans la depression majeure: Ralentissement clinique et inhibition cognitive. *Can. J. Psychol.* 1992 46:41-52.

Bergy EJ, Cho MI, Mammarskjold ML. Aggregation of human immunodeficiency virus type 1 by human salivary secretions. *Crit. Rev. Oral. Bio. Med.* 1993 4:467-74.

Beral V, Peterman T, Berkleman R, et al. AIDS_associated non-hodgkin's lymphoma. *Lancet* 1991 337:805-9.

Biglino A, Limone P, Forno B, Pollono A, Cariti G, Molinatti GM, Gioannini. Altered adrenocorticotropin and cortisol response to corticotropin-releasing hormone in HIV-1 infection. *Eur. J. Endocrinol.* 1995 133:173-9.

Birdsall HH, Siwak EB, Trial J, Rodriguez-Barradas M, White AC Jr, Wietgrefe S, Rossen RD. Transendothelial migration of leukocytes carrying infectious HIV-1: an indicator of adverse prognosis. *AIDS.* 2002 16:5-12.

Black B. HIV/AIDS and the Church: Kenyan religious leaders become partners in prevention. *Aidscaptions.* 1997, 4:23-6.

Bouten M. Sharing the pain: response of the churches in Papua New Guinea to the AIDS pandemic. *P. N. G. Med. J.* 1996 39:220-4.

Carli G Suman AL Biasi G Marcolongo R. Reactivity to superficial and deep stimuli in patients with chronic musculoskeletal pain. *Pain* 2002 100 259-69.

Carr A, Samaras K, Chisholm D, Cooper DA. Pathogenesis of HIV-1-protease inhibitor-associated peripheral lipodystrophy, hyperlipidaemia, and insulin resistance. *Lancet* 1998, 351:1881-3.

Catania A, Manfredi MG, Airaghi L, Vivirito MC, Milazzo F, Zanussi C. Evidence for an impairment of the immune-adrenal circuit in patients with acquired immunodeficiency syndrome. *Horm. Metab. Res.* 1990 22:597-8.

Catania A, Manfredi MG, Airaghi L, Vivirito MC, Milazzo F, Lipton JM, Zanussi C. Delayed cortisol response to antigenic challenge in patients with acquired immunodeficiency syndrome. *Ann. N. Y. Acad. Sci.* 1992 650:202-4.

Catania A, Airaghi L, Manfredi MG, Vivirito MC, Milazzo F, Lipton JM, Zanussi C. Proopiomelanocortin-derived peptides and cytokines: relations in patients with acquired immunodeficiency syndrome. *Clin. Immunol. Immunopathol.* 1993 66:73-9.

Catania A, Manfredi MG, Airaghi L, Vivirito MC, Capetti A, Milazzo F, Lipton JM, Zanussi C. Plasma concentration of cytokine antagonists in patients with HIV infection. *Neuroimmunomodulat.* 1994, 1:42-9.

Centers for Disease Control. 1993 revised classification system for HIV infection and expanded case definition for AIDS among adolescents and adults. *Morb. Mort. Weekly Rep.* 1993; 41 (RR-17):1-19.

Chen JJ, Huang J, Shirtliff M, Briscoe E, Ali S, Cesani F, Paar D, Cloyd MW. Transendothelial migration of leukocytes carrying infectious HIV-1: an indicator of adverse prognosis. *AIDS.* 2002 16:5-12.

Chiappelli F. Immunophysiological role and clinical implications of non-immunoglobulin soluble products of immune effector cells. *Adv. Neuroimmunol,* 1991, 1:234-40.

Chiappelli F, Yamashita N, Faisal M, Kemeny M, Bullington R, Nguyen L, Clement LT, Fahey JL. Differential effect of β-endorphin on three human cytotoxic cell populations. *Int. J. Immunopharmacol,* 1991, 13:291-7.

Chiappelli F, Kavelaars A, Heijnen CJ. β-endorphin effects on membrane transduction in human lymphocytes. *Ann. N.Y. .Acad. Scien,* 1992, 650:211-7.

Chiappelli F Trignani S. Neuroendocrine-immune interactions: implications for clinical research. In: *Primary and secondary eating disorders: A psychoneuroendocrine and metabolic approach.* E Ferrari, F Brambilla, SB Solerte eds. 1994; Pergamon Press, London: PP. 185-198.

Chiappelli F, Prolo P, Cajulis E, Harper S, Sunga E, Concepcion E. Consciousness, emotional self-regulation, and the psychosomatic network: Relevance to Oral Biology and Medicine. In *Consciousness, Emotional Self-regulation and the Brain*; M. Beauregard, Ed. Advances in Consciousness Research, John Benjamins Publishing Company, 2004a; Chapter 9, pp. 253-74.

Chiappelli F, Prolo P, Negoatis N, Lee A, Milkus V, Bedair D, Delgodei S, Concepcion E, Crowe J, Termeie D, Webster R. Tools and Methods for Evidence-Based Research in Dental Practice: Preparing the Future. *J. Eviden. Based Dent. Pract,* 2004b 4:16-23.

Chiappelli F, Cajulis OS. Psychobiological views on "stress-related oral ulcers". *Quintess. Intern,* 2004, 35:223-7.

Chrousos GP. Gold PW. The concepts of stress and stress system disorders. Overview of physical and behavioral homeostasis. *JAMA,* 1992, 267:1244-52.

Cole SW, Kemeny ME, Taylor SE. Social identity and physical health: Accelerated HIV progression in rejection-sensitive gay men. *J. Person Social Psychol.* 1997, 72:32-35.

Cole S, Kemeny M, Fahey J, Zack J, Naliboff B.Psychological risk factors for HIV pathogenesis: Mediation by the autonomic nervous system. *Biol. Psychiat.* 2003 54:1444-56.

Christeff N, De Truchis P, Melchior JC, Perronne C, Gougeon ML. Longitudinal evolution of HIV-1-associated lipodystrophy is correlated to serum cortisol:DHEA ratio and IFN-alpha. *Eur. J. Clin. Invest.* 2002 32:775-84.

Chrousos GA, Kattah JC, Beck RW, Cleary PA and the Optic Neuritis Study Group. Side effects of glucocorticoid treatment. *JAMA* 1993 269:2110-2.

Crombie R, Silverstein RL, et al. Identification of a CD36-related thrombospondin 1-binding domain in HIV-1 envelope glycoprotein gp120: relationship to HIV-1 specific inhibitory factors in human saliva. *J. Exp. Med.* 1998 198:25-35.

Croxson TS, Chapman WE, Miller LK, Levit CD, Senie R, Zumoff B. Changes in the hypothalamic-pituitary-gonadal axis in human immunodeficiency virus-infected homosexual men. *J. Clin. Endocrinol. Metab.* 1989 68:317-21.

Cruess DG, Antoni MH, Gonzalez J, Fletcher MA, Klimas N, Duran R, Ironson G, Schneiderman N. Sleep disturbance mediates the association between psychological distress and immune status among HIV-positive men and women on combination antiretroviral therapy. *J. Psychosom. Res.* 2003 54:185-9.

d'Ettorre G, Forcina G, Lichtner M, Mengoni F, D'Agostino C, Massetti AP, Mastroianni CM, Vullo V. Interleukin-15 in HIV infection: immunological and virological interactions in antiretroviral-naive and -treated patients. *AIDS.* 2002 16:181-8.

Dobs AS, Dempsey MA, Ladenson PW, Polk BF. Endocrine disorders in men infected with human immunodeficiency virus. *Am. J. Med.* 1988 84:611-6.

Dodd CL, Greenspan D, Katz MH et al. Oral candidiasis in HIV infection: pseudomembranous and erythematous candidiasis show similar rates of progression to AIDS. *AIDS* 1991 5:1339-43.

Dodd CL, Greenspan D, Westhouse JL et al. Xerostomia associated with didanosine [letter]. *Lancet* 1992 340:790.

EC-Clearinghouse on Oral Problems Related to HIV Infection. WHO Collaborating Centre on Oral Manifestations of the Human Immunodeficiency Virus. Classification and diagnostic criteria for oral lesions in HIV infection. *J. Oral. Path. Med.* 1993; 22:289-291.

Engle GL. A unified concept of health and disease. *Persp. Biol. Medicine.* 1960, 3:459-85.

Epstein JB, Priddy RW, Sherlock CH. Hairy leukoplakia-like lesions in immunosuppressed patients following bone marrow transplantation. *Transplantation* 1988 46: 462-4.

Epstein JB, Silverman Jr. S. Head and neck malignancy associated with HIV infection. *Oral Surg, Oral. Med, Oral. Pathol.* 1992 73:193-200.

Eyeson JD, Warnakulasuriya K, Johnson NW. Prevalence and incidence of oral lesions- the changing scene. *Oral. Dis.* 2000 6:367-273.

Feigal DW, Katz MH, Greenspan D et al. The Prevalence of oral lesions in HIV-infected homosexual and bisexual men: three San Francisco epidemiologic cohorts. *AIDS* 1991; 5:519-25.

Feligioni M, Raiteri L, Pattarini R, Grilli M, Bruzzone S, Cavazzani P, Raiteri M, Pittaluga A. The human immunodeficiency virus-1 protein Tat and its discrete fragments evoke selective release of acetylcholine from human and rat cerebrocortical terminals through species-specific mechanisms. *J. Neurosci.* 2003 Jul 30;23(17):6810-8.

Ficarra G, Berson AM, Silverman S, Quivey JM, Lozada-Nur F, Sooy DD, Migliorati CA. Kaposi's sarcoma of the oral cavity: A study of 134 patients with a review of the pathogenesis, epidemiology, clinical aspects and treatment. *Oral Surg, Oral. Med, Oral Pathol.* 1988 66: 543-50.

Ficcara G, Chiodo M, Morfini M et al. Oral lesions among HIV-infected hemophiliacs. A study of 54 patients. *Haematologica.* 1994 79:148-53.

Fisher LM, Freed DM, Corkin S. Stroop Color-Word Test performance in patients with Alzheimer's disease. *J. Clin. Exp. Neuropsychol.* 1990 12:745-58.

Freeman R, Roberts MS, Friedman LS, Broadridge C. Autonomic function and human immunodeficiency virus infection *Neurol.* 1990, 40:575-80.

Futterman, AD, Kemeny, ME, Shapiro, D and Fahey, JL. Immunological and physiological changes associated with induced positive and negative moods. *Psychosom. Medicine,* 1994, 56:499-511.

Gesch D Bernhardt O Kirbschus A. Association of malocclusion and functional occlusion with tempomandibular disorders (TMD) in adults: A systematic review of population-based studies. *Quintessence Int.* 2004 35: 211-21.

Glick M, Muzyka BC. Alternate therapies for major aphthous ulcers in AIDS patients. *J. Am. Dent. Assoc.* 1992 123:61-5.

Gottilieb MS, Schroff R, Schauber HM, et al.. Pneumocystis carinii pneumonia and mucosal candidiasis in previously healthy homosexual men. *N Engl J Med.* 1981 305: 1425-31.

Green G. Social support and HIV. *AIDS Care.* 1993, 5:87-104.

Greenspan D, Schiødt M, Greenspan JS, et al. *AIDS and the mouth: Diagnosis and management of oral lesions, 1990.* Chicago: Mosby Year Book, Inc

Greenspan, D, Greenspan JS, Conant M, et al. Oral hairy leukoplakia in male homosexuals: Evidence of association with both papillomavirus and a herpes-group virus. *Lancet* 1984 3: 831-4.

Greenspan D, Greenspan JS, DeSouza YG, et al. Oral hairy leukoplakia in an HIV-negative renal transplant recipient. *J. Oral Pathol. Med.* 1989; 18: 32-4.

Greenspan D, Canchola AJ, MacPhail LA, Cheikh B, Greenspan JJ. Effect of highly active antiretroviral therapy on frequency of oral warts. *Lancet* 2001 357:1411-2.

Gilguin J, Weiss L, Kazatchkine MD. Genital and oral erosions induced by foscarnet. *Lancet* 1990 335: 287.

Gujuluva C, Burns AR, Pushkarsky T, Popik W, Berger O, Bukrinsky M, Graves MC, Fiala M. HIV-1 penetrates coronary artery endothelial cells by transcytosis. *Mol. Med.* 2001 7:169-76

Gustafson DH, Hawkins RP, Boberg EW, Bricker E, Pingree S, Chan CL. The use and impact of a computer-based support system for people living with AIDS and HIV infection. *Proc. Annu. Symp. Comput. Appl. Med. Care.* 1994, 604-8.

Hinkle LE Jr. Human ecology and psychosomatic medicine. *Psychosom. Med.* 1967; 29: 391–5.

Iribarren J, Prolo P, Neagos N, Chiappelli F. Post-Traumatic Stress Disorder: Research in the Third Millennium. *Evidence-Based Complementary and Alternative Medicine,* 2004 (In press, pending revisions)

Irwin M. Effects of sleep and sleep loss on immunity and cytokines. *Brain Behav. Immun.* 2002 16:503-12.

Jones M. Olafson K. Del Bigio MR. Peeling J. Nath A. Intraventricular injection of human immunodeficiency virus type 1 (HIV-1) Tat protein causes inflammation, gliosis, apoptosis, and ventricular enlargement. *J. Neuropathol. Exp. Neurol.* 1998 57:563-70.

Kabani S, Greenspan D, DeSouza Y, et al. Oral hairy leukoplakia with extensive oral mucosal involvement. *Oral Surg, Oral Med, Oral Pathol.* 1989 67:411-5.

Kandanearatchi A, Williams B, Everall IP. Assessing the efficacy of highly active antiretroviral therapy in the brain. *Brain. Pathol.* 2003 13:104-10.

Katz MH, Greenspan D, Westenhouse J. Progression to AIDS in HIV infected homosexual and bisexual men with hairy leukoplakia and oral candidiasis. *AIDS* 1992 6: 95-100.

Kiecolt-Glaser JK, McGuire L, Robles TF, Glaser R. Psychoneuroimmunology and psychosomatic medicine: back to the future. *Psychosom. Medicine,* 2002, 64:15-28.

Kino T, Gragerov A, Kopp JB, Stauber RH, Pavlakis GN, Chrousos GP. The HIV-1 virion-associated protein vpr is a coactivator of the human glucocorticoid receptor. *J. Expt. Med.* 1999, 189:51-62.

Klein RS, Harris CA, Small CR et al. Oral candidiasis in high-risk patients as the initial manifestation of acquired immunodeficiency syndrome. *N. Eng. J. Med.* 1984: 311:354-8.

Koutkia P, Mylonakis E, Levin RM. Human immunodeficiency virus infection and the thyroid. *Thyroid.* 2002 12:577-82.

Koutkia P, Canavan B, Breu J, Johnson ML, Depaoli A, Grinspoon SK. Relation of leptin pulse dynamics to fat distribution in HIV-infected patients. *Am. J. Clin. Nutr.* 2004 79:1103-9.

Kumar M, Kumar AM, Waldrop D, Antoni MH, Schneiderman N, Eisdorfer C. The HPA axis in HIV-1 infection. *J. Acquir. Immune. Defic. Syndr.* 2002 31S:89-93.

Kunz-Ebrecht SR, Mohamed-Ali V, Feldman PJ, Kirschbaum C, Steptoe A. Cortisol responses to mild psychological stress are inversely associated with proinflammatory cytokines. *Brain Behav. Imm.* 2003 17:373-83.

Kusdra L, McGuire D, Pulliam L. Changes in monocyte/macrophage neurotoxicity in the era of HAART: implications for HIV-associated dementia. *AIDS.* 2002 16:31-8.

Liu NQ, Lossinsky AS, Popik W, Li X, Gujuluva C, Kriederman

Lambert M. Thyroid dysfunction in HIV infection. *Baillieres Clin. Endocrinol. Metab.* 1994 8:825-35.

Lapossy E Glasser P Hrycaj P Dubler B Samborski W Muller W. Cold induced vasospasm in patients with fibromyalgia and and chronic low back pain in comparison to healthy subjects. *Clin. Rheumatol.* 1994 13:442-5.

Licinio J, Gold PW, Wong ML. A molecular mechanism for stress-induced alterations in susceptibility to disease. *Lancet* 1995, 346:104-6.

Lee A, Prolo P, Cruz Rosenblum M, Neagos N, Chiappelli F. Does Mindfulness Meditation Stress Reduction and Music Therapy Work in Dentistry? – A Systematic Evaluation of the Literature by Means of an Evidence-Based Research Approach. 2004 American Association of Public Health Dentistry and Association of State and Territorial Dental Directors National Oral Health Conference, May 3-5, 2004, Los Angeles , CA

Lo R. The use of prayer in spiritual care. *Aust. J. Holist. Nurs.* 2003, 10:22-9.

Lo R, Brown R. Holistic care and spirituality: potential for increasing spiritual dimensions of nursing. *Aust. J. Holist. Nurs.* 1999, 6:4-9.

Luc G, Bard JM, Juhan-Vague I, Ferrieres J, Evans A, Amouyel P, Arveiler D, Fruchart JC, Ducimetiere P. PRIME Study Group. C-reactive protein, interleukin-6, and fibrinogen as predictors of coronary heart disease: the PRIME Study. *Arterioscler. Thromb. Vasc. Biol.* 2003 23:1255-61.

Lupien SJ, McEwen BS. The acute effects of corticosteroids on cognition: integration of animal and human model studies. *Brain Res. Brain Res. Rev.* 1997, 24:1-27.

Lutgendorf SK, Costanzo ES. Psychoneuroimmunology and health psychology: An integrative model. *Brain Behav. Immunity.* 2003, 17:225-32.

Maden C, Hopkins SG, Lafferty WE. Progression to AIDS or death following diagnosis with a Class IV non-AIDS disease: utilization of a surveillance database. *J. Acquir. Immune. Def. Syndr.* 1994 7:972-7

Maekawa K Twu C Lotaif A Chiappelli F Clark GT. Function of β-Adrenergic receptors on mononuclear cells in female patients with fibromyalgia. *J. Rheumatol.* 2003 30:364-8.

Malamud D, Davis C, Berthold P, et al. Human submandibular saliva aggregates HIV. *AIDS Res. Human Retro. Vir.* 1993 9:633-7.

Manfredi B, Sacerdote P, Bianchi M, Locatelli L, Veljic-Radulovic J, and Panerai AE. Evidence for an opioid inhibitory effect on T cell proliferation. *J. Neuroimmunol.* 1993 44:43-8.

Manfredi B, Clementi E, Sacerdote P, Bassetti M, and Panerai AE. Age related changes in mitogen induced ß-endorphin release from human peripheral blood mononuclear cells. *Peptides* 1995 16:699-706.

Mason JW. Organization of psychoendocrine mechanisms. *Psychosom. Med.* 1968 30S): 565–808.

Masur H, Michelis MA, Greene JB, et al. An outbreak of community-acquired Pneumocystis carinii pneumonia: Initial manifestation of cellular immune dysfunction. *N. Engl. J. Med.* 1981 305: 1431-8.

McArthur JC, Haughey N, Gartner S, Conant K, Pardo C, Nath A, Sacktor N. Human immunodeficiency virus-associated dementia: an evolving disease. *J. Neurovirol.* 2003 9:205-21

McCarthy GM. Host factors associated with HIV related oral candidiasis. A review. *Oral Surg, Oral Med, Oral. Pathol.* 1992 73:181-6.

McEwen B, Wingfield JC. The concept of allostasis in biology and biomedicine. *Hormones Behav.* 2003, 43:2-15.

McNeely MC, Yarchoan R, Broder S, et al. Dermat0ologic complications associated with administration of 2', 3'-dideoxycytidine in patients with human immunodeficiency virus infection. *J. Acad. Dermatol.* 1989 21:1213-7.

Mc Neeley TB, Dealy M, et al. Secretory Leukocyte Protease Inhibitor: A human saliva protein exhibiting anti-HIV activity in vitro. *Clin. Invest.* 1995 96:456-64.

Mirani M, Elenkov I, Volpi S, Hiroi N, Chrousos GP, Kino T. HIV-1 protein Vpr suppresses IL-12 production from human monocytes by enhancing glucocorticoid action: potential implications of Vpr coactivator activity for the innate and cellular immunity deficits observed in HIV-1 infection. *J. Immunol.* 2002 169:6361-8.

Mirsattari, S. M., Power, C., Nath, A. 1998. Parkinsonism with HIV infection. *Mov. Disord.* 13:684-9.

Moore LVH, Moore WEC, Riley C, et al. Periodontal microflora Of HIV positive subjects with gingivitis or adult periodontitis. *J. Periodontol.* 1993; 64:48-56.

Mulder CL. Psychosocial correlates and the effects of behavioral interventions on the course of human immunodeficiency virus infection in homosexual men. *Patient. Educ. Couns.* 1994, 24:237-47.

Müller F, Frøland SS, et al. Both Ig A subclasses are reduced in parotid saliva in patients with *AIDS.Clin. Exp. Immunol.* 1991 91:83:203.

Munck A, Guyre PM. Glucocorticoid physiology, pharmacology and stress. *Adv. Exp. Med. Biol*, 1986, 196:81-96.

Myburgh NG, Hobdell MH, Lalloo R. African countries propose a regional oral health strategy: The Dakar Report from 1998. *Oral Dis.* 2004 10:129-37.

Myers ABR. *On the etiology and prevalence of diseases of the heart among soldiers.* London, J. Churchill, 1870.

Nakashima H, Yamatmoto N, et al. Defensins inhibit HIV replication in vitro. *AIDS* 1993 7:1129.

Naidu S. Differing religious views on the AIDS epidemic. *Posit. Outlook.* 1997 4:28-9.

Narayanasamy A. Spiritual coping mechanisms in chronically ill patients. *Br. J. Nurs.* 2002, 11:1461-70.

Nath, A., Haughey, N. J., Jones, M., Anderson, C., Bell, J. E., Geiger, J. D. Synergistic neurotoxicity by human immunodeficiency virus proteins Tat and gp120: protection by memantine. *Ann. Neurol.* 2000, 47:186-94.

Nath A, Jones M, Maragos W, Booze RM, Mactutus C, Bell J, Mattson M. Neurotoxicity and Dysfunction of Dopaminergic Systems Associated with AIDS Dementia. *J. Psychopharmacology.* 2004, In Press

Navazesh M, Mulligan R, Barron Y, Redford M, Greenspan D, Alves M, Phelan J; Women's Interagency HIV Study participants. A 4-year longitudinal evaluation of xerostomia and salivary gland hypofunction in the Women's Interagency HIV Study participants. *Oral Surg, Oral Med, Oral Pathol, Oral Radiol, Endod.* 2003 95:693-8

Nicolatou-Galitis O, Velegraki A, Paikos S, Economopoulou P, Stefaniotis T, Papanikolaou IS, Kordossis T. Effect of PI-HAART on the prevalence of oral lesions in HIV-1 infected patients. A Greek study. *Oral Dis.* 2004 10:145-50.

Nowak MD D, Peesapati MD SK, Jeet MD A, Moktan MD S, Kudej MD M, Martin-Naar MD MA, Trauber MD D, Renedo MD MF. Serum leptin concentration in patients infected with human immunodeficiency virus. *Endocr. Pract.* 1999, 5:124-8.

Odden K, Schenck K, Koppang HS, et al. Candidal infection in the gingiva of HIV-infcted persons. *J. Oral Pathol. Med* 1994: 23:178-83.

Panerai AE, Manfredi B, Granucci F, and Sacerdote P. The beta-endorphin inhibition of mitogen-induced splenocytes proliferation is mediated by central and peripheral paracrine/autocrine. *J. Neuroimmunol.* 1995 58:71-76.

Panerai AE, Sacerdote P. β-Endorphin in the immune system: a role at last? *Immunol. Today.* 1997 18: 317-9.

Patel T, Park SH, Lin L, Chiappelli F, Huang GT-J. Substance P induces interleukin-8 production from human dental pulp cells. *Oral Surgery, Oral Medicine, Oral Pathology, Oral Radiology, and Endodontics*, 2003, 96:478-85.

Patton LL, McKaig R, Eron JJ Jr. et al. Oral hairy leukoplakia and oral candidiasis as predictors of HIV viral load. *IADS* 1999 13:2174-5

Patton LL, McKaig R, Strauss R, Rogers D, Eron JJ Jr. Changing prevalence of oral manifestations of human immunodeficiency virus in the era of protease inhibitor therapy. *Oral Surg, Oral Med, Oral Pathol, Oral Radiol, Endod.* 2000 89:299-304.

Patton LL, Phelan JA, Ramos-Gomez FJ, et al. Prevalence and classification of HIV-associated oral lesions. *Oral Dis.* 2002 8S:98-109.

Phelan JA, Saltzman BR, Friedland GH, et al. Oral findings in patients with acquired immunodeficiency syndrome. *Oral Surg, Oral Med, Oral Pathol.* 1987 64:50-6.

Phelan, JA, Klein RS. Resolution of oral hairy leukoplakia during treatment with azidothymidine. *Oral Surg, Oral Med, Oral Pathol.* 1988 65:717-20

Phelan JA, Eisig S, Freedman PD, et al. Major aphthous-like ulcers in patients with AIDS. *Oral Surg, Oral Med, Oral Pathol.* 1991 71:68-72.

Penneys NS, Hick B. Unusual cutaneous lesions associated with acquired immune deficiency syndrome. *J. Am. Acad. Dermatol.* 1985 13: 845-52.

Piluso S, Di Lollo S, Baroni G, Leoncini F, Gaglioti D, Saccardi A,Ficcara G. Unusual clinical aspects of oral Non-H odgkins Lymphomas in patients with HIV infection. *Oral Oncol, Eur. J. Cancer.* 1994 30B:61-4.

Pinheiro A, Marcenes W, Zakrzewska JM, Robinson PG. Dental and oral lesions in HIV infected patients: a study in Brazil. *Int. Dent. J.* 2004 54:131-7.

Pollack JJ, Santarpia RP, Heller HM, et al. Determination of salivary anticandidal activities in healthy adults and patients with AIDS: a pilot study. *J. Acq. Immun. Def. Syn.* 1992 5:610-8.

Prolo P, Wong M-L, Licinio J. Molecules in focus: leptin. *Int J Biochem Cell Biol* 1998 30:1285-90.

Prolo P, Chiappelli F, Fiorucci A, Dovio A, Sartori ML, Angeli A. Psychoneuroimmunology: New avenues of research for the 21st Century. *Ann. N.Y. Acad. Scien*, 2002, 966:400-8.

Prolo P. Iribarren J. Neagos N, Chiappelli F. Role of pro-inflammatory cytokines in sleep disorders. In *Neuroendocrine Correlates of Sleep and Wakefulness.* S.R. Pandi-Perumal and D.P. Cardinali, Eds. 2004 (in press).

Rabkin JG, Rabkin R, Wagner G. Testosterone replacement therapy in HIV illness. *Gen. Hosp. Psychiat.* 1995 17:37-42.

Redfield RR, Wright DC, Tramont EC. The Walter Reed staging classification for HTLV-III/LAV infection. *N. Eng. J. Med.* 1986 314:131-2

Reichart PA, Khongkhunthian P, Bendick C. Oral manifestations in HIV-infected individuals from Thailand and Cambodia. *Med. Microbiol. Immunol. (Berl).* 2003 192:157-60.

Rose S, Bisson J, Wessely S. A systematic review of single-session psychological interventions ('debriefing') following trauma. *Psychother. Psychosom.* 2003, 72:171-5

Rosenstein DI, Chiodo DT, Bartley MH. Treating recurrent aphthous ulcers in patients with AIDS. *J. Am. Dent. Assoc.* 1991 122:64-8.

Rufman JP. Gastrointestinal Manifestations of AIDS. *Clinics of North America* 1988 17:599-614.

Ryan J, Colman J, Pedersen J, et al Thalidomide to treat esophageal ulcer in AIDS. *New Eng. J. Med.* 1992 16:208.

Sacerdote P, Ruff MR, Pert CB. Vasoactive intestinal peptide 1-12: a ligand for the CD4 (T4)/human immunodeficiency virus receptor. *J. Neurosci. Res.* 1987, 18:102-7

Sacerdote P, Ruff MR, Pert CB. VIP1-12 is a ligand for the CD4/human immunodeficiency virus receptor. *Ann. N. Y. Acad. Sci.* 1988, 527:574-8.

Sacerdote P, Breda M, Barcellini W, Meroni PL, and Panerai AE. Age-related changes of beta-endorphin and cholecystokinin in human rat mononuclear cells. *Peptides* 1991a 12:1353-6.

Sacerdote P, Rubboli F, Locatelli L, Ciciliato IMP, and Panerai AE. Pharmacological modulation of neuropeptides in peripheral mononuclear cells. *J. Neuroimmunol.* 1991b 32:35-4

Sacerdote P, Manfredi B, Bianchi M, and Panerai AE. Intermittent but not continuous inescapable footshock stress affects immune responses and immunocyte beta-endorphin concentrations. *Brain-Behav-Immun.* 1994a 8:251-60.

Sacerdote P, Bianchi M, Manfredi B, and Panerai AE. Intracerebroventricular interleukin-1 alpha increases immunocyte beta-endorphin concentrations in the rat: involvement of corticotrophin-releasing-hormone, catecholamines and serotonin. *Endocrinology.* 1994b 135:1346-52.

Sanders EC 2nd. New insights and interventions: churches uniting to reach the African American community with health information. *J. Health Care Poor. Underserved.* 1997 8:373-5.

Schiødt M, Pindborg JJ. AIDS and the oral cavity. Epidemiology and clinical oral manifestations of human immunodeficiency virus infection: a review. *Int. J. Oral. Maxillofac. Surg.* 1987 16:1-14.

Schiødt M, Dodd CL, Greenspan D, et al. Natural History of HIV-associated salivary gland disease. *Oral Surg, Oral Med, Oral Pathol.* 1992 7:326-31

Schiødt M, Nørgaard T, Greenspan JS. Oral hairy leukoplakia in an HIV-negative woman with Behçet's syndrome. *Oral Surg, Oral Med, Oral Pathol.* 1995 79:53-6.

Schulkin J. Allostasis: a neural behavioral perspective, *Hormones Behav* 2003, 43: 21-27

Schwarzer R, Dunkel-Schetter C, Kemeny M. The multidimensional nature of received social support in gay men at risk of HIV infection and AIDS. *Am. J. Community Psychol.* 1994, 22:319-39.

Sciolla A. Sleep disturbance and HIV disease. *Focus.* 1995 10:1-4.

Scott LV, Dinan TG. Vasopressin and the regulation of hypothalamic-pituitary-adrenal axis function: implications for the pathophysiology of depression. *Life Sci.* 1998, 62:1985-98.

Seligman ME. Learned helplessness. *Annu. Rev. Med.* 1972, 23:407-12.

Shiboski CH, Hilton JF, Greenspan D et al. HIV-related oral manifestations in two cohorts of women in San Francisco. *J. Acquir. Immune. Def. Syndr.* 1994 7:1964-71.

Silverman S Jr., Magliorati CA, Lozada-Nur F, Greenspan D, Conant M. Oral findings in peoples with or at risk for AIDS: a study of 375 homosexual males. *J. Am. Den. Assoc.* 1986 112:415-25.

Singh RB, Kartik C, Otsuka K, Pella D, Pella J. Brain-heart connection and the risk of heart attack. *Biomed. Pharmacother.* 2002, 56S:257-65.

Speransky AD. *Basis for theory in medicine*. International Publisher, New York, 1943.

Sokol-Anderson ML, Prelutsky DJ, Westblom TU. Giant esophageal aphthous ulcers in AIDS patients: treatment with low-dose corticosteroids. *AIDS* 1991 5: 1537-8.

Solomon GF. Psychoneuroimmunology: Interactions between central nervous system and immune system. *J. Neuroscien. Res.* 1987, 18:1-9.

Solomon GF, Moos RH. Emotions, immunity, and disease. *Arch. Gen. Psychiat.* 1964, 11:657-74.

Solomon GF, Ironson GH, Balbin EG. Psychoneuroimmunology and HIV/AIDS. *Ann. N. Y. Acad. Sci.* 2000, 917:500-4.

Solomon S. Religious beliefs and HIV / AIDS / STD health promotion. *AIDS STD. Health. Promot. Exch.* 1996, 5:1-3.

Somlai AM, Heckman TG, Kelly JA, Mulry GW, Multhauf KE. The response of religious congregations to the spiritual needs of people living with HIV/AIDS. *J. Pastoral. Care.* 1997, 51:415-26.

Sterling P and Eyer J. Allostasis: A new paradigm to explain arousal pathology. In: S. Fisher and J. Reason, Editors, *Handbook of Life Stress, Cognition, and Health*, Wiley, New York 1988.

Stolarczyk R, Rubio SI, Smolyar D, Young IS, Poretsky L. Twenty-four-hour urinary free cortisol in patients with acquired immunodeficiency syndrome. *Metabolism.* 1998 47:690-4.

Sulis E, Floris C, Sulis ML, Zurrida S, Piro S, Pintus A, Contu L. Interferon administration intralesionally in skin and oral cavity lesions in heterosexual drug addicted patients with AIDS-related Kaposi's Sarcoma. *Eur. J. Clin. Oncol.* 1989 25:759-61.

Sweet SP, Rahman D, Challacombe. IgA subclasses in HIV disease: dichotomy between raised levels in serum and decreased secretion rates in saliva. *Immunol.* 1995 86:556-9.

Syrjänen S, Laine P, Happonen RP, et al. Oral hairy leukoplakia is not a specific sign of HIV infection but related to suppression in general. *J. Oral Pathol. Med.* 1989; 18: 28-31.

Tesoriero JM, Parisi DM, Sampson S, Foster J, Klein S, Ellemberg C. Faith communities and HIV/AIDS prevention in New York State: results of a statewide survey. *Public Health. Rep.* 2000 15:544-56.

Teoh SK, Mendelson JH, Mello NK, Skupny A. Alcohol effects on naltrexone-induced stimulation of pituitary, adrenal and gonadal hormones during the early luteal phase, *J. Clin. Endocr. Metab.* 1988 66, 1181-6

Valentine C, Deenmamode J, Sherwood R. Xerostomia associated with didanosine. *Lancet* 1992 340:1542-3.

Van Der Merwe LJ, Walsh C, Hattingh Z, Bester I, Veldman D. Serum leptin levels, BMI and fat percentage of HIV positive women (25 - 44 years)in Mangaung, South Africa. *Asia Pac. J. Clin. Nutr.* 2004, 13S:173

Velegraki A, Nicolatou O, Theodoridou M, et al. Psediatric AIDS-related linear gingival Erythema: a form of erythematous candidiasis? *J. Oral Pathol.* 1999; 28:178-82.

Verges B, Chavanet P, Desgres J, Vaillant G, Waldner A, Brun JM, Putelat R. Adrenal function in HIV infected patients. *Acta Endocrinol.* 1989, 121:633-7.

Vgontzas AN, Papanicolaou DA, Bixler EO, Lotsikas A, Zachman K, Kales A, Wong M-L, Licinio J, Prolo P, PW Gold PW, Hermida RC, Mastorakos G, Chrousos GP: Circadian interleukin-6 secretion and quantity and depth of sleep. *J. Clin. Endocrinol. Metabol.* 1999 84:2603-07.

Vgontzas AN, Bixler EO, Lin H-M, Prolo P, Mastorakos G, Vela-Bueno A, Kales A, Chrousos GP 2001 Chronic insomnia is associated with nyctohemeral activation of the hypothalamic-pituitary-adrenal axis: clinical implications. *J. Clin. Endocrinol. Metab.* 2001 86:3787–94.

Vgontzas AN, Zoumakis M, EBixler EO, Lin HM, Prolo P, Vela-Bueno A Kales A, Chrousos GP. Impaired Nighttime Sleep In Healthy Old Vs. Young Adults is Associated with Elevated Plasma IL-6 and Cortisol Levels: Physiologic and Therapeutic Implications. *J. Clin. Endocrinol. Metab.* 2003 88: 2087-95.

Vitillo RJ. The Catholic Church's response to the pandemic of HIV / AIDS. *Child Worldw.* 1993, 20:18-9.

Wong M-L, Webster EL, Spokes H, Phu P, Ehrhart-Bornstein M, Bornstein S, Park C-S, Rice KC, Chrousos GP, Licinio J, Gold PW. Chronic administration of the non-peptide CRH type 1 receptor antagonist Antalarmin does not blunt hypothalamic-pituitary-adrenal axis responses to acute immobilization stress. *Life Sci.*1999, 65:PL53-8.

World Health Organization. Acquired Immunodeficiency Syndrome(AIDS): interim proposal for a WHO staging system for HIV infection and Disease. *Wkly. Epidemiol. Rec.* 1990; 65:221-228.

Wright AN Gatchel RJ Wildenstein L Riggs R Bushang P Elleis III E. Biopsychosocial differences between high-risk and low-risk patients with acute TMD-related pain. *JADA* 2004 135:474-83

Yamaguchi Y, Semmel M, et al. Virucidal effects of glucose oxidase and peroxidase or their protein conjugates on Human Immunodeficiency virus type 1. *Antimicrob. Agents Chemo.* 1993 37:26-31.

Youle M, Clarbour J, Farthing C, et al. Treatment of resistant aphthous ulceration with thalidomide in patients positive for HIV antibody. *British. Med. J.* 1989 298: 432.

Younai FS, Marcus M, Freed JR, et al. Self-reported oral dryness and HIV disease in a national sample of patients receiving medical care. *Oral Surg, Oral Med, Oral Pathol, Oral Radiol, Endodontics.* 2001;92:629-36.

Younai, FS. Oral HIV Transmission. *CDA Journal.* 2001; 29: 142-8.

In: Neuro-AIDS
Editors: A. Minagar and P. Shapshak, pp. 165-184

ISBN: 1-59454-610-X
© 2006 Nova Science Publishers, Inc.

Chapter VII

Cerebrovascular Disease in HIV-Infected Patients

*Alejandro A. Rabinstein**

Department of Neurology, Mayo Clinic College of Medicine
Rochester, MN USA

Abstract

Stroke in patients with human immunodeficiency virus (HIV) infection and advanced immunosuppression are mainly related to opportunistic infections, cardiac embolism from cardiomyopathy, and probably hypercoagulability. High-activity antiretroviral therapy (HAART) may now considerably limit or effectively halt the progression of immunosuppression. However, the use of protease inhibitors is associated with metabolic derangements -including dyslipidemia, lipodystrophy and insulin resistance- that might result in accelerated atherosclerosis. Therefore, patients receiving HAART may be at risk for premature vascular events, such as cerebral infarctions. In addition, a small vessel arteriopathy has been documented in HIV-infected patients and impaired vasomotor reactivity might compromise cerebral perfusion, especially as these patients age. Future studies should examine if the prevalence and mechanisms of stroke in HIV-infected patients change as the use of effective antiviral treatment continues to grow.

Keywords: HIV – Stroke – Cerebral Infarction – Mechanisms – Vasculitis – Hypercoagulability – Atherosclerosis - Hemorrhage

Thanks to the therapeutics applications resulting from indefatigable research, the burden of disease caused by human immunodeficiency virus (HIV) infection has changed dramatically over the last decade. It is fair to say today that the course of HIV infection is

---

* Correspondence concerning this article should be addressed to Alejandro A. Rabinstein, MD 200 First Strret SW, Mayo W8B. Rochester, Minnesota, 55905. Telephone: (507) 538-1036; Fax: (507) 266-4419; E-mail: rabinstein.alejandro@mayo.edu.

primarily determined by where the patient lives. In third-world countries, where access to even rudimentary forms of treatment remains a luxury, AIDS continues to wreak havoc among patients of all ages and strokes may still be mostly the result of opportunistic infections. Conversely, in developed countries, where highly active antiretroviral therapies (HAART) are available, HIV infection has been transformed into a chronic disease. Compliant patients with access to HAART are much less likely to develop cerebrovascular complications from opportunistic infections. Yet, they may be at risk of having stroke and myocardial infarction from accelerated atherosclerosis or other forms of intrinsic vascular disease, either due to the HIV virus itself or to the drugs used for its treatment.

Stroke is both an old foe and a looming threat for HIV-infected patients. It is commonly recognized that immunodepressed HIV-infected patients have increased risk of stroke due to opportunistic co-infections with vascular involvement, greater incidence of dilated cardiomyopathy, and a prothrombotic diathesis. Cocaine and heroine use further augment that risk. More recently, the long-term effects of HIV itself on the cerebral vasculature and the atherogenic potential of new antiretroviral drugs have emerged as growing threats to the HIV population.

Throughout this chapter I will try to provide update information on the relationship between HIV infection and cerebrovascular disease. The role of traditional causes of stroke, infections, and emergent pathophysiological mechanisms will be discussed. But first, it is essential to start by defining the scope of the problem.

The Prevalence of Stroke in HIV Infection: Necropsy Studies and Clinical Series

The prevalence of cerebral infarction has ranged between 6% and 34% (Pinto, 1996; Berger, 1990; Anders, 1986, Mizusawa, 1988; Moskowitz, 1984; Kieburtz, 1993; Connor, 2000; Rosemberg, 1996) in necropsy studies of HIV-infected brains. Pathologic findings have been often considered asymptomatic (Pinto, 1996; Kieburtz, 1993; Connor, 2000). In fact, the rates of stroke-like presentations in different cohorts of patients with HIV infection have not exceeded 5% (Pinto, 1996; Snider, 1983; Koppel, 1985; Berger, 1987; McCarthur, 1987; Engstrom, 1989; Levy, 1988), confirming the subclinical nature of some of the lesions noted on necropsy. Table 1 summarizes the most relevant clinical series and necropsy studies devoted to the evaluation of stroke in the HIV population.

In a comprehensive literature review, Pinto summarized the results of 11 necropsy studies and 6 clinical series of patients evaluated between 1979 and 1990 (Pinto, 1996). Only half of the clinical series were prospective (Snider, 1983; Berger, 1987; McCarthur, 1987), and most lacked control groups. The majority of patients were in advanced stages of the disease, and only 12% of all patients were asymptomatic. Overall, the prevalence of presentation with stroke syndrome was 1.3%. Ischemic infarctions were consistently more common than intracerebral hemorrhages (68% versus 32%), but still the proportion of hemorrhagic events was slightly greater than that observed in the general population given that subarachnoid hemorrhages were excluded from the analysis. Both types of stroke were frequently thought to be caused by underlying HIV-related conditions. Thrombocytopenia, primary CNS lymphoma, and metastatic Kaposi's sarcoma were associated with intracerebral hemorrhages. Concomitant opportunistic infections and nonbacterial thrombotic endocarditis were often identified in patients with cerebral infarction. The author concluded that, given the limitations of the data, it was not clear whether there was an association between AIDS and stroke.

Some studies, however, suggest that HIV-infected patients have an increased risk of stroke. Engstrom et al. retrospectively identified 12 cases of ischemic stroke among 1,600 AIDS patients studied over a 5-year period. The annual risk of stroke in these patients (0.75%) was substantially higher than that expected in the general population younger than 45 years of age (0.025%) (Engstrom, 1989; Grindal, 1978). Yet, one must recognize the caveat that while the risk for HIV patients was defined from a highly selected cohort (cases identified through hospital registries and neuropathological reports), the comparison was made with incidence estimates from the general population.

Case-control studies should be helpful in determining if strokes are actually more frequent in the HIV population. Berger et al (Berger, 1990) compared necropsies from 181 patients dying of complications of AIDS with 111 age-matched patients dying of other conditions between 1983 and 1987. Thirteen subjects (7%) with AIDS had evidence of a stroke within a week of their demise, compared to 25 (23%) in the control group. Among the 10 patients with ischemic strokes, four cases were ascribed to thrombosis, four to cardiac embolism and the remaining two to vasculitis. Cardiac pathology was present in 8/13 AIDS patients with stroke. Opportunistic infections and tumors were very prevalent in this population as well as thrombocytopenia. Conversely, traditional risk factors for atherosclerosis were distinctly uncommon in this young population.

Qureshi et al. conducted a retrospective, case-control study to evaluate the relationship between HIV infection and stroke in young patients from a single large inner-city hospital (Qureshi, 1997). The researchers assessed 236 patients aged 19 to 44 years admitted with a diagnosis of stroke between 1990 and 1994. Serologic HIV status was known in 113 patients, of whom 25 were seropositive (10 had AIDS). The control group consisted of age- and sex-matched patients with known HIV status admitted with the diagnosis of status epilepticus. The results indicated that HIV infection was associated with the occurrence of stroke (odds ratio [OR], 2.3; 95% confidence interval [CI], 1.0-5.3; $P = 0.05$) and particularly with cerebral infarction (OR, 3.4; 95% CI, 1.1-8.9; $P = 0.03$) after adjustment for several cerebrovascular risk factors. Among patients with stroke, cerebral infarction was more frequent in those who were seropositive (80% vs. 56%). In addition, seropositive patients had a higher frequency of cerebral infarction associated with meningitis ($P < 0.001$) and protein S deficiency ($P = 0.06$, NS) compared with the seronegative group. In fact, the association between HIV infection and cerebral infarction was not statistically significant if all cases with meningitis and protein S deficiency were excluded, suggesting that most of the excess risk of stroke in HIV patients could be mediated by these two mechanisms. Strokes of undetermined cause were not more common in the group of HIV-infected patients, in contrast to the findings of previous studies (Levy, 1988; Engstrom, 1989). Unfortunately, the researchers did not provide information about serum lipid levels, antiretroviral regimens used (although PIs had not yet been released when these data were collected), or subtypes of ischemic stroke (the authors only mention, somewhat surprisingly, that no cardioembolic strokes were observed in HIV-infected patients).

Hoffmann et al. found no significant overall increase in stroke rate in their retrospective, case-control study of black HIV-infected Africans from KwaZulu Natal, South Africa (Hoffmann, 2000). However, there was a higher rate of large-vessel cryptogenic stroke in the HIV population. The authors suspected that a possible underlying prothrombotic state could have been responsible for this finding.

Another study of black South African heterosexual HIV-infected patients with stroke showed no major differences, according to the investigators' interpretation, in the distribution of risk factors and pathophysiological mechanisms when compared with young African HIV-negative patients with stroke (Mochan, 2003). However, careful review of the data seems to contradict this conclusion. In this series of 35 HIV-infected patients with stroke (33/35 with ischemia; 40% with CD4+ T lymphocyte count < 200 cells/mm^3), hypertension and cardiac embolism were uncommon (prevalence below 10%) while meningitis (26%) and coagulopathies (49%) were quite frequent. Protein S deficiency was once again the coagulopathy most often diagnosed (11/35 cases) followed by antiphospholipid antibodies (5/35). Vasculopathy/vasculitis was deemed responsible for the stroke in four patients. No cause was found in five others (14%). Due to lack of corresponding epidemiological data on the general young population of the region, this study does not allow to draw any conclusions in regards to whether the overall risk of stroke is increased in HIV-infected patients.

In a cohort study from Germany, 15 of 772 HIV-infected patients had documented cerebrovascular events (Evers, 2003). The resulting prevalence was 1.9% with an annual incidence rate of 216 per 100,000 infected individuals. However, these data should be judged cautiously, since it is extracted from a selected population of patients attending special HIV neurology clinics. Strokes were typically seen in later stages of the infection (average CD4+ T lymphocyte count 142 cells per mm^3). Among the 9 patients with stroke, 3 were considered to have probable vasculitis (based on suggestive angiographic changes, elevated serum inflammatory markers, and intrathecal production of immunoglobulins) and 2 had documented cardioembolic sources (including 1 patient with protein S deficiency). The rest of the cases, including all patients with transient ischemic attacks, were classified as cryptogenic (10/15; 66%). As acknowledge by the researchers, incomplete evaluations may have contributed to the diagnostic uncertainty in several of these cryptogenic cases.

The radiological patterns of infarction were studied in a retrospective analysis of 71 abnormal magnetic resonance scans of HIV-infected patients (Gillams, 1997). Twenty-two infarctions were identified in 13 of these patients. Basal ganglia involvement was documented in 15 cases and median lesion size was only 2 cm. Concurrent intracerebral opportunistic infections were present in 5 (38%) patients and 8 (61%) had history of intravenous drug abuse. Magnetic resonance angiography was performed in 8 cases and was suggestive of vasculitis in 2 of them.

Table 1: Selected case series and necropsy studies reporting stroke rates in HIV-infected patients.

Study	Type	N	Stroke, n (%)	Stroke type	Proven causes
Snider '83	Case series	160	6 (4)	Ischemic 3 Hemorrhagic 3	NBTE Ramsay-Hunt syndrome CNS lymphoma Thrombocytopenia
Guarda '84	Necropsy	13	1 (8)	Ischemic	NBTE
Moskowitz '84	Necropsy	52	3 (6)	Ischemic 2 Hemorrhagic 1	None proven
Koppel '85	Case series	121	1 (0.8)	Hemorrhagic	Toxoplasmosis
Anders '86	Necropsy	89	18 (20)	Ischemic 13 Hemorrhagic 5	NBTE DIC
Berger '87	Case series	132	4 (3)	NA	NBTE Thrombocytopenia
McArthur '87	Case series	186	1 (0.5)	Ischemic	Cardioembolism
Levy and Bredesen '88	Case series	1286	20 (1.6)	Ischemic 15 (6 with TIA) Hemorrhagic 5	NBTE Eosinophilic vasculitis CNS lymphoma
Mizusawa '88	Necropsy	83	28 (34)	Ischemic 24 Hemorrhagic 4	Opportunistic infections Thrombocytopenia
Engstrom '89	Case series	1600	12 (0.75)	All ischemic	Cryptococcal meningitis HZ vasculitis Disseminated TB NBTE
Berger '90	Necropsy	181	13 (7)	All ischemic	Thrombosis (4 cases) Cardioembolism (4 cases) Vasculitis (2 cases)
Kieburtz '93	Necropsy	70	14 (20)	All ischemic	Opportunistic vasculitis or vasculopathy (3 cases) Cardioembolism (4 cases)
Gillams '97	Case series	71*	22 (31)	All ischemic	Opportunistic infections (5 cases) IVDA (6 cases)
Qureshi '97	Case series†	25	20 (80)	All ischemic	Meningitis (5 cases) Protein S deficiency (4 cases)
Roquer '98	Case series	790	8 (1)	Hemorrhagic**	Toxoplasmosis (2) Thrombocytopenia (2) Tuberculosis (1) Hypertension (1)
Connor '00	Necropsy	183	10 (5.5)	All ischemic	HIV vasculopathy
Hoffmann '00	Case series†	1298	25 (1.9)	All ischemic	Large vessel cryptogenic ?? prothrombotic state
Mochan '03	Case series	NA	35	Ischemic 33 Hemorrhagic 2	Coagulopathy (17) Meningitis (8) Vasculopathy/vasculitis (4) Cardioembolism (3) Hypertension (2) Meningitis (1) Hypertension (1)
Evers '03	Case series	772	15 (1.9)	All ischemic (6 with TIA)	Vasculitis (3) Cardioembolic (2)

*Patients with abnormal brain MRI
† Case-control study among all patients with documented stroke over the study period
**Cases designed to report only cases of intracerebral hemorrhage
††Only includes cases with ischemia in the absence of opportunistic infections or tumors.

DIC, disseminated intravascular coagulation; HZ, herpes zoster; IVDA, intravenous drug abuse; NBTE, non-bacterial throbotic endocarditis; TB, tuberculosis; TIA, transient ischemic attack.

It is important to notice that most of these clinical studies were performed before the introduction of PIs and the emergence of combination drug regimens known as HAART. The availability of PIs and HAART have revolutionized the therapy of HIV and changed the outlook of infected patients. Many adequately treated, compliant patients with HIV can now expect to lead long, healthy lives. This creates a new population of HIV-infected individuals who are middle age and older, have a controlled infection, and whose age puts them at a higher risk for vascular disease. In addition, recent evidence suggests that either HIV infection or the drugs used to treat it could increase the risk of premature vascular events, although this evidence remains mostly anecdotal at this stage (Henry, 1998; Behrens, 1998; Vittecoq, 1998; Laurence, 1998; Maggi, 2000). Therefore, as HIV infection is successfully treated in more patients, clinicians now face the challenge of preventing long-term health problems in these patients, particularly accelerated atherosclerosis.

Mechanisms of Ischemic Stroke in HIV-Infected Patients

Formerly, most ischemic strokes in HIV-infected patients were reported to be caused by cardioembolism or opportunistic diseases of the central nervous system (Pinto, 1996; Berger 1990; Berger, 1987; McCarthur, 1987; Levy, 1988; Engstrom, 1989). Prothrombotic states were also frequently implicated (Qureshi, 1997; Brew, 1996). Intravenous drug abuse has been associated with strokes in HIV-infected patients (Pinto, 1996; Berger, 1990; Gillams, 1997), although the strength of such association is not well defined (Qureshi, 2001). The proportion of cerebral infarcts classified as cryptogenic varies fairly widely across different clinical series (Pinto, 1996; Kieburtz, 1993; Engstrom, 1989; Hoffmann, 2000). The existence of an HIV-related vasculopathy in patients free of concomitant opportunistic illnesses is supported by recent evidence (Connor, 2000; Brilla, 1999). Additionally, PIs have been associated with an increased risk of vascular events, including stroke (The Writing Committee, 2004).

Traditional and new proposed stroke mechanisms are discussed in the following sections. These mechanisms are listed in Table 2.

Traditional Mechanisms

Cardiac Embolism

Cardiac disease is common in HIV-infected patients (Berger, 1990; Roldan, 1987; Cardoso, 1998) and typically has been the main cause of embolic stroke in this population (Berger, 1990). Roldan et al. found pathologic changes in the heart in 55% of patients who died of AIDS (Roldan, 1987). Cardiac lesions included lymphocytic myocarditis, marantic endocarditis, toxoplasmic endocarditis, and bacterial endocarditis. A more recent prospective case-control study evaluated the left ventricular function of 98 consecutive HIV-infected patients by echocardiography (Cardoso, 1998). Diastolic dysfunction was found in 63% of seropositive patients and depressed left ventricular ejection fraction in 32%, with an 8% rate of symptomatic congestive heart failure. Echocardiographic abnormalities were significantly more frequent in HIV-infected patients than in controls, and the difference could not be explained by any confounding factors. Cardiac dysfunction was more common in more advanced stages of the infection but was also present in asymptomatic HIV-positive patients.

Table 2. Proposed mechanisms of ischemic stroke in HIV-infected patients

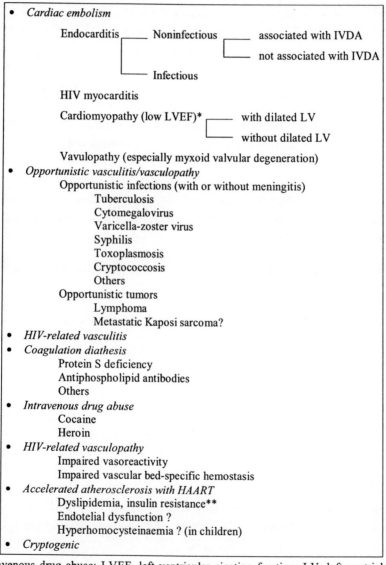

IVDA, intravenous drug abuse; LVEF, left ventricular ejection fraction; LV, left ventricle; HAART, highly active antiretroviral therapy
* May be associated with mural thrombi
** These metabolic disturbances have been documented with regimens containing protease inhibitors and nucleoside analogue reverse transcriptase inhibitors.

Nonbacterial thrombotic (marantic) endocarditis and bacterial endocarditis (both with and without history of intravenous drug abuse) have been reported as causes of ischemic stroke in HIV-infected patients (Berger, 1990; Snider, 1983; Levy, 1988; Engstrom, 1989; Mesquita, 1996). Other cardiac conditions related to stroke in HIV patients include dilated cardiomyopathy, atrial and ventricular mural thrombi, myxoid degeneration of valves, and more questionably, HIV myocarditis (Berger, 1990; Evers, 2003). Aortic root dilatation associated with left ventricular dilation, increased viral load, and lower CD4 cell count has been documented in HIV-infected children (Lai, 2001).

Dilated cardiomyopathy was the most prevalent cardiac condition associated with ischemic strokes before the introduction of HAART. However, the increased incidence of coronary events in patients treated with HAART (Rickerts, 2000) may lead myocardial infarctions to become the most frequent cause of cerebral embolism.

Opportunistic Vasculitis or Vasculopathy

Several opportunistic infections have been implicated in the development of vascular disease associated with ischemic strokes. They include tuberculosis (Berger, 1990; Engstrom, 1988; Gillams, 1997), cytomegalovirus (Berger, 1990; Kieburtz, 1993), varicella-zoster virus (Engstrom, 1989; Eidelberg, 1986), herpes simplex virus (Engstrom, 1989), syphilis (Johns, 1987; Kase, 1988), cryptococcosis (Engstrom, 1989; Gillams, 1997), candidiasis (Kieburtz, 1993), and lymphoma (Kieburtz, 1993). Other potential causes in this category are toxoplasmosis (Berger, 1990; Engstrom, 1989; Brew, 1996; Gillams, 1997), mucormycosis (Berger, 1990), aspergillosis (Berger 1990; Gillams, 1997), and, more questionably, coccidiodomycosis and trypanosomiasis (Brannagan, 1999).

Case reports of opportunistic vasculitis with cerebral involvement vary in the modalities used for diagnostic confirmation and the degree of associated systemic disease. Most often, infectious cerebral vasculitis by opportunistic agents are seen in patients with advanced immunosuppression. However, we have observed isolated cases of cerebral vasculitis, for example caused by varicella-zoster virus, is patients with relatively preserved immune markers. In these cases, the occurrence of vasculitis portends worsening immune status and poor overall prognosis.

The actual incidence of stroke in HIV-infected patients with these opportunistic diseases involving the central nervous system is unknown but most likely low (Chetty, 2001). These causes should generally be considered when the cerebral infarction occurs in an HIV-infected patient with advanced immunodeficiency. Fortunately, the current use of HAART has dramatically decreased the frequency of these conditions.

Hypercoagulable Conditions

Various haemostatic abnormalities have been documented in HIV-infected patients with ischemic stroke. The most consistently reported prothrombotic states have been protein S deficiency (Qureshi, 1997; Brew, 1996; Evers, 2003), and antiphospholipid antibodies (Brew, 1996; Abuaf, 1997). In their 3-year prospective study of 27 patients without opportunistic disease presenting with transient neurologic deficits, Brew et al. found a high prevalence of IgG anticardiolipin antibodies (70%) and protein S deficiency (53%) (Brew, 1996).

In terminally ill patients, stroke can be precipitated by disseminated intravascular coagulation (Berger, 1990; Anders, 1986) or cerebral venous thrombosis as a consequence of dehydration and cachexia (Berger, 1990). Hyperviscosity has been reported in AIDS (Martin, 1989) and could represent a potential cause of cerebral infarction. In transsexual men, use of estrogens might favor the occurrence of thrombotic strokes (deMarinis, 1978).

Unrecognized prothrombotic states have been suspected responsible for the high incidence of "cryptogenic strokes" (Hoffmann, 2000), but no proof has been offered to support this hypothesis. New varieties of antiphospholipid antibodies have been described recently and should be studied in HIV-infected patients. Other forms of hypercoagulability have also been observed in HIV-infected patients, but whether their frequency is higher than that in the normal population has not been assessed (Saif, 2001).

Intravenous Drug Abuse

Although infrequently reported as causes of cerebral infarction in HIV-infected patients, active use of cocaine and heroin increases the risk of stroke. However, it is inappropriate to assume that a stroke is due to substance abuse just based on a positive toxicological test or the mere history of drug addiction. This conclusion can only be reached after thorough exclusion of other pathophysiological mechanisms.

The mechanism of ischemia in cocaine-induced stroke is unclear. Vasoconstriction, increased platelet aggregation, and apparent vasculitis have been postulated (Caplan, 2000; Heesch, 2000; Herning, 1999). In my experience, cocaine abusers tend to have relatively small subcortical infarctions in the territory of penetrating arterial branches. In heroin users, strokes usually occur following reintroduction of the drug after a period of abstinence, suggesting that the underlying mechanism could be immunologic (Caplan, 2000; Caplan, 1982).

Possible New Mechanisms

HIV-Related Vasculopathy

Growing evidence supports the occurrence of a disease involving small vessels in the central nervous system in HIV-infected patients who are free of other risk factors for these vascular changes. The autopsy study on the Edinburgh HIV cohort revealed the presence of an asymptomatic vasculopathy characterized by small-vessel wall thickening, perivascular space dilatation, rarefaction and pigment deposition with vessel wall mineralization, and occasional perivascular inflammatory cell infiltrates without definitive evidence of vasculitis. These findings were detected in all patients with hypoxic/ischemic pathologic lesions who had no intercurrent central nervous system opportunistic diseases or potential embolic sources (10 cases; 5.5% of the total cohort) (Connor, 2000). The vascular changes were similar to those found in cases of cerebral arteriolosclerosis in elderly, hypertensive, and diabetic patients. However, Edinburgh patients were young (range, 22-47 years) and mostly free of traditional vascular risk factors (although 48% of the cohort were intravenous drug users, including 5 of the 10 patients with vasculopathy). Neither the degree of vasculopathy nor the extent of cerebral infarction was associated with the viral load; however, all patients were severely immunodepressed. None of these patients had been exposed to PIs, and there was no evidence of systemic embolism in other organs.

In their autopsy series, Mizusawa et al. noted multiple subclinical cerebral infarcts involving cortex, striatum, and brainstem in 29% of cases. Mural thickening of small vessels was present in half of these patients (Mizusawa, 1988). A vasculopathy mediated primarily by HIV was thought to be responsible in 6 of 14 cases of cerebral infarction in another autopsy study (Kieburtz, 1993). Other pathologic abnormalities observed in isolated cases such as eosinophilic (Schwartz, 1986), necrotizing (Vinters, 1988), or granulomatous (Yanker, 1986) vasculitis appear to be exceptional. Histologically proven cases of isolated central nervous system vasculitis in HIV-infected patients without opportunistic infectious or tumors are rare (Nogueras, 2002). The pathogenic role of HIV in these patients has not been clarified (Nogueras, 2002).

The clinical relevance of HIV-related vasculopathy is still a matter of debate. However, some data suggest that cerebrovascular hemodynamic function may be impaired in HIV-infected patients. Abnormalities of cerebral perfusion have been documented in asymptomatic HIV-infected patients using ^{113}Xe single-photon emission computed tomography (Tran Dinh, 1990). Brilla et al. examined 31 HIV-positive patients (7 with AIDS; mean time since diagnosis, 4 years; mean ± SD age, 39 ±11 years) using transcranial Doppler imaging to evaluate cerebrovascular reserve capacity (CRC) (Brilla, 1999). These patients had reduced baseline blood flow velocity and significantly diminished CRC after the administration of acetazolamide compared with controls. No relationship with CD4 cell count or duration of seropositivity could be demonstrated, although CRC was slightly worse in AIDS patients. Unfortunately, the study did not provide any information on the antiretroviral regimens administered. Transcranial Doppler imaging also has been used to monitor the progression of a reversible form of symptomatic cerebral vasospasm observed in a few HIV-infected patients with presumed underlying HIV-related vasculopathy (Zunker, 1996). The cause for this impaired vasoreactivity remains to be established but the disorder appears to be confined to small cerebral arterioles, the same vessels showing pathologic changes in the autopsy studies discussed above.

Accelerated Atherosclerosis and the Use of HAART

Clinically manifest atherosclerotic disease was not commonly documented in HIV-infected patients in the pre-PI era, although this low incidence of atherosclerosis may have been related to the reduced life expectancy of these patients (Passalaris, 2000). The marked reduction in the incidence of comorbid conditions and premature mortality afforded by the use of HAART may account for a growing prevalence of atherosclerosis in an aging HIV population. Underlying pro-atherosclerotic effects of HIV infection itself, such as endothelial dysfunction, may also become clinically significant as HIV-infected individuals grow older (Lafeuillade, 1992; Blann, 1998; Stein, 2001).

Carotid intima-media thickness, a reliable marker of atherosclerosis, has consistently been shown to be higher in HIV-infected patients than in matched controls (Seminari, 2002; Hsue, 2004). Intima-media thickness at baseline and also progression of disease at one year were greater among the HIV-infected in a recent study (Hsue, 2004). In this cohort,, progression of atherosclerosis correlated with the presence of traditional vascular risk factors and was more prominent in patients with lower CD4+ count (Hsue, 2004).

PIs can induce a variety of metabolic abnormalities, including hypertriglyceridemia, hypercholesterolemia, increased serum insulin and peptide C levels with proven insulin resistance, and peripheral lipodystrophy (Carr 1998). Marked lipid abnormalities may be present in 24% to 64% of patients treated with PIs (Henry, 1998; Carr, 1998; Tsiodras, 2000). Overall, the largest published studies on the metabolic effects of PIs have shown an average increase of total cholesterol and serum triglyceride levels of 28% and 96% respectively, compared with either pretreatment values or matched PI-naïve HIV-infected controls (Passalaris, 2000).

Treatment with PIs has been associated with severe premature atherosclerotic vascular disease (Henry, 1998; Behrens, 1998; Vittecoq, 1998; Laurence, 1998; The Writing Committee, 2004; Friis-Moller, 2003; Holmberg, 2002; Escaut, 2003), although this association has not been uniformly found (Bozzette, 2003). In these reports, patients were mostly young and had few or no traditional risk factors for atherosclerosis, with the exception of the metabolic derangements occurring after the initiation of PIs (Henry, 1998; Behrens, 1998; Vittecoq, 1998; Laurence, 1998). Myocardial infarction has been the vascular event observed in most cases (Holmberg, 2002; Escaut, 2003; Friis-Moller, 2003), but the incidence of stroke is also increased (The Writing Committee, 2004). In a collaborative international study that followed prospectively more than 23.000 HIV-infected patients for up to 3 years, the incidence of myocardial infarction increased by 26% among patients treated with combination antiretroviral therapy including a PI (used in 67% of patients) or a non-nucleoside reverse transcriptase inhibitor (Friis-Moller, 2003). The risk of a first stroke in these patients was 5.7 per 1000 person-years and it correlated with the duration of exposure to combination antiretroviral therapy (The Writing Committee, 2004). It is essential to emphasize that in these studies, the benefit of combination antiretroviral therapy clearly continued to outweigh the risks of vascular disease observed.

Whether any particular PI drug or combination of PI agents is more atherogenic remains unclear. Different studies have preferentially implicated different PIs (most frequently ritonavir), but all available PIs can induce potentially atherogenic metabolic derangements (Tsiodras, 2000; Graham, 2000; Periard, 1999). Furthermore, information has emerged linking treatment with nucleoside reverse transcriptase inhibitors in PI-naïve HIV-infected patients to similar changes in body habitus and metabolic abnormalities observed in PI-treated patients (Galli, 2002).

Flow-mediated vasodilation but not nitroglycerin-induced vasodilation is impaired in nonsmoking subjects treated with PIs compared with nonsmoking, PI-naïve HIV-infected controls, indicating an underlying endothelial dysfunction (Stein, 2001). This could be the effect of the metabolic abnormalities produced by PIs (dyslipidemia, insulin resistance). In addition, an increased prevalence of premature carotid atherosclerosis in HIV-infected individuals treated with PI-containing regimens for at least 12 months has been shown by ultrasonography (Maggi, 2000). Fifty-three percent of these patients presented acquired lesions of the carotid wall (presence of plaque or intimal-media thickness > 1 mm) compared with 15% of PI-naïve HIV-infected subjects and less than 7% of healthy non-HIV-infected controls. However, the study failed to reveal significant differences in hemodynamic variables such as pulsation index, resistance index, and peak, minimal and mean speeds. Another case-control study using ultrasonography to identify early signs of atherosclerosis in femoral and carotid arteries of HIV-infected individuals showed that a larger proportion of patients in the HIV-infected group had atherosclerotic plaques. However, the presence of plaques was not associated the use of PIs, but rather with classic vascular risk factors, especially smoking (Depairon, 2001).

The management of HIV-infected individuals treated with PIs should include close monitoring of lipid and glucose levels (Dubé, 2000; Wanke, 2000). Diet and exercise should always be the first focus of attention. Risk factors for atherosclerosis should be assessed and, if present, aggressively modified. If hyperlipidemia is present despite non-pharmachologic interventions, a statin drug that is not metabolized by CYP3A4, such as pravastatin, probably would be the first choice for drug therapy. A fibrate can be useful if triglyceride elevation is the primary concern; fenofibrate alone or the addition of a statin would be indicated if there is coexistent elevation in LDL-cholesterol level (Passalaris, 2000). The safety and efficacy of lipid-lowering agents in HIV-infected patients remains under scrutiny (Dubé, 2000). Drug interactions are a reason for concern since they can potentially result in potential muscle toxicity and liver dysfunction. Simvastatin and lovastatin are extensively metabolized by CYP3A4 and should probably be avoided in patients receiving PIs (CYP3A4 inhibitors) since the interaction could promote excessive levels of the statin and increase the risk of severe rhabdomyolysis (Dubé, 2000; Omar, 2001). This risk would be even larger if a fibrate is also part of the therapeutic regimen (Omar, 2001). The possibility of muscle damage is particularly worrisome in HIV-infected who may develop hyperlactatemia and, occasionally, severe muscle injury from mitochondrial toxicity induced by nucleoside analog reverse transcriptase inhibitors (Boubaker, 2001). Switching from PI to nevirapine could lead to partial reversion of the metabolic disorder with sustained virological suppression (Martinez, 1999). Switching to a different PI is a largely unproven strategy. The results of ongoing clinical trials will help define the safest and most effective therapeutic approach to this problem.

Intracerebral Hemorrhage
in HIV-Infected Patients

Intracerebral hemorrhages (ICH) in HIV-infected patients are usually associated with opportunistic diseases in the central nervous system, such as lymphoma, toxoplasmosis, cerebral tuberculosis and metastatic Kaposi sarcoma (Pinto, 1996; Snider, 1983; Koppel, 1985; Levy, 1988; Roquer, 1996; Roquer, 1998). Another frequently implicated cause of ICH is thrombocytopenia (Pinto, 1996; Snider, 1983; Berger, 1987; Roquer, 1998). Other potential causes include disseminated intravascular coagulation and ruptured mycotic aneurysms, the latter known to occur more frequently in intravenous drug users. Mortality tends to be high (Roquer, 1998).

Overall, it is unclear whether hemorrhagic stroke is more frequent in the HIV-infected population (Pinto, 1996; Qureshi, 1997), but some authors have suggested that could be the case (Roquer, 1998). Moreover, because most of the conditions conferring an increased risk of ICH have shown a declining incidence in recent years (Ammassari, 2000), we may expect a concomitant decline in the number of new cases of ICH.

Stroke in HIV-Infected Children

The incidence of symptomatic cerebrovascular disease in pediatric AIDS is 1.3% per year, but cerebrovascular lesions have been documented in 25% of autopsies (Burns 1992; Park, 1990). The increased incidence of cerebrovascular disease is seen especially in children with severe immunosuppression and with vertically acquired infection or neonatal exposure to the virus (Patsalides, 2002). Reported mechanisms have included septic or thrombotic embolism in association with cardiomyopathy or endocarditis, thrombocytopenia, and infectious vasculitis of intracranial vessels caused by cytomegalovirus, varicella-zoster virus, or mycobacterial or fungal infections (Park, 1990).

A T-cell-mediated vasculitis/perivasculitis has been recognized in children with HIV encephalitis and concurrent ischemic stroke (Legido, 1999; Joshi, 1987). Fibrosis and calcification of the media with variable luminal narrowing is also characteristically present (Joshi, 1987). In addition, a form of cerebral aneurysmal arteriopathy has been observed in the major vessels of the circle of Willis of these HIV-infected children (Dubrovsky, 1988; Philippet, 1994; Patsalides, 2002). These aneurysmal dilatations are seen in conjunction with medial fibrosis, intimal hyperplasia, and vascular occlusion leading to areas of infarction. Inflammation involving the vasa vasorum and leading to vessel wall ischemia (Kabus, 1991) and transendothelial migration of HIV-infected monocytes (Persidsky, 1997) have been quoted as potential mechanisms for the production of these aneurysms. The pathology may be related to concomitant varicella-zoster virus infection or HIV-1 virus itself (Dubrovsky, 1988).

Other recent findings of yet unproven clinical relevance deserve mention. Aortic root dilatation associated with left ventricular dilation, increased viral load, and lower CD4 cell count has been documented in HIV-infected children (Lai, 2001). Hyperhomocysteinaemia has been observed in HIV-infected children on antiretroviral therapy, particularly when PIs are used (Vilaseca, 2001). This phenomenon is probably the consequence of underlying folate deficiency. Whether these children have increased risk of premature stroke remains to be studied.

Finally, endothelial dysfunction has also been documented in HIV-infected children without risk factors for early atherosclerosis (Bonnet, 2004). The long-term clinical significance of this finding remains presently unclear.

Conclusions

The relationship of HIV-infection with stroke, once thought to be of rather marginal clinical relevance and only applicable to patients with advanced immune suppression, is undergoing remarkable changes. These changes parallel those observed in the management and prognosis of HIV infection itself and relate to the increased survival of HIV-infected patients and the metabolic effects of the drugs used for treatment. While strokes associated with opportunistic infections or tumors may be showing a declining incidence, clinicians should remain alert to the possibility of a growing overall incidence of stroke in the HIV-infected population due to the emergence of new mechanisms such as possible accelerated atherosclerosis in patients treated with HAART and a form of HIV-related vasculopathy with endothelial dysfunction. Studies supporting the role of these novel mechanisms are available but information on their clinical impact is still lacking. Although new combination antiretroviral regimens may increase the risk of premature vascular events, the benefits of such regimens clearly predominate. As epidemiological studies further define the magnitude of the risk of vascular disease in general and stroke in particular in HIV-infected patients under treatment with HAART, interventional trials testing strategies to minimize such risk will be needed.

References

Abuaf N, Laperche S, Rajoely B, Carsique R, Deschaps A, Rouquette AM, et al. Autoantibodies to phospholipids and to the coagulation proteins in AIDS. *Thromb. Haemost.* 1997;77:856-861.

Ammassari A, Cingolani A, Pezzotti P, De Luca A, Murri R, Giancola L, et al. AIDS-related focal brain lesions in the era of highly active antiretroviral therapy. *Neurology* 2000;55;1194-1200.

Anders KH, Guerra WF, Tomiyasu U, Vinters HV. The neuropathology of AIDS: UCLA experience and review. *Am. J. Pathol.* 1986;124:537-558.

Behrens G, Schmidt H, Meyer D, Stoll M, Schmidt RE. Vascular complications associated with the use of HIV protease inhibitors. *Lancet* 1998;351:1958.

Berger JR, Harris JO, Gragorios J, Norenberg M. Cerebrovascular disease in AIDS: a case-control study. *AIDS* 1990;4:239-244.

Berger JR, Moskowitz L, Fischl M, Kelley RE. Neurological disease as the presenting manifestation of acquired immunodeficiency syndrome. *South Med. J.* 1987;80:683-686.

Blann A, Constans J, Dignat-George F, Seigneur M. The platelet and endothelium in HIV infection. *Br. J. Hematol.* 1998;100:613-614.

Bonnet D, Aggoun Y, Szezepanski I, Bellal N, Blanche S. Arterial stiffness and endothelial dysfunction in HIV-infected children. *AIDS* 2004;18:1037-1041.

Boubaker K, Flepp M, Sudre P, Furrer H, Haensel A, Hirschel B, et al. Hyperlactatemia and antiretroviral therapy: The Swiss HIV Cohort Study. *Clin. Infect. Dis.* 2001;33:1931-1937.

Bozzette SA, Ake CF, Tam HK, Chang SW, Louis TA. Cardiovascular and cerebrovascular events in patients treated for human immunodeficiency virus infection. *N. Engl. J. Med.* 2003;348:702-710.

Brannagan TH III. Retroviral-associated vasculitis of the nervous system. *Neurol. Clin.* 1999;15:927-944.

Brew BJ, Miller J. Human immunodeficiency virus type 1-related transient neurological deficits. *Am. J. Med.* 1996;101:257-261.

Brilla R, Nabavi DG, Schulte-Altedorneburg G, Kemény V, Reichelt D, Evers S et al. Cerebral vasculopathy in HIV infection revealed by transcranial Doppler: a pilot study. *Stroke* 1999;30:811-813.

Burns DK. The neuropathology of pediatric acquired immunodeficiency syndrome. *J. Child. Neurol.* 1992;7:332-346.

Caplan LR, Hier DB, Banks G. Current concepts in cerebrovascular disease-stroke: stroke and drug abuse. *Stroke* 1982;13:869-872.

Caplan LR, Nonatherosclerotic vasculopahties. In: Caplan LR (ed) *Caplan's Stroke. A clinical approach.* Boston, MA: Butterworth Heinemann; 2000:321-322.

Cardoso JS, Moura B, Martins L, Mota-Miranda A, Rocha-Goncalves F, Lecour H. Left ventricular dysfunction in human immunodeficicency virus (HIV)-infected patients. *Int. J. Cardiol.* 1998;63:37-45.

Carr A, Samaras K, Burton S, Freund J, Chisholm DJ, Cooper DA. A Syndrome of peripheral lipodystrophy, hyperlipidemia and insulin resistance in patients receiving HIV protease inhibitors. *AIDS* 1998;12:F51-F58.

Chetty R. Vasculitides associated with HIV infection. *J. Clin. Pathol.* 2001;54(4):275-278.

Connor MD, Lammie GA, Bell JE, Warlow CP, Simmonds P, Brettle RD. Cerebral infarction in adult AIDS patients: observations form the Edimburgh HIV autopsy cohort. *Stroke* 2000;31:2117-2126.

deMarinis M, Arnett EN. Cerebrovascular occlusion in a transsexual man taking mestranol. *Arch. Intern. Med.* 1978;138:1732-1733.

Depairon M, Chessex S, Sudre P, Rodondi N, Doser N, Chave P, et al. Premature atherosclerosis in HIV-infected individuals – focus on protease inhibitor therapy. *AIDS* 2001;15:329-334.

Dubé MP, Sprecher D, Henry WK, Aberg JA, Torriani FJ, Hodis HN, et al. Preliminary guidelines for the evaluation and management of dyslipidemia in adults infected with human immunodeficiency virus and receiving antiretroviral therapy: Recommendations of the adult AIDS Clinical Trial Group Cardiovascular Disease Focus Group. *Clin. Infect. Dis.* 2000;31:1216-1224.

Dubrovsky T, Curless R, Scott G, Chaneles M, Post MJD, Altman N, et al. Cerebral aneurysmal arteriopathy in childhood AIDS. *Neurology* 1988;51:560-565.

Eidelberg D, Sotrel A, Horoupian DS, Neumann PE, Pumarola –Sune T, Price RW. Thrombotic cerebral vasculopathy associated with herpes zoster. *Ann. Neurol.* 1986;19:7-14.

Engstrom JW, Lowenstein DH, Breseden DE. Cerebral infarctions and transient neurological defifcits associated with acquired immunodeficiency syndrome. *Am. J. Med.* 1989;86:528-532.

Escaut L, Monsuez JJ, Chironi G, Merad M, Teicher E, Smadja D, Simon A, Vittecoq D. Coronary artery disease in HIV infected patients. *Intensive Care Med.* 2003;29:969-973.

Evers S, Nabavi D, Rahmann A, Heese C, Reichelt D, Husstedt I-W. Ischaemic cerebrovascular events in HIV infection. A cohort study. *Cerebrovasc. Dis.* 2003;15:199-205.

Friis-Moller N, Sabin CA, Weber R, d'Arminio Monforte A, El-Sadr WM, Reiss P, Thiebaut R, Morfeldt L, De Wit S, Pradier C, Calvo G, Law MG, Kirk O, Phillips AN, Lundgren

JD; Data Collection on Adverse Events of Anti-HIV Drugs (DAD) Study Group. Combination antiretroviral therapy and the risk of myocardial infarction. *N. Engl. J. Med.* 2003;349:1993-2003.

Galli M, Ridolfo AL, Adorni F, Gervasoni C, Ravasio L, Corsico L, et al. Body habitus changes and metabolic alterations in protease inhibitor-naïve HIV-1-infected patients treated with two nucleoside reverse transcriptase inhibitors. *J. Acquir. Immune. Defic. Syndr.* 2002;29:21-31

Gillams AR, Allen E, Hrieb K, Venna N, Craven D, Carter AP. Cerebral infarction in patients with AIDS. *AJNR Am. J. Neuroradiol.* 1997;18:1581-1585.

Graham NM. Metabolic disorders among HIV-infected patients treated with protease inhibitors: a review. *JAIDS* 2000; 5:S4-S11.

Grindal AB, Cohen RJ, Saul RF, Taylos JR. Cerebral infarction in young adults. *Stroke* 1978;9:39-42.

Guarda LA, Luna MA, Smith JL Jr, Mansell PW, Gyorkey F, Roca AN. Acquired immune deficiency syndrome: postmortem findings. *Am. J. Clin. Pathol.* 1984;81:549-557.

Heesch CM, Wilhelm CR, Ristich J, Adnane J, Bontempo FA, Wagner WR. Cocaine activates platelets and increases the formation of circulating platelet containing microaggregates in humans. *Heart.* 2000;83:688-695.

Henry K, Melroe H, Heubesch J, Hermundson J, Levine C, Swensen L, Daley J. Severe premature coronary artery disease with protease inhibitors. *Lancet* 1998;351:1328.

Herning RI, Better W, Nelson R, Gorelick D, Cadet JL. The regulation of cerebral blood flow during intravenous cocaine administration in cocaine abusers. *Ann. N. Y. Acad. Sci.* 1999;890:489-94.

Hoffmann M, Berger JR, Nath A, Rayens M. Cerebrovascular disease in young, HIV-infected, black Africans in the KwaZulu Natal province of South Africa. *J. Neurovirol.* 2000;6:229-236.

Holmberg SD, Moorman AC, Williamson JM, Tong TC, Ward DJ, Wood KC, Greenberg AE, Janssen RS; HIV Outpatient Study (HOPS) investigators. Protease inhibitors and cardiovascular outcomes in patients with HIV-1. *Lancet.* 2002;360:1747-1748.

Hsue PY, Lo JC, Franklin A, Bolger AF, Martin JN, Deeks SG, Waters DD. Progression of atherosclerosis as assessed by carotid intima-media thickness in patients with HIV infection. *Circulation.* 2004;109:1603-1608.

Husson RN, Salni R, Lewis LL, Butler KM, Patronas N, Pizzo PA. Cerebral artery aneurysms in children infected with human immunodeficiency virus. *J. Pediatr.* 1992;121:927-930.

Johns DR, tiernet M, Felsenstein D. Alteration in the natural history of neurosyphilis by concurrent infection with the human immunodeficiency virus. *N. Engl. J. Med.* 1987;316:1569-1572.

Joshi VV, Pawel B, Connor E, Sharer L, Oleske JM, Morrison S, Marin-Garcia J. Arteriopathy in children with acquired immunodeficiency syndrome. *Pediatr. Pathol.* 1987;7:261-275.

Kabus D, Greco MA. Arteriopathy in children with AIDS: microscopic changes in the vasa vasorum with gross irregularities of the aortic intima. *Pediatr. Pathol.* 1991;11:793-795.

Kase CS, Levitz SM, Wolinsky JS, Sulis CA. Pontine pure motor hemiparesis due to meningovascular syphilis in human immunodeficiency virus-positive patients. *Arch. Neurol.* 1988;45:823.

Kieburtz KD, Eskin TA, Ketonen L, Tuite MJ. Opportunistic cerebral vasculopathy and stroke in patients with AIDS. *Arch. Neurol.* 1993;50:430-432.

Kieburtz KD, Eskin TA, Ketonen L, Tuite MJ. Opportunistic cerebral vasculopathy and stroke in patients with the acquired immunodeficiency syndrome. *Arch. Neurol.* 1993;50:430-432.

Koppel BS, Wormser GP, Tuchman AJ, Maayan S, Hewlett D Jr, Daras M. Central nervous system involvement in patients with acquired immune deficiency syndrome (AIDS). *Acta Neurol. Scand.* 1985;71:337-353.

Koppel BS, Wormser GP, Tuchman AJ, Maayan S, Hewlett D Jr. Daras M. Central nervous system involvement in patients with acquired immunodeficiency syndrome (AIDS). *Acta Neurol. Scand* 1985;71:337-353.

Lafeuillade A, Alessi MC, Poizot-Martin I, Boyer-Neumann C, Zandotti C, Gastaut JA, et al. Endothelial cell dysfunction in HIV infection. *J. Acquir. Immune. Defic. Syndr.* 1992;5:127-131.

Lai WW, Colan SD, Easley KA, Lipshultz SE, Starc TJ, Bricker JT et al. Dilatation of the aortic root in children infected with human immunodeficiency virus type1: the prospective P2 C2 HIV multicenter study. *Am. Heart J.* 2001;141:661-701.

Laurence J. Vascular complications associated with the use of HIV protease inhibitors. *Lancet* 1998;351:1960.

Legido A, Lischner HW, de Chadarevian J-P, Katsetos CD. Stroke in pediatric HIV infection. *Pediatr. Neurol.* 1999;21:588.

Levy RM, Bredesen DE, Rosenblum ML. Neurological manifestations of the acquired immunodeficiency syndrome (AIDS): experience at UCSF and review of the literature. *J. Neurosurg.* 1985;62:475-495.

Levy RM, Breseden DE. CNS dysfunction in AIDS. *J. Acquir. Immune. Defic. Syndr.* 1988;1:41-64.

Maggi P, Serio G, Epifani G, Fiorentino G, Saracino A, Fico C et al.. Premature lesions of the carotid vessels in HIV-infected patients treated with protease inhibitors. *AIDS* 2000;14:123-128.

Martin CM, Matlow AG, Chew E, Sutton D, Pruzanski W. Hyperviscosity syndrome in a patient with acquired immunodeficiency syndrome. *Arch. Intern. Med.* 1989;149:1435-1436.

Martinez E, Conget I, Lozano L, Csamitjana R, Gatell JM. Reversion of metabolic abnormalities after switching from HIV-1 pretease inhibitors to nevirapine. *AIDS* 1999;13:805-810.

McArthur JC. Neurological manifestations of AIDS. *Medicine.* 1987;66:407-437.

Mesquita ET, Ramos RG, Ferrari AH, Martins W, da Cruz GG. Rheumatic heart disease and infective endocarditis in a patient with acquired immunodeficiency syndrome. *Arq. Bras. Cardiol.* 1996;67:255-257.

Mizusawa H, Hirano A, Llena JF, Shintaku M. Cerebrovascular lesions of AIDS. *Acta Neuropathol.* 1988;76:451-457.

Mizusawa H, Hirano A, Llena JF, Shintaku M. Cerebrovascular lesions in acquired immune deficiency syndrome (AIDS). *Acta Neuropathol. (Berl)*. 1988;76:451-457.

Mochan A, Modi M, Modi G. Stroke in black South African HIV-positive patients. A prospective analysis. *Stroke* 2003;34:10-15.

Moskowitz LB, Hensley GT, Chan JC, Gregorios J, Conley FK. The neuropathology of acquired immunodeficiency syndrome. *Arch. Pathol. Lab. Med.* 1984;108:867-872.

Moskowitz LB, Hensley GT, Chan JC, Gregorios J, Conley FK. The neuropathology of acquired immune deficiency syndrome. *Arch. Pathol. Lab. Med.* 1984;108:867-872.

Nogueras C, Sala M, Sasal M, Vinas J, Garcia N, Bella MR, et al. Recurrent stroke as a manifestation of primary angiitis of the central nervous system in a patient infected with human immunodeficiency virus. *Arch. Neurol.* 2002;59:468-473.

Omar MA, Wilson JP, Cox TS. Rhabdomyolysis and HMG-CoA reductase inhibitors. *Ann. Pharmacother.* 2001;35:1096-1107.

Park YD, Belman AL, Kim TS, Kure K, Llena JF, Lantos G, et al. Stroke in pediatric acquired immunodeficiency syndrome. *Ann. Neurol.* 1990;28:303-311.

Passalaris JD, Sepkowitz KA, Glesby MJ. Coronary artery disease and human immunodeficiency virus infection. *Clin. Infec. Dis.* 2000;31:787-797.

Patsalides AD, Wood LV, Atac GK, Sandifer E, Butman JA, Patronas NJ. Cerebrovascular disease in HIV-infected pediatric patients: neuroimaging findings. *AJR. Am. J. Roentgenol.* 2002;179:999-1003.

Periard D, Telenti A, Sudre P, Cheseaux J-J, Halfon P, Reymond MJ, et al. Atherogenic dyslipidemia in HIV-infected individuals treated with protease inhibitors. *Circulation* 1999;100:700-705.

Persidsky Y, Stins M, Way D, Witte MH, Weinand M, Kim KS, Bock P, Gendelman HE, Fiala M. A model for monocyte migration through the blood-brain barrier during HIV-1 encephalitis. *J. Immunol.* 1997 Apr 1;158(7):3499-510.

Philippet P, Blanche S, Sebag G, Rodesh G, Griscelli C, Tardieu M. Stroke and cerebral infarcts in children infected with human immunodeficiency virus. *Arch. Pediatr. Adolesc. Med* 1994;148:965-970.

Pinto AN. AIDS and cerebrovascular disease. *Stroke* 1996;27:538-543.

Qureshi AI, Janssen RS, Karon JM, Weissman JP, Akbar MS, Safdar K, Frankel MR. Human immunodeficiency virus infection and stroke in young patients. *Arch. Neurol.* 1997;54:1150-1153.

Qureshi AI, Suri MF, Guterman LR, Hopkins LN. Cocaine use and the likelihood of nonfatal myocardial infarction and stroke: data from the Third National Health and Nutrition Examination Survey. *Circulation.* 2001;103:502-506.

Rickerts V, Brodt H, Staszewski S, Stille W. Incidence of myocardial infarctions in HIV-infected patients between 1983 and 1998: the Frankfurt HIV-cohort study. *Eur J Med Res* 2000;5:329-333.

Roldan EO, Moskowitz L, Hensley GT. Pathology of the heart in AIDS. *Arch. Pathol. Lab. Med.* 1987;111:943-946.

Roquer J, Palomeras E, Knobel H, Pou A. Intracerebral haemorrhage in AIDS. *Cerebrovasc. Dis.* 1998;8:222-227.

Roquer J, Palomeras E, Pou A. AIDS and cerebrovascular disease. *Stroke* 1996;27:1694.

Rosemberg S, Lopes MBS, Tsanadis AM. Neuropathology of acquired immunodeficiency syndrome (AIDS): analysis of 22 Brazilian cases. *J. Neurol. Sci.* 1986;76:187-198.

Saif MW, Greenberg B. HIV and thrombosis: a review. *AIDS Patient Care STDS* 2001;15:15-24.

Schwartz ND, So YT, Hollander H, Allen S, Fye KH. Eosinophilic vasculitis leading to amaurosis fugax in a patient with acquired immunodeficiency syndrome. *Arch. Intern. Med.* 1986:146:2059-2060.

Seminari E, Pan A, Voltini G, Carnevale G, Maserati R, Minoli L, Meneghetti G, Tinelli C, Testa S. Assessment of atherosclerosis using carotid ultrasonography in a cohort of HIV-positive patients treated with protease inhibitors. *Atherosclerosis.* 2002;162:433-438.

Shah SS, Zimmerman RA, Rorke LB, Vezina LG. Cerebrovascular complications of HIV in children. *AJNR Am. J. Neuroradiol.* 1996;17:1913-1917.

Snider WD, Simpson DM, Nielsen S, Gold JW, Metroka CE, Posner JB. Neurological complications of acquired immune deficiency syndrome: analysis of 50 patients. *Ann. Neurol.* 1983;14:403-418.

Snider WD, Simpson DM, Nielsen S, Gold JWM, Metroka CE, Posner JB. Neurological complications of the acquired immunodeficiency syndrome: analysis of 50 patients. *Ann. Neurol.* 1983;14:403-418.

Stein JH, Klein MA, Bellehumeur JL, McBride PE, Wiebe DA, Otvos JD, Sosman JM. Use of human immunodeficiency virus-1 protease inhibitors is associated with atherogenic lipoprotein changes and endothelial dysfunction. *Circulation* 2001;104:257-262.

The neuropathology of AIDS. UCLA experience and review. The neuropathology of AIDS. UCLA experience and review. *Am. J. Pathol.* 1986;124:537-558.

The Writing Committee. Cardio- and cerebrovascular events in HIV-infected persons. *AIDS.* 2004;18:1811-1817.

Tran Dinh YR, Mamo H, Cervoni J, Caulin C, Saimot AC. Disturbances in the cerebral perfusion of HIV-1 seropositive asymptomatic subjects: a quantitative tomography study of 18 cases. *J. Nucl. Med.* 1990;31:1601-1607.

Tsiodras S, Mantzoros C, Hammer S, Samore M. Effects of protease inhibitors on hyperglycemia, hyperlipidemia, and lipodystrophy: a 5-year cohort study. *Arch. Intern. Med.* 2000;160:2050-2056.

Vilaseca MA, Sierra C, Colome C, Artuch R, Valls C, Munoz-Almagro C, et al. Hyperhomocysteinaemia and folate deficiency in human immunodeficiency virus-infected children. *Eur. J. Clin. Invest.* 2001;31:992-998.

Vinters HV, Guerra WF, Eppolito L, Keith PE. Necrotizing vasculitis of the nervous system in a patient with AIDS-related complex. *Neuropathol. Appl. Neurobiol.* 1988;14:417-424.

Vittecoq D, Escaut L, Monsuez JJ. Vascular complications associated with the use of HIV protease inhibitors. *Lancet* 1998;351:1958-1959.

Wanke CA, Falutz JM, Shevitz A, Phair JP, Kotler DP. Clinical evaluation and management of metabolic and morphologic abnormalities associated with human immunodeficiency virus. *Clin. Infect. Dis.* 2000;34:248-259.

Yanker BA, Skolnik PR, Shoukimas GM, Gabuzda DH, Sobel RA, Ho DD. Cerebral granulomatous angiitis associated with isolation of human T-lymphotropic virus type III from the central nervous system. *Ann. Neurol.* 1986;20:362-364.

Zunker P, Nabavi DG, Allardt A, Husstedt IW, Schuierer G. HIV-associated stroke: report of two unusual cases. *Stroke* 1996;27:1694-1695.

In: Neuro-AIDS
Editors: A. Minagar and P. Shapshak, pp. 185-198

ISBN: 1-59454-610-X
© 2006 Nova Science Publishers, Inc.

Chapter VIII

Varicella Zoster Virus Infection in HIV-Positive and AIDS Patients

Steven B. Deitch[1] and Donald H. Gilden[1,2,]*
Departments of [1]Neurology and [2]Microbiology, University of Colorado
Health Sciences Center, Denver, CO. USA.

Abstract

Varicella zoster virus (VZV) is an exclusively human neurotropic alphaherpesvirus. Primary infection causes chickenpox (varicella), after which virus becomes latent in ganglia along the entire neuraxis. Virus reactivation usually produces shingles (zoster) and other serious neurologic disorders. In HIV+ and AIDS patients of any age, virus reactivation is more frequent, more protracted and dissemination is more common. Neurologic complications due to VZV in AIDS patients have been found to be as high as 59%. Management of VZV infections in HIV-infected patients often requires prolonged antiviral therapy with hospitalization. Despite immunosuppression, most HIV+ and AIDS patients who develop serious neurological complications due to VZV can be treated successfully, if monitored closely and provided with aggressive antiviral therapy early in the course of infection.

Keywords: VZV, HIV, AIDS, Varicella Zoster Virus, Shingles, Chickenpox, Encephalitis, Myelitis, Vasculopathy, Retinal Necrosis,

[*] Correspondence concerning this article should be addressed to Donald H. Gilden, M.D. Department of Neurology University of Colorado Health Sciences Center. 4200 E. 9th Avenue, Mail Stop B182 Denver, CO   80262. Telephone: 303-315-8281; Fax: 303-315-8720; Email: don.gilden@uchsc.edu.

Introduction

Varicella zoster virus (VZV) is an exclusively human neurotropic alphaherpesvirus. Primary infection produces about 4 million cases of chickenpox (varicella) annually in the United States. After chickenpox, VZV becomes latent in cranial nerve, dorsal root and autonomic nervous system ganglia along the entire neuraxis (Gilden et al., 1983, 2001; Mahalingam et al., 1990). Virus reactivation results in shingles (zoster), characterized by severe, sharp, lancinating radicular pain and rash restricted to 1-3 dermatomes. In more than 40% of zoster patients over age 60, pain persists for months and sometimes years, so-called postherpetic neuralgia (PHN). Although neither the pain of zoster nor the more chronic pain of PHN is life-threatening, it is difficult to manage. Less often, after VZV reactivates from ganglia, virus spreads to the spinal cord causing myelitis, or to cerebral arteries producing a vasculopathy that affects large and small cerebral vessels. Compared to zoster and PHN, VZV myelitis and vasculopathy are more serious, causing considerable neurologic deficit and sometimes death. Compared to immunocompetent individuals, HIV-infected people of any age are at risk for developing more frequent and severe illness after varicella or zoster. Management of VZV infections in HIV-infected patients requires prolonged antiviral therapy and often hospitalization.

Epidemiology of VZV in HIV

HIV currently infects 40.3 million people worldwide (Fig. 1; UNAIDS, 2005). Infection is acquired by heterosexual or homosexual contact, exposure to contaminated blood or perinatally. Heterosexual contact is now the most common mode of transmission. Seroprevalence studies indicate that in tropical regions where HIV is highly endemic, susceptibility to primary VZV infection (varicella) is more common among adults than children (World Health Organization Weekly Epidemiological Record, 1998). Thus, adults in tropical areas have a higher risk of developing varicella once immunocompromised from HIV infection. In contrast, before varicella vaccine was available in the United States, 95% of cases occurred among infants, children and adolescents under age 15. In adults who have previously had chickenpox, the risk of zoster increases with advancing age due to a natural decline in cell-mediated immunity to VZV. Accordingly, HIV-infected patients of any age are at greater risk than age-matched, non-HIV-infected individuals to develop zoster (Margolis et al., 1991). Furthermore, HIV-infected children with a low CD4 count at the time of varicella are more likely to develop zoster (Benson et al., 2004). In areas with a high prevalence of HIV, there is an increased incidence of zoster, and disease is recurrent and more protracted than in non-HIV infected individuals (Colebunders et al., 1988). Compared to immunocompetent individuals, VZV myelopathy in AIDS patients is more insidious, progressive and can be fatal (Gilden et al., 1994). Finally, VZV multifocal vasculopathy in AIDS patients is chronic and may occur without rash (Gilden, 2002).

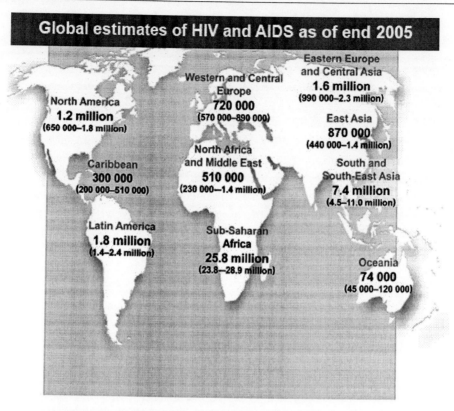

Figure 1. The number of HIV and AIDS patients by geographic region. Reprinted with permission of UNAIDS.

Host Immunosuppression and Virus Reactivation

Zoster occurs most often in elderly and immunocompromised individuals, usually due to a VZV-specific host immunodeficiency. Cases of zoster and its neurological complications are expected to increase in the United States for several reasons. First, the aging population continues to grow, and there is a natural decline in cell-mediated immunity (CMI) to VZV with advancing age (Berger et al., 1981; Miller, 1980). Second, the number of patients being treated with cytotoxic drugs and X-irradiation, including immunosuppressed organ transplant recipients, is increasing. Third, zoster is common in AIDS patients. Zoster may herald the onset of disease, occur later, and may recur. With improved treatment regimens for AIDS and a greater survival time of AIDS patients, the frequency of zoster is likely to increase. Overall, zoster may be viewed in the context of a continuum in immunodeficient individuals, ranging from a natural decline in VZV-specific immunity with age, to more serious immune deficits seen in cancer patients and transplant recipients, and ultimately to patients with AIDS. The remainder of this chapter is devoted exclusively to VZV infection in HIV-positive individuals and patients with AIDS.

Overview

A study of 3,231 patients with acute central nervous system (CNS) symptoms of suspected viral origin revealed that VZV was the most common agent associated with encephalitis, as well as meningitis and myelitis (Koskiniemi et al., 2001). VZV comprised 29% of all confirmed or probable causative etiologic agents. In adults with HIV infection, neurologic complications due to VZV were studied clinically with magnetic resonance imaging (MRI) and cerebrospinal fluid (CSF) exam. Diagnosis was confirmed by positive polymerase chain reaction (PCR) for VZV DNA in CSF. At diagnosis, 59% had AIDS. A history of zoster was found in 35% of cases. A concomitant zoster rash and/or acute retinal necrosis were noted in 71% and 12% of patients, respectively. In decreasing order, neurologic diseases were characterized mostly by encephalitis, myelitis, radiculitis and meningitis. After intravenous antiviral therapy, 53% of patients recovered, 29% developed serious sequelae and 18% died. Severe symptoms and a low CD4 cell count were associated with serious sequelae and death. VZV should be considered a possible cause of encephalitis, myelitis, radiculitis or meningitis in HIV-infected patients, especially in patients with a history of or concomitant zoster, or with acute retinal necrosis. VZV PCR in CSF allows rapid diagnosis and early specific antiviral treatment (De La Blanchardiere et al., 2000). Another review of 23 AIDS patients with VZV infection of the CNS (Chretien et al., 1997) revealed that multifocal vasculopathy was the most common presentation. Ventriculitis with infected ependymal cells was common. Focal necrotizing encephalitis and myelitis were also seen, including vasculopathy involving leptomeningeal arteries.

Clinical Manifestations of Zoster in HIV-Infected Individuals

In non-HIV-infected individuals, zoster is usually characterized by a painful, blistery red rash, which is restricted to one to three dermatomes. In HIV-infected individuals, zoster is more serious. One AIDS patient had zoster that lasted 104 days (Matsuo et al., 2001). Multiple dermatomes and bilateral involvement are common. Pain lasts longer and the risk of neurologic complications is greater (Gnann, 2002). Furthermore, zoster recurs in 13 to 26% of HIV-infected individuals (Colebunders et al., 1988; Glesby et al., 1993; Veenstra et al., 1996) compared to 3 to 5% of immunocompetent people (Benson et al., 2004). Skin lesions are verrucous and persist. Chronic skin lesions are frequently associated with resistance to thymidine kinase (TK)-dependent antiviral drugs.

Increased Incidence of Zoster in HIV-Infected Individuals, Including Children

Compared to HIV-negative adolescents and adults, the incidence of zoster is 15 to 25 times greater in HIV-infected adolescents and adults, and 3 to 7 times greater in HIV-infected elderly individuals than in HIV-negative elderly individuals (Benson et al., 2004). A study at the Baragwanath Hospital clinic in Johannesburg, Africa, revealed that of 181 HIV-positive black adults 16 to 66 years old, zoster was the first sign of HIV infection in 13% of patients (Karstaedt, 1992). At the skin clinic of the Kilimanjaro Christian Medical Centre in Africa, all of 200 consecutive 20- to 40-years-old patients with zoster tested positive for HIV infection (Naburi and Leppard, 2000). Although most non-HIV infected children are not affected by zoster, HIV-infected children are at risk for developing zoster. Zoster in children is often the first sign of undiagnosed HIV infection (Leppard and Naburi, 1998). The rate of zoster was 70% in children with HIV-induced low levels of CD4+ lymphocytes at the time of primary varicella infection (Gershon et al., 1997).

HAART[1] Therapy and Increased Incidence of Zoster

Severe immunosuppression correlates with a higher incidence of zoster. However, HAART therapy, which lowers HIV load and increases CD8+ T-lymphocytes numbers is paradoxically associated with an increased incidence of opportunistic infections, particularly zoster (Martinez et al., 1998; Jacobson, 2001). Identified risks for developing zoster after HAART therapy are: (1) low blood CD4+ and CD8+ counts before treatment; (2) low serum VZV-specific Ig levels before and after treatment; and (3) successful therapy that produces an increase in CD8+ T lymphocytes while lowering the HIV load (Tangsinmankong et al., 2004). Importantly, although zoster occurs after HAART, Domingo et al. (2001) found that none of the HIV-infected individuals who had received HAART therapy developed disseminated zoster or progressive outer retinal necrosis.

VZV Myelitis

VZV myelitis in AIDS patients differs from the myelitis after varicella or zoster in immunocompetent patients. In the latter, myelitis may complicate acute varicella or zoster, usually 1-2 weeks after rash. Clinical features are paraparesis with impaired sensory level and sphincter function. The CSF is either normal or shows mild pleocytosis with a normal to mild elevation of protein. MRI reveals T2-weighted hyperintense lesions, sometimes with focal cord swelling. Most patients improve significantly, but some experience persistent lower extremity stiffness and weakness. Because most immunocompetent patients survive, the pathology of this form of VZV-associated transverse myelitis is unknown. Moreover, virological and immunological verification is wanting; VZV cannot usually be cultured from CSF, although PCR has revealed VZV DNA in CSF. VZV myelitis has classically been diagnosed by its close temporal relationship with rash.

---

[1] HAART is defined as a treatment regimen using 3 or more antiretroviral drugs for at least 6 months, with no interruption of more than 2 months in the first 6 months of treatment.

In AIDS patients, the development of myelopathy is often more insidious, progressive and sometimes fatal. Spinal cord MRI scanning shows focal or longitudinal serpiginous enhancing lesions (Fig. 2) (Hwang et al., 1991; Gilden et al., 1994). Autopsy studies have demonstrated spinal cord necrosis and intense inflammation with frank parenchymal invasion by VZV, findings similar to those described in patients who died of VZV myelitis after long-term, low-dose steroid use (Hogan and Krigman, 1973; Tako and Rado, 1965). A fatal VZV myelitis in one AIDS patient was preceded by five episodes of thoracic-distribution zoster, one of which disseminated, all within 12 months (Gilden et al., 1994). An early search for VZV DNA or VZV antibody in CSF is essential for diagnosis, particularly since aggressive treatment with acyclovir, even in AIDS patients, may produce a favorable response (Lionnet et al., 1996; de Silva et al., 1996). Finally, myelopathy may occur before zoster rash in AIDS patients (Gómez-Tortosa et al., 1994).

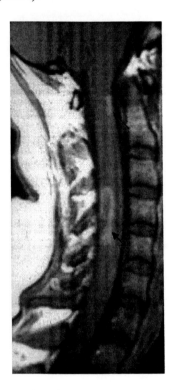

Figure 2. Magnetic resonance imaging of the spinal cord in an AIDS patient with myelitis shows enhancing lesions at the cervicomedullary junction (top arrow) and in the mid-cervical region (bottom arrow). Reprinted with permission of Neurology.

VZV Vasculopathy

Two clinical presentations are apparent. The first is a unifocal vasculopathy, formerly called granulomatous arteritis, which predominates in elderly immunocompetent adults and is characterized by acute focal deficit that develops weeks to months after contralateral trigeminal distribution zoster. Vasculopathy is usually restricted to 1-3 large cerebral arteries of either the anterior (Gilden, 2002) or posterior (Russman et al., 2003) circulation. The second is VZV multifocal vasculopathy, most often seen in immunocompromised individuals, particularly AIDS patients, which usually produces headache, fever, mental status changes and focal deficit. A CSF mononuclear pleocytosis is usually present in both unifocal and multifocal vasculopathy. Brain MRI scanning reveals a single large infarct in unifocal vasculopathy, whereas in multifocal vasculopathy, ischemic and hemorrhagic infarcts are seen in both cortex and subcortical areas (Fig. 3). Cerebral angiography reveals focal arterial stenosis (Fig. 4). Pathological changes in affected arteries include multinucleated giant cells, Cowdry A inclusion bodies and herpesvirus particles (hallmarks of human herpesvirus infection), and virological analysis reveals both VZV DNA and antigen in affected vessels (Fig. 5). Recent clinical virological correlations have revealed that the manifestations of VZV vasculopathy are protean, and that both unifocal and multifocal vasculopathy can occur without rash. Vasculopathy may be recurrent and present with transient ischemic attacks remote from and months after acute zoster, including posterior ischemic optic neuropathy (Gilden, 2002).

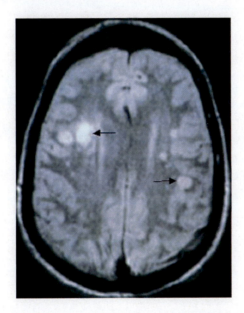

Figure 3. Brain magnetic resonance imaging scan of a patient with VZV multifocal vasculopathy reveals multiple large (arrows) and small areas of infarction in both cerebral hemispheres. Reprinted with permission of Neurology.

Unifocal large vessel infarcts follow trigeminal-distribution zoster and are presumed to result from transaxonal transport of virus from trigeminal afferent fibers that innervate anterior circulation vessels (Mayberg et al., 1981). Similarly, smaller infarcts in deep white and gray matter may reflect transport of VZV from trigeminal or cervical afferent fibers to smaller branches of posterior circulation vessels (Mayberg et al., 1981; Saito and Moskowitz, 1989).

During the time from zoster rash until the development of vasculopathy, virus reactivated from ganglia is presumed to actively travel along transaxonal pathways to arteries in which virus remains productive. Diagnosis is verified by the detection of VZV DNA in CSF. Because infection is active and often protracted, anti-VZV IgM or IgG antibody in CSF with reduced serum/CSF ratios of VZV antibody compared to total IgG or albumin is found (Gilden et al., 1998). The detection of antibody to VZV in CSF, even without amplifiable VZV DNA, can be diagnostic. Recognition of the wide spectrum of VZV vasculopathy and its proclivity to recur is essential, since effective antiviral therapy can be curative. Finally, oral antiviral treatment is insufficient to treat VZV vasculopathy; intravenous acyclovir is required and repeated treatment may be needed if ischemia recurs.

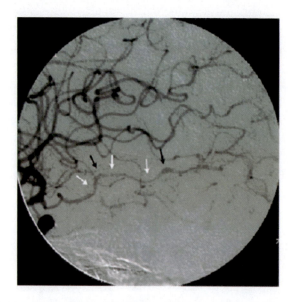

Figure 4. Cerebral angiogram from a patient with VZV vasculopathy without rash shows focal area of stenosis (white arrows) and post-stenotic dilatation (black arrows) involving the right posterior cerebral artery. Reprinted with permission of American Medical Association.

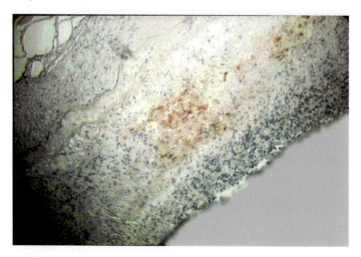

Figure 5. Immunohistochemical analysis of cerebral artery from a patient with VZV vasculopathy. VZV antigen (red staining) is detected after incubation of artery with rabbit antiserum directed against the VZV gene 63 protein. X86. Reprinted with permission of Journal of NeuroVirology.

Retinal Necrosis

VZV retinitis has been estimated to occur in 0.6% of patients with HIV infection. Two clinical syndromes develop. The first is acute retinal necrosis, which is seen in both immunocompetent and immunocompromised hosts. Both herpes simplex virus and VZV cause acute retinal necrosis. AIDS patients also develop progressive outer retinal necrosis (PORN), which is almost exclusively caused by VZV (Fig. 6). PORN is usually bilateral (Moorthy et al., 1997) and occurs in patients with CD4 counts typically less than 50. PORN may be preceded by retrobulbar optic neuritis and aseptic meningitis (Franco-Paredes, et al., 2002), central retinal artery occlusion, or ophthalmic distribution zoster (Menerath et al., 1995), and may occur with multifocal vasculopathy or myelitis. Retinal detachment often follows VZV necrotizing retinopathy. Proof that VZV causes PORN has come from both the detection of amplifiable VZV DNA in both aqueous and vitreous biopsies (Tran et al., 2003), as well as by histological examination of necropsy specimens from eyes and brain combined with *in situ* hybridization (van der Horn et al., 1996). Treatment with acyclovir is often not adequate. Patients with PORN who were treated with a combination of ganciclovir and foscarnet or with ganciclovir alone had a better final visual acuity than those treated with either acyclovir or foscarnet (Moorthy et al., 1997). In one instance, oral bromovinyldeoxyuridine treatment was successful when acyclovir failed (Dullaert et al., 1996).

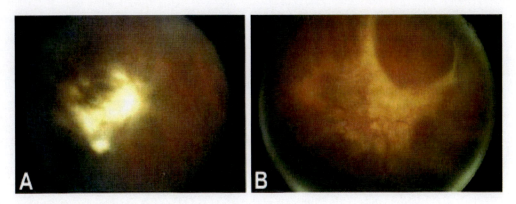

Figure 6. Funduscopic photographs of an AIDS patient show a peripheral chorioretinal lesion (A); 6 weeks later, the patient developed a complicated retinal detachment (B). At the time or surgical repair, a vitreous sample was positive for amplifiable VZV DNA. Reprinted with permission of Ophthalmology.

Mixed Syndromes

Not surprisingly, multiple neurologic complications due to VZV may occur in HIV-infected patients. One AIDS patient developed a sixth cranial nerve palsy followed by progressive fatal myelopathy; at autopsy, findings included ventriculoencephalitis and vasculitis with transverse infarction of the spinal cord without evidence of direct infection of the spinal cord parenchyma. Spinal cord infarction secondary to VZV vasculitis is an unusual cause of myelopathy in immunosuppressed patients (Kenyon et al., 1996). Another report describes 11 AIDS patients who developed productive VZV infection of the CNS (Gray et al., 1994). Zoster was seen in only 4 patients, while multifocal vasculopathy, predominantly involving white matter, was the most common finding. Ventriculitis was also seen, as well as hemorrhagic meningomyeloradiculitis with necrotizing vasculitis. Focal necrotizing myelitis was observed in one case.

Treatment

The following guidelines for treatment of HIV-infected individuals with zoster are currently endorsed by the Centers for Disease Control, National Institutes of Health, The United States Public Health Service, and The Department of Health and Human Services (Benson et al., 2004). HIV-infected patients with zoster require immediate antiviral treatment. For localized zoster, oral treatment with famciclovir or valacyclovir is usually adequate, whereas patients with disseminated zoster require treatment with intravenous acyclovir (Table 1). No drug has been shown to prevent recurrent zoster in HIV-infected individuals (Benson et al., 2004).

Table 1. Treatment of Herpes Zoster in HIV-Infected and AIDS patients

Signs	Treatment	Dose/Duration
restricted dermatomal skin lesion	famciclovir or valacyclovir	500 mg PO TID 7-10d; 1 gm PO TID 7-10d
disseminated skin lesions and/or visceral disease	Acyclovir	10 mg/kg IV q8h; continued until all signs of skin lesions and/or visceral disease have resolved
progressive outer retinal necrosis (PORN)	acyclovir and	10 mg/kg IV q8h (infuse at a constant rate for 1 hour) for 7-14d
	foscarnet	60 mg/kg IV q8h slowly for 1-2 hr (no faster than 1 mg/kg/minute) for 7-14 days
	- concomitant laser retinal photocoagulation may be necessary to prevent retinal detachments	In one series, patients treated with ganciclovir and foscarnet or with ganciclovir alone had a better final visual acuity than those treated with either acyclovir or foscarnet; in one instance, oral bromovinyldeoxyuridine treatment was successful when acyclovir failed.

If skin lesions become verrucous or do not resolve with oral famciclovir or valacyclovir, treatment with acyclovir intravenously is recommended. If an HIV-positive or AIDS patient does not respond to 10-14 days of treatment with intravenous acyclovir, intravenous treatment can be continued for an extended time, sometimes for a total of one month, followed by oral famiclovir or valaciclovir. If prolonged treatment fails, then treatment with foscarnet should be considered.

Conclusion

Zoster is more common in HIV-infected individuals (Verroust et al., 1987) and patients with AIDS (Friedman-Klein et al., 1986). These patients can ultimately manifest a more severe form of VZV than immunocompetent individuals. In immunocompromised patients, zoster progresses to myelopathy more often than in immunocompetent individuals, and myelopathy is more protracted and sometimes fatal. Similarly, immunocompromised patients more often develop multifocal vasculopathy characterized by mental status changes and focal deficit with ischemic and hemorrhagic infarcts. Despite immunosuppression, most HIV-positive and AIDS patients who develop serious neurological complications due to VZV can have a favorable outcome, if monitored closely and provided with aggressive antiviral therapy early in the course of infection.

Acknowledgements

This work was supported in part by Public Health Service grants AG 06127 and NS 32623 from the National Institutes of Health. Steven Deitch is supported by Public Health Service grant NS 07321 from the National Institutes of Health. We thank Marina Hoffman for editorial assistance and Cathy Allen for manuscript preparation.

References

Benson, C., Kaplan, J.E., Masur, H., Pau, A., and Holmes, K.K. (2004). Treating opportunistic infections among HIV-infected adults and adolescents. Recommendations from CDC, the National Institutes of Health, and the HIV Medicine Association/Infectious Diseases Society of America. *Morbidity and Mortality Weekly Report, 53(RR15),* 1-112.

Berger, R., Florent, G., and Just, M. (1981). Decrease of the lymphoproliferative response to varicella-zoster virus antigen in the aged. *Infection and Immunity, 32,* 24-27.

Chretien, F., Belec, L., Lescs, M.C., Authier, F.J., De Truchis, P., Scaravilli, F., and Gray, F. (1997). Central nervous system infection due to varicella and zoster virus in AIDS. *Archives d Anatomie et de Cytology Pathologiques, 45,* 142-152.

Colebunders, R., Mann, J.M., Francis, H., Bila, K., Izaley, L., Ilwaya, M., Kakonde, N., Quinn, T.C., Curran, J.W., and Piot, P. (1988). Herpes zoster in African patients: a clinical predictor of human immunodeficiency virus infection. *Journal of Infectious Diseases, 157,* 314-318.

De La Blanchardiere, A., Rozenberg, F., Caumes, E., Picard, O., Lionnet, F., Livartowski, J., Coste, J., Sicard, D., Lebon, P., and Salmon-Ceron, D. (2000). Neurological complications of varicella-zoster virus infection in adults with human immunodeficiency virus infection. *Scandinavian Journal of Infectious Diseases, 32,* 263-269.

de Silva, S.M., Mark, A.S., Gilden, D.H., Mahalingam, R., Balish, M., Sandbrink, F., and Houff, S. (1996). Zoster myelitis: Improvement with antiviral therapy in two cases. *Neurology, 47,* 929-931.

Domingo, P., Torres, O.H., Ris, J., and Vazquez, G. (2001). Herpes zoster as an immune reconstitution disease after initiation of combination antiretroviral therapy in patients with human immunodeficiency virus type-1 infection. *American Journal of Medicine, 110,* 605-609.

Dullaert, H., Maudgal, P.C., Leys, A., Dralands, L., and Clercq, E. (1996). Bromovinyldeoxyuridine treatment of outer retinal necrosis due to varicella-zoster virus: a case report. *Bulletin de la Societe Belge d Ophthalmologie, 262,* 107-113.

Franco-Paredes, C., Bellehemeur, T., Merchant, A., Sanghi, P., DiazGranados, C., and Rimland, D. (2002). Aseptic meningitis and optic neuritis preceding varicella-zoster progressive outer retinal necrosis in a patient with AIDS. *AIDS, 16,* 1045-1049.

Friedman-Kien, A.E., Lafleur, F.L., Gendler, E., Hennessey, N.P., Montagna, R., Halbert, S., Rubinstein, P., Krasinski, K., Zang, E., and Poiesz, B. (1986). Herpes zoster: a possible early clinical sign for development of acquired immunodeficiency syndrome in high-risk individuals. *Journal of the American Academy of Dermatology, 14,* 1023-1028.

Gershon, A.A., Mervish, N., LaRussa, P., Steinberg, S., Lo, S.H., Hodes, D., Fikrig, S., Bonagura, V., and Bakshi, S. (1997). Varicella-zoster virus infection in children with underlying human immunodeficiency virus infection. *Journal of Infectious Diseases, 176,* 1496-1500.

Gilden, D.H. (2002). Varicella zoster virus vasculopathy and disseminated encephalomyelitis. *Journal of Neurological Sciences, 195,* 99-101.

Gilden, D.H., Vafai, A., Shtram, Y., Becker, Y, Devlin, M., and Wellish, M. (1983). Varicella-zoster virus DNA in human sensory ganglia. *Nature, 306,* 478-480.

Gilden, D.H., Beinlich, B.R., Rubinstein, E.M., Stommel, E., Swenson, R., and Rubinstein, D. (1994). Varicella zoster virus myelitis: an expanding spectrum. *Neurology, 44,* 1818-1823.

Gilden, D.H., Bennett, J.L., Kleinschmidt-DeMasters, B.K., Song, D.D., Yee, A.S., and Steiner, I. (1998). The value of cerebrospinal fluid antiviral antibody in the diagnosis of neurologic disease produced by varicella zoster virus. *Journal of Neurological Sciences, 149,* 140-144.

Gilden, D.H., Gesser, R, Smith, J., Wellish, M., LaGuardia, J.J., Cohrs, R.J., and Mahalingam, R. (2001). Presence of VZV and HSV-1 DNA in human nodose and celiac ganglia. *Virus Genes, 23,* 145-147.

Glesby, M.J., Moore, R.D., and Chaisson, R.E. (1993). Herpes zoster in patients with advanced human immunodeficiency virus infection treated with zidovudine. Zidovudine Epidemiology Study Group. *Journal of Infectious Diseases, 168,* 1264-1268.

Gnann, J.W. Jr. (2002). Varicella-zoster virus: atypical presentations and unusual complications. *Journal of Infectious Diseases, 186, Suppl.* 1, S91-98.

Gómez-Tortosa, E., Gadea, I., Gegúundez, M.I., Esteban, A., Rábano, J., Fernández-Guerrero, M.L., and Soriano, F. (1994). Development of myelopathy before herpes zoster rash in a patient with AIDS. *Clinical Infectious Diseases, 18,* 810-812.

Gray, F., Belec, L., Lescs, M.C., Chretien, F., Ciardi, A., Hassine, D., Flament-Saillour, M., de Truchis, P., Clair, B., and Scaravilli, F. (1994). Varicella-zoster virus infection of the central nervous system in the acquired immune deficiency syndrome. *Brain, 117,* 987-999.

Hogan, E.L., and Krigman, M.R. (1973). Herpes zoster myelitis: Evidence for viral invasion of spinal cord. *Archives of Neurology, 29,* 309-313.

Hwang, Y.M., Lee, B.I., Chung, J.W., Ahn, J.H., Kim, K.W., and Kim, D.I. (1991). A case of herpes zoster myelitis: positive magnetic resonance imaging finding. *European Neurology, 31,* 164-167.

Jacobson, M.A. (2001). Human immunodeficiency virus-associated immune reconstitution disease. *American Journal of Medicine, 110,* 662-663.

Karstaedt, A.S. (1992). AIDS--the Baragwanath experience. Part III. HIV infection in adults at Baragwanath Hospital. *South African Medical Journal, 82,* 95-97.

Kenyon, L.C., Dulaney, E., Montone, K.T., Goldberg, H.I., Liu, G.T., and Lavi, E. (1996). Varicella-zoster ventriculo-encephalitis and spinal cord infarction in a patient with AIDS. *Acta Neuropathologica (Berlin), 91,* 202-205.

Koskiniemi, M., Rantalaiho, T., Piiparinen, H., von Bonsdorff, C.H., Farkkila, M., Jarvinen, A., Kinnunen, E., Koskiniemi, S., Mannonen, L., Muttilainen, M., Linnavuori, K., Porras, J., Puolakkainen, M., Raiha, K., Salonen, E.M., Ukkonen, P., Vaheri, A., Valtonen, V., and Study Group. (2001). Infection of the central nervous system of suspected viral origin: a collaborative study from Finland. *Journal of Neurovirology, 7,* 400-408.

Leppard, B., and Naburi, A.E. (1998). Herpes zoster: an early manifestation of HIV infection. *African Health, 21,* 5-6.

Lionnet, F., Pulik, M., Genet, P., Petitdidier, C., Davous, P., Lebon, P., and Rozenberg, F. (1996). Myelitis due to varicella-zoster virus in two patients with AIDS: successful treatment with acyclovir. *Clinical Infectious Diseases, 22,* 138-140.

Mahalingam, R., Wellish, M., Wolf, W., Dueland, A.N., Cohrs, R., Vafai, A., and Gilden, D.H. (1990). Latent varicella zoster virus DNA in human trigeminal and thoracic ganglia. *New England Journal of Medicine, 323,* 627-631.

Margolis, T.P., Lowder, C.Y., Holland, G.N., Spaide, R.F., Logan, A.G., Weissman, S.S., Irvine, A.R., Josephberg, R., Meisler, D.M., and O'Donnell, J.J. (1991). Varicella-zoster virus retinitis in patients with the acquired immunodeficiency syndrome. *American Journal of Ophthalmology, 112,* 119-131.

Martinez, E., Gatell, J., Moran, Y., Aznar, E., Buira, E., Guelar, A., Mallolas, J., and Soriano, E. (1998). High incidence of herpes zoster in patients with AIDS soon after therapy with protease inhibitors. *Clinical Infectious Diseases, 27,* 1510-1513.

Matsuo, K., Honda, M., Shiraki, K., and Niimura, M. (2001). Prolonged herpes zoster in a patient infected with the human immunodeficiency virus. *Journal of Dermatology, 28,* 728-733.

Mayberg, M., Langer, R.S., Zervas, N.T., and Moskowitz, M.A. (1981). Perivascular meningeal projections from the cat trigeminal ganglia: possible pathway for vascular headaches in man. *Science, 213,* 228-230,

Menerath, J.M., Gerard, M., Laurichesse, H., Goldschmidt, P., Peigue-LaFeuille, H., Rozenberg, F., and Beytout, J. (1995). Bilateral acute retinal necrosis in a patient with acquired immunodeficiency syndrome. *Journal Francais d Ophthalmologie, 18,* 625-633.

Miller, A.E. (1980). Selective decline in cellular immune response to varicella-zoster in the elderly. *Neurology, 30,* 582-587.

Moorthy, R.S., Weinberg, D.V., Teich, S.A., Berger, B.B., Minturn, J.T., Kumar, S., Rao, N.A., Fowell, S.M., Loose, I.A., and Jampol, L.M. (1997). Management of varicella zoster virus retinitis in AIDS. *British Journal of Ophthalmology, 81,* 189-194.

Naburi, A.E., and Leppard, B. (2000). Herpes zoster and HIV infection in Tanzania. *International Journal of STD and AIDS, 11,* 254-256.

Russman, A.N., Lederman, R.J., Calabrese, L.H., Embi, P.J., Forghani, B., and Gilden, D.H. (2003). Multifocal varicella zoster virus vasculopathy without rash. *Archives of Neurology, 60,* 1607-1609.

Saito, K., and Moskowitz, M.A. (1989). Contributions from the upper cervical dorsal roots and trigeminal ganglia to the feline circle of Willis. *Stroke, 20,* 524-526.

Tako, J., and Rado, J.P. (1965). Zoster meningoencephalitis in a steroid-treated patient. *Archives of Neurology, 12,* 610-612.

Tangsinmankong, N., Kamchaisatian, W., Lujan-Zilbermann, J., Brown, C.L., Sleasman, J.W., and Emmanuel, P.J. (2004). Varicella zoster as a manifestation of immune restoration disease in HIV-infected children. *Journal of Allergy and Clinical Immunology, 113,* 742-746.

Tran, T.H., Rozenberg, F., Cassoux, N., Rao, N.A., LeHoang, P., and Bodaghi, B. (2003). Polymerase chain reaction analysis of aqueous humour samples in necrotizing retinitis. *British Journal of Ophthalmology, 87,* 79-83.

UNAIDS. (2005). 2005 Report on the global AIDS epidemic: executive summary. UNAIDS, p. 10.

van den Horn, G.J., Meenken, C., and Troost, D. (1996). Association of progressive outer retinal necrosis and varicella zoster encephalitis in a patient with AIDS. *British Journal of Ophthalmology, 80,* 982-985.

Veenstra, J., Krol, A., van Praag, R.M., Frissen, P.H., Schellekens, P.T., Lange, J.M., Coutinho, R.A., and van der Meer, J.T. (1995). Herpes zoster, immunological deterioration and disease progression in HIV-1 infection. *AIDS, 9,* 1153-1158.

Verroust, F., Lemay, D., and Laurian, Y. (1987). High frequency of herpes zoster in young hemophiliacs. *New England Journal of Medicine, 15,* 166-167.

World Health Organization Weekly Epidemiological Record. (1998). Varicella vaccines. *World Health Organization Weekly Epidemiological Record, 73,* 241-248.

In: Neuro-AIDS
Editors: A. Minagar and P. Shapshak, pp. 199-223

ISBN: 1-59454-610-X
© 2006 Nova Science Publishers, Inc.

Chapter IX

Imaging of the Central Nervous System Complications of HIV and AIDS Related Illnesses

Rohit Bakshi[1],* and Leena Ketonen[2]

[1]Departments of Neurology and Radiology, Brigham and Women's Hospital, Harvard Medical School, Boston, MA, USA;
[2]Department of Radiology, University of Rochester Medical Center, Rochester, NY, USA.

Abstract

Neuroimaging technology provides a continuously expanding array of techniques to non-invasively study the living nervous system. In patients infected with human immunodeficiency virus (HIV) or acquired immunodeficiency syndrome (AIDS), neurologic complications represent potentially treatable manifestations requiring early and accurate diagnosis. Many of the central nervous system (CNS) complications are associated with significant morbidity or death if left unrecognized. We shall provide an overview of neuroimaging methods and their role in the evaluation of patients with HIV and AIDS related CNS disorders. Emphasis will be placed on structural magnetic resonance imaging (MRI) and functional imaging. Neuroimaging is a key tool in the clinical management of this population such as in the early detection of HIV or opportunistic infections, tumors, or cerebrovascular disorders. Applications of neuroimaging in this population also include the ability to monitor treatment effects. In addition, through a variety of advanced imaging strategies, the underlying neurochemistry, metabolism, and blood flow of lesions can be studied to aid the differential diagnosis of lesions and guide further management. The authors' aim is for

---

* Correspondence concerning this article should be addressed to Rohit Bakshi, MD, FAAN, Associate Professor of Neurology & Radiology, Brigham & Women's Hospital, Harvard Medical School. 77 Avenue Louis Pasteur – HIM 730, Boston, MA 02115, USA. Voice: 617-525-5788, Fax: 617-525-5223; Email: rbakshi@bwh.harvard.edu.

this chapter to be useful to trainees and practitioners in the clinical and imaging fields of general medicine, infectious diseases, and clinical neurosciences.

Keywords: Human immunodeficiency virus, Acquired immunodeficiency syndrome, Neuroimaging, Magnetic resonance imaging, Magnetic resonance spectroscopy

Neuroimaging Techniques

The mainstream neuroimaging modalities include computed tomography (CT), magnetic resonance imaging (MRI), single photon emission computed tomography (SPECT), positron emission tomography (PET), ultrasound/neurosonology (carotid and transcranial Doppler), myelography, and catheter (conventional) angiography. MRI methods include conventional (T1-weighted vs. T2-weighted, spin-echo vs. gradient echo) and advanced (echoplanar, diffusion, perfusion, spectroscopy, magnetization transfer) techniques. Computerized tomography (CT) produces images by detection of the attenuation of X-rays through tissue. MRI is based on the magnetic resonance spin and relaxation properties of protons. Compared to MRI, CT has the disadvantage of ionizing radiation, decreased signal to noise, artifacts related to bone, and the inability to characterize neurochemistry and diffusion-related changes. CT is being rapidly replaced by MRI for most neuroimaging indications in the HIV/AIDS population. Thus, in this review the author will focus on MRI rather than CT.

The conventional MRI techniques include spin-echo or gradient-echo methods typically featuring T1-weighted and T2-weighted pulse sequences. T1-weighted images (T1WI) are sensitive to anatomic changes such as mass effect, midline shift, or sulcal effacement and also to certain forms of hemorrhage, calcification or adipose. T2-weighted images (T2WI) and their variations (e.g. proton-density images) are sensitive to nearly all CNS pathologies due to their sensitivity to prolongation of dephasing of water protons. Most CNS diseases are characterized by increased water content reflecting pathologic processes such as edema, demyelination, inflammation, gliosis, tract degeneration, and necrosis. Short-tau inversion recovery (STIR) for the spine and fluid-attenuated inversion-recovery (FLAIR) for the brain are techniques that combine T2-weighting and inversion recovery pulses that suppress CSF and provide higher sensitivity than conventional sequences. For example, FLAIR images provide high sensitivity for intracranial disease in the HIV/AIDS population (Thurnher, et al., 1997a) and other neurologic diseases (Bakshi, et al., 2001), but also present a unique set of technical challenges (Bakshi, et al., 2000).

Developed in the past decade, echoplanar MRI allows ultrafast scanning times and a range of new pulse sequences such as diffusion-weighted (DWI) and perfusion-weighted (PWI) MRI (Bammer et al., 2005). These techniques can detect ischemia and tissue at risk for infarction more sensitively than conventional MRI and CT (Sorensen, et al., 1996; Xavier, et al., 2003). In addition, both techniques have applications to the HIV and AIDS population. DWI is based on the use of specialized gradients and echoplanar scanning capability in the detection of water diffusion. Water molecules in healthy tissue are in a state of constant random diffusion (Brownian motion). Apparent diffusion coefficient (ADC) maps can be calculated which provide a physiologic estimate of the water velocity. DWI and ADC maps of the brain can be obtained in approximately 30 seconds on echoplanar platforms (Bammer et al., 2005). Causes of restricted diffusion include cytotoxic edema, inflammation/pus, high viscosity, and spongiform change. Causes of elevated diffusion include cystic change, vasogenic edema and necrosis. DWI is useful in the HIV/AIDS population to study intracranial infectious vs. neoplastic mass lesions and for the early detection of stroke (e.g. due to vasculitis or meningitis). PWI scans depict perfusion of the brain microvasculature after a rapid intravenous bolus of gadolinium contrast (Sorensen, et al., 1996; Keston, et al., 2003; Bammer et al, 2005). PWI is useful in the HIV/AIDS population to examine the blood flow and, in turn, the metabolic characteristics of intracranial mass lesions and regional changes related to cognitive dysfunction (Keston, et al., 2003). Proton magnetic resonance spectroscopy (MRS) can non-invasively image the neurochemical profile of brain tissue (Lin et al. 2005). As recently reviewed from a technical standpoint (Drost, et al., 2002; Lin et al. 2005), most MRS studies of the brain are obtained by proton spectroscopy with water suppression and either a single-voxel or multi-voxel technique with peaks expressed as parts per million (ppm). In a clinical MRS brain study the metabolites of interest are myo-inositol (3.6 ppm), choline (3.25 ppm), creatine (3.0 ppm), glutamine/glutamate (2.2 to 2.4 ppm), N-acetyl-aspartate (NAA, 2.0 ppm), and lactate/lipids (1.33-0.9 ppm). NAA is a marker of neuronal and axonal integrity. Choline is thought to represent phospholipid membrane biosynthesis and cellular proliferation. Creatine (Cr) reflects cellular energy and typically acts as a reference peak. Increased macromolecular (lipid and lactate) peaks indicate areas of necrosis and anaerobic metabolism. The most common clinical role of MRS in the HIV/AIDS population is the discrimination of neoplastic from nonneoplastic processes (Leclerc, et al., 2002) and early detection of HIV brain infection (Bakshi, 2004).

Functional MRI is based on the detection of changes in blood oxygenation related to cerebral activation (Bammer et al., 2005), and has a research role in the HIV/AIDS population at present. PET and SPECT are collectively known as nuclear imaging techniques, based on the radioactive tagging of molecules administered and imaged through the physiologic and pathologic uptake of these tracers by living tissue (Brooks, 2005). Their major role is to characterize metabolic changes in the brain related to mass lesions or cognitive changes in the HIV/AIDS population.

HIV Encephalopathy

Direct HIV infection of the brain (HIV encephalitis) typically occurs in two stages. The first stage occurs at the time of initial HIV infection and is often subclinical (Sidtis, et al., 1990; Trotot, et al., 1997), characterized by multifocal <1 cm white matter lesions that are hyperintense on T2WI. Such lesions are reported in about one-third of seropositive asymptomatic patients (Bakshi, 2004). The second stage is a progressive subacute encephalitis with brain atrophy. This second stage is also known as HIV encephalopathy, the AIDS dementia complex, HIV-1-associated dementia, or HIV-1-associated cognitive/motor complex (Sidtis, et al., 1990; Trotot, et al., 1997; Avison, et al., 2002; Balakrishnan, et al., 1990; Chang, et al., 1999; Chang, et al., 2000; Chang, et al., 1997; Chrysikopoulos, et al., 1990; Flowers, et al., 1990; Hawkins, et al., 1993; Jordan, et al., 1991; Miller, et al., 1997;

Navia, et al., 1997; Olsen, et al., 1988; Post, et al., 1988; Simone, et al., 1998). Brain atrophy, a common feature of symptomatic HIV encephalitis (Bakshi, 2004; Chrysikopoulos, et al., 1990; Post, et al., 1988; Heyes, et al., 2001), is most prominent in central regions (ventricular enlargement) to a greater extent than cortical atrophy (sulcal prominence) (Figure 1). The white matter lesions of HIV encephalitis have been correlated with multinucleated giant cells, microglial nodules, demyelination and vacuolation (Hawkins, et al., 1993). Such lesions are typically hypodense on CT scans and essentially isointense on T1WI and hyperintense on T2WI (Figure 1) without mass effect or gadolinium enhancement. The white matter lesions of early HIV encephalitis typically affect the periventricular white matter and centrum semiovale with sparing of the subcortical (arcuate) U-fibers. The lesions are characteristically symmetric, "fluffy" or "cotton-like," typically becoming confluent and diffuse as the disease progresses (Figure 1). In later stages the lesions typically extend to the internal capsules, basal ganglia, thalamus, and cerebral peduncles (Trotot, et al., 1997; Chrysikopoulos, et al., 1990; Hawkins, et al., 1993). The lack of significant hypointensity on T1WI is helpful in differentiating HIV encephalitis from more aggressive conditions such as progressive multifocal leukoencephalopathy.

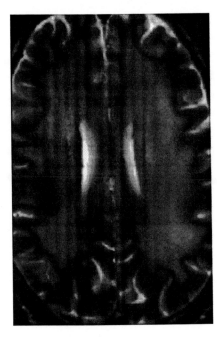

Figure 1. HIV encephalitis in a 36-year-old man who presents with memory loss. A conventional spin-echo T2-weighted axial image is shown. Hyperintense lesions are present in the periventricular and lobar white matter, with relative sparing of the subcortical (arcuate) U-fibers, and no associated mass effect. The morphology of the lesions is typical for HIV encephalitis with a "cotton-like" or "fluffy" appearance. The lesions are diffuse, poorly circumscribed and show confluence. Enlargement of the subarachnoid spaces (cortical sulci) and lateral ventricles is suggested for the patient's age, consistent with diffuse brain atrophy. The white matter lesions were isointense on T1WI (not shown) and non-enhancing (not shown).

Newer imaging techniques appear to play a role in the evaluation of HIV encephalitis. PWI has shown that patients with symptomatic HIV encephalitis have decreased cerebral perfusion in the bilateral inferior lateral frontal and medial parietal cortex and increased perfusion in the posterior inferior parietal white matter (Chang, et al., 2000). These regional blood flow changes correlate with the level of neuropsychologic dysfunction. One MRS study showed a decreased NAA/Cr ratio in the frontal gray matter in early symptomatic HIV encephalitis (Navia, et al., 1997). Another study showed higher Choline/Cr and myo-inositol/Cr in the basal ganglia and significantly reduced NAA/Cr and significantly higher myo-inositol/Cr in the frontal white matter (Lee et al., 2003). White matter lesions of HIV encephalitis are reported to show increased myo-inositol, increased choline, and decreased NAA (Chang, et al., 1999). Chang et al. (1999) showed that highly active antiretroviral therapy (HAART) led to a reversal of initially increased choline and myoinositol. Using MRS of the centrum semiovale, Simone et al. (1998) reported decreased NAA and increased choline in all 60 HIV seropositive patients vs. normal controls. However, the NAA/Cr ratio was significantly lower in lymphoma and progressive multifocal leukoencephalopathy than in HIV encephalitis and toxoplasmosis. A lipid peak was associated with lymphomas while a lactate peak was associated with progressive multifocal leukoencephalopathy. MRS is more sensitive than conventional MRI in detecting subclinical HIV encephalitis (Suwanwelaa, et al., 2000). DWI has sensitivity to the altered integrity of white matter fibers in the early stage of HIV encephalitis (Pomara, et al., 2001). Functional imaging techniques (i.e. SPECT and PET) have shown that metabolic abnormalities precede both the structural and clinical effects of the disease (Navia, et al., 1997). An fMRI study of 13 patients infected with HIV and 7 healthy control subjects showed increases in cerebral blood volume in the deep and cortical gray matter in the HIV group (Tracey et al., 1998). Deep gray matter changes were particularly well associated with cognitive impairment. In one patient, these fMRI abnormalities reversed and paralleled cognitive improvement after initiation of ant-retroviral monotherapy.

HIV and the Spinal Cord

Spinal cord involvement in the HIV/AIDS population may occur from a variety of sources, such as vacuolar myelopathy (VM), opportunistic infection, or neoplastic disease (Berger, et al., 2002 ; Eggers, 2002; Rottnek, et al., 2002; Bhigjee, et al., 2001; Di Rocco, et al., 1998; Thurnher, et al., 1997b; Chong, et al., 1999; Sartoretti-Schefer, et al., 1997; Quencer, et al., 1997; Anneken et al., in press). The etiology of VM may be linked to direct infection of the cord by HIV. This is the most common cause of spinal cord disease in patients with HIV/AIDS. The pathology of VM is characterized by patchy vacuolation and pallor of the lateral and posterior columns with the later appearance of gliosis, demyelination and necrosis. Spinal MRI typically shows cord atrophy involving the thoracic cord more commonly than the cervical cord (Chong, et al., 1999; Sartoretti-Schefer, et al., 1997; Quencer, et al., 1997). Frank intramedullary cord lesions are seen less commonly than atrophy and are hyperintense on T2WI, isointense to madly hypointense on T1WI, and non-enhancing with gadolinium. Lesions may be diffuse (Chong, et al., 1999) or isolated to the posterior columns (Sartoretti-Schefer, et al., 1997). The cord lesions of VM likely represent extensive vacuolation (Sartoretti-Schefer, et al., 1997). Some authors have argued that direct infection of the cord by HIV (HIV myelitis) is distinct from VM (Quencer, et al., 1997) with the former characterized by lesions involving both the gray and white matter of the spinal cord (Quencer, et al., 1997). A normal MRI may be seen in VM such as in the early clinical stage (Chong, et al., 1999). Other causes of myelopathy in this population include cancer (e.g. meningeal or intramedullary lymphoma, extradural leiomyoma), bone disease (epidural masses, spine infection), and opportunistic neural infections (e.g. cytomegalovirus polyradiculitis, herpes radiculitis/myelitis, tuberculosis, toxoplasmosis, fungal infection) (Thurnher, et al., 1997b; Quencer, et al., 1997).

Toxoplasmosis

Toxoplasma gondii brain infection typically affects immunocompromised hosts such as those with HIV/AIDS (Bakshi, 2004; Porter, et al., 1992; Luft, et al., 1993; Laissy, et al., 1994; Issakhanian, et al., 2001; Revel, et al., 1992; Ramsey, et al., 1997) or other immunocompromised states (Ionita, et al., 2004). Cerebral toxoplasmosis is the most common opportunistic CNS infection in patients with AIDS and the most common cause of intracranial mass lesions in this population. The spinal cord is affected much less commonly than the brain (Thurnher, et al., 1997b; Quencer, et al., 1997; Vyas, et al., 1996). Cerebral toxoplasmosis typically presents as an acute illness with fever, confusion, headache, seizures, and focal neurologic signs. In the emergency room, CT is often used as the initial neuroimaging study, although MRI is clearly more sensitive for detection of the disease (Figure 2) (Porter, et al., 1992; Luft, et al., 1993). On noncontrast CT scans, acute or subacute lesions typically appear hypodense (Figure 2) (Porter, et al., 1992). Chronic lesions appear calcified (hyperdense) on CT scans, especially after treatment (Revel, et al., 1992). On MRI (Figure 2), multiple lesions are seen commonly and affect the cortical gray-white junction and deep central gray nuclei (Bakshi, 2004; Porter, et al., 1992; Luft, et al., 1993; Laissy, et al., 1994; Issakhanian, et al., 2001; Revel, et al., 1992; Ramsey, et al., 1997; Ionita, et al., 2004). However, solitary toxoplasmosis may also occur. Other common locations include the periventricular white matter, posterior fossa, and cerebral cortex. Toxoplasmosis lesions typically appear isointense to hypointense on T1WI but are variable on T2WI. Prominent edema and mass effect are typically seen with edema disproportionately large relative to the size of the nidus. Non-edematous lesions without mass effect may be seen occasionally, especially in the non-AIDS setting (Ionita, et al., 2004). On T2WI, the lesions may be difficult to distinguish from the surrounding edema (both are hyperintense). Alternatively, a "target" appearance may be seen (central isointense or hypointense core) (Figure 2). Gadolinium administration is the mainstay of conventional imaging in toxoplasmosis because the lesions typically enhance robustly (Ramsey, et al., 1997). The enhancement patterns are typically ringlike, heterogeneous, or nodular (Figure 2), while smaller lesions may show homogeneous uptake. One caveat is that fulminant involvement may occur despite a relative lack of enhancement (Ionita, et al., 2004). MRI is a key tool for the longitudinal therapeutic monitoring of cerebral toxoplasmosis (Porter, et al., 1992; Luft, et al., 1993; Laissy, et al., 1994; Ramsey, et al., 1997). MRI improvement is typically noted 14 days after treatment. The role of advanced imaging techniques in the diagnosis of toxoplasmosis is discussed below.

Toxoplasmosis: *2 cases*

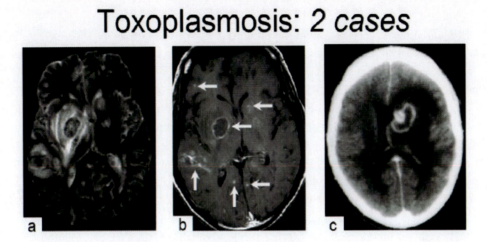

Figure 2. Toxoplasmosis in two patients with AIDS. (A, B): MRI scans are shown of a 38-year-old man with AIDS and a CD4 count of 209 who presented with four days of decreased mentation, poor oral intake, ataxia, and nonfluent speech. He developed new onset seizures. MRI of the head was performed; representative T2-weighted (A) and post-contrast T1-weighted (B) images are shown. Note the asymmetric involvement of the basal ganglia, gray-white junction, and cerebral cortex with enhancement of many of the lesions (B, arrows). Associated moderate to severe mass effect and surrounding edema is present. The concentric hyperintensity and hypointensity (target appearance) of the basal ganglia lesion on the T2-weighted image (A) is characteristic of toxoplasmosis. The patient's serum toxoplasmosis IgG was highly positive and he clinically improved 8 days after antitoxoplasma medical therapy. (C): Post-contrast CT scan is shown from another patient with AIDS. Note the typical findings of toxoplasmosis including mass effect and ringlike enhancement with an "eccentric target" sign. The patient received antitoxoplasma medical therapy and 10 days later the lesion and edema improved significantly on a repeat CT scan (not shown).

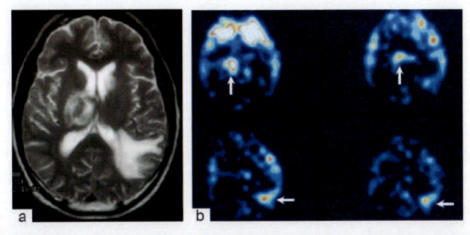

Figure 3. Primary CNS lymphoma in AIDS. Axial T2-weighted image (A) shows multiple lesions, the largest in the right basal ganglia and left parietal area with a smaller lesion in the left caudate head. The core of the right basal ganglia lesion is hypointense. Thallium (Tl 201) SPECT (B) shows increased abnormal tracer uptake in the right basal ganglia and left parietal lesions (arrows). There is prominent bilateral frontal uptake (normal findings) on the SPECT scans due to calibration necessary to visualize the periphery of the right basal ganglia lesions. Biopsy confirmed the diagnosis of primary CNS lymphoma.

Lymphoma

Primary central nervous system lymphoma (PCNSL) is a lymphocytic cancer typically of non-Hodgkin B-cell origin (Hochberg, et al., 1988). This is the most common intracranial neoplasia and the second most common cause of cerebral mass lesions in the HIV/AIDS population. While PCNSL afflicts immunocompromised patients, such as those with AIDS (Hochberg, et al., 1988; Taiwo, 2000; Ruiz, et al., 1997; Thurnher, et al., 2001; Cordoliani, et al., 1992), it also occurs in immunocompetent hosts (Coulon, et al., 2002; Bakshi, et al., 1999a; Giglio, et al., 2002). CT typically shows the tumor as hypodense or hyperdense on noncontrast images and enhancing after contrast administration (Thurnher, et al., 2001). MRI typically shows PCNSL as hypointense or isointense on T1WI and hypointense to slightly hyperintense on T2WI (Figure 3). The masses are characteristically associated with less edema and mass effect than expected based on tumor size (Figure 3). MRI with gadolinium contrast administration is a key tool in the evaluation of PCNSL - intense contrast enhancement is noted in at least 75% of cases (Bakshi, 2004; Thurnher, et al., 2001; Bakshi, et al., 1999a; Giglio, et al., 2002). However, occasional cases have been reported showing little or no enhancement (Bakshi, 2004; Thurnher, et al., 2001; Bakshi, et al., 1999a; Giglio, et al., 2002). Enhancement patterns are variable, ranging from homogeneous to nodular and ringlike patterns. Lymphoma has a propensity to spread along CSF pathways leading to subependymal or leptomeningeal enhancement and additional diagnostic specificity. Highlighting the need for early diagnosis, the doubling time of tumor volume in untreated patients is approximately 14 days. While solitary PCNSL may occur, multiple lesions are the rule (Figure 3). Differential diagnosis in the HIV/AIDS setting includes opportunistic infection, most notably toxoplasmosis (see below). Unusual manifestations of PCNSL include temporal cortical disease mimicking viral encephalitis (Giglio, et al., 2002) or non-enhancing diffuse infiltration of the neuraxis (Thurnher, et al., 2001; Bakshi, et al., 1999a). Spinal PCNSL, such as osseous, epidural, meningeal, radicular, or intramedullary involvement, occurs in 2-4% of the HIV/AIDS population (Thurnher, et al., 1997b; Quencer, et al., 1997). As discussed below, advanced imaging techniques play a role in the evaluation of PCNSL (Figures 3, 4).

Toxoplasmosis vs. Lymphoma

The main diagnostic dilemma of an intracranial mass lesion in the HIV/AIDS population is to differentiate toxoplasmosis from PCNSL (Figure 4). Conventional MRI is not reliable for distinguishing the two entities (Figure 4). PCNSL is favored by a solitary lesion, ventricular encasement, subependymal enhancement or homogeneous enhancement (in lesions larger than 1 x 1 cm), and hypointensity of the nidus on T2WI (Figures 3, 4). MRI findings suggesting toxoplasmosis include multiple lesions, basal ganglia/thalamic involvement, copious edema, hemorrhage, and a hyperintensity of the core on T2WI (Figure 2). In a body of research that continues to unfold, newer imaging methods have shed light on the evaluation of mass lesions in this population (Figures 3, 4) (Camacho, et al., 2003;

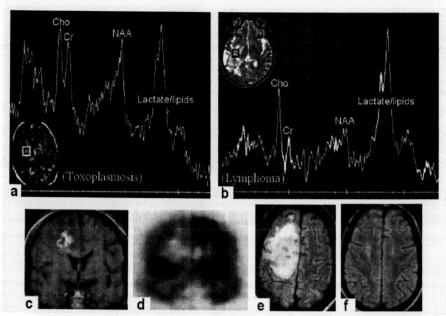

Figure 4. Toxoplasmosis vs. primary CNS lymphoma in AIDS: advanced imaging methods in 3 patients. Reproduced with permission (Bakshi, 2004). A-B. Single-voxel MRS and representative thumbnail MRI slices with voxel localizer of patients with toxoplasmosis (A) and primary CNS lymphoma (B). In patient A, a mild increase in choline (Cho) to creatine (Cr) ratio, a moderate reduction in NAA/Cr, and lactate/lipid peaks are present. In patient B, a marked increased Cho/Cr, marked decreased NAA/Cr, and lactate/lipid peaks are present. The latter findings of severe Cho and NAA changes are consistent with malignancy rather than an infectious or inflammatory process such as toxoplasmosis. C-F. Solitary toxoplasmosis – role of functional imaging. A 32 year-old man with AIDS developed acute headache, fever, leg weakness, and new onset seizures. MRI shows a solitary heterogeneously enhancing lesion (C) in the frontal lobe that is isointense to hyperintense on proton density images (E) with copious surrounding edema. The differential diagnosis includes toxoplasmosis and primary CNS lymphoma. For further clarification, a resting brain neurolite (perfusion) SPECT scan (D) was performed and shows that the lesion is "cold" due to marked hypoperfusion (white areas). Thus, a presumptive diagnosis of toxoplasmosis was made and the patient received anti-toxoplasmosis treatment. Follow-up MRI (F) shows resolution of the lesion.

Chang, et al., 1995; Walot, et al., 1996; Ketonen, et al., 1998; Chinn, et al., 1995; De La Pena, et al., 1998; Sugahara, et al., 1999; Ruiz, et al., 1994; Villringer, et al., 1995; Naddaf, et al., 1998; Pomper, et al., 2002). On MRS studies, toxoplasmosis appears to be associated with modest increases in choline, moderate decreases in NAA and pathologic macromolecular (lactate/lipid) peaks (Figure 4) while PCNSL is reported to show macromolecular peaks but also dramatically elevated choline and severely decreased NAA (Bakshi, 2004; Chang, et al., 1997; Simone, et al., 1998; Ramsey, et al., 1997; Chang, et al., 1995; Walot, et al., 1996; Chinn, et al., 1995; Pomper, et al., 2002) (Figure 4). Nuclear neuroimaging techniques clearly have a role in differentiating PCNSL from toxoplasmosis (Figures 3, 4) (Ramsey, et al., 1997; Ketonen, et al., 1998; De La Pena, et al., 1998; Ruiz, et al., 1994; Villringer, et al., 1995; Naddaf, et al., 1998; Pomper, et al., 2002). One early study showed that SPECT with thallium had a 94% positive predictive value in diagnosing PCNSL, seen as "hot" lesion (high tracer uptake) (Figure 3) (Ruiz, et al., 1994). FDG-PET showed 90% accuracy in differentiating toxoplasmosis ("cold") from PCNSL ("hot") (Villringer, et al., 1995). Another study of two SPECT techniques showed no false-negative cases of

PCNSL (sensitivity 100%) and a specificity of 54% to 69% (Naddaf, et al., 1998). Ketonen et al. (1998) have asserted that MRI and thallium-SPECT are complementary tests for the distinction between PCNSL and toxoplasmosis. False negative PCNSL lesions are likely to be necrotic with a thin enhancing rim on MRI. To minimize false negative thallium-SPECT studies, the SPECT scan should be read in conjunction with MRI. The simultaneous use of thallium and sestamibidi can also help differentiate PCNSL from benign brain lesions in patients with AIDS (De La Pena, et al., 1998). Taken together, the above findings suggest that hypermetabolic ("hot") lesions on nuclear neuroimaging studies are the best candidates for biopsy prior to the onset of therapy in patients with HIV/AIDS and enhancing brain masses (Figure 3). In contrast, antitoxoplasma therapy with expectant follow-up is a reasonable approach to those with hypometabolic ("cold") lesions (Figure 4).

Progressive Multifocal Leukoencephalopathy

An opportunistic infection caused by the JC virus, progressive multifocal leukoencephalopathy (PML) is a progressive, demyelinating CNS disorder. Structural neuroimaging studies (Bakshi, 2004; Garrels, et al., 1996; Kastrup, et al., 2002; Power, et al., 1997; Rosas, et al., 1999; Shapiro, et al., 2001; Whiteman, et al., 1993; Lizerbram, et al., 1997; Post, et al., 1999; Iranzo, et al., 1999) of PML show the lesions as multifocal, asymmetric, severely hypodense on CT scans, severely hypointense on T1WI, and hyperintense on T2WI, with a surprising paucity of mass effect (Figure 5). Histologic correlation indicates that lesions seen by imaging are correlated with areas of demyelination and axonal loss (Whiteman, et al., 1993). Post-contrast CT or MRI shows that lesions are usually nonenhancing or, less commonly, minimally enhancing. However, in the age of HAART, robustly enhancing PML may be seen in patients experiencing immune reconstitution (Hoffman et al., 2003). Early PML is characterized by lesions in the occipitoparietal lobar white matter abutting the gray-white junction with involvement of the subcortical (arcuate) U-fibers but sparing of the cortical ribbon. This results in a classic "scalloped" appearance of lesions known as the "heart of the gyrus" sign (Figure 5). In later stages the disease typically extends to the anterior lobes, corpus callosum, deep gray nuclei, posterior fossa, and spinal cord (Bakshi, 2004; Garrels, et al., 1996; Whiteman, et al., 1993). MRI has a key role in the longitudinal monitoring of the therapeutic outcome of PML (Garrels, et al., 1996; Power, et al., 1997; Shapiro, et al., 2001). Elevated choline, reduced NAA, and the presence of macromolecular (lactate/lipids) (Figure 5) have been reported in the disease on MRS studies (Simone, et al., 1998; Iranzo, et al., 1999).

Neuroimaging of Meningitis

The lack of bone artifact makes MRI far superior to CT for the evaluation of meningeal disease (Chang, et al., 1990a). However, the diagnosis of meningitis should of course rely on clinical and CSF data as the sensitivity and specificity of MRI remains questionable (Chang,

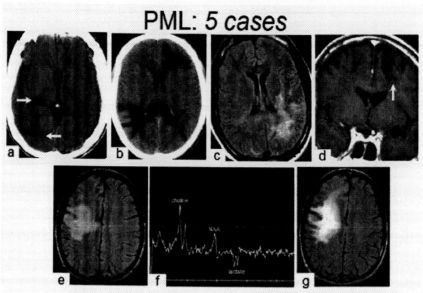

Figure 5. Progressive multifocal leukoencephalopathy (PML) in five patients with AIDS. Noncontrast CT of one patient (A) shows hypodensity of the posterior white matter in the occipitoparietal and internal capsule region (arrows). Noncontrast CT of another patient (B) shows bilateral posterior and anterior subcortical hypodensities including multifocal white matter lesions in the left frontal and (right greater than left) occipitoparietal area with involvement of the splenium of corpus callosum. Note the typical sparing of the cerebral cortex. FLAIR image (C) shows another patient with posterior predominant lesions confined largely to white matter but extending to the gray-white junction and arcuate (U) fibers. Coronal T1-weighted post-contrast image (D) of a fourth patient demonstrates marked hypointensity of bilateral asymmetric lesions. The sparing of the overlying cortex leads to a "heart of the gyrus" sign (arrow), characteristic of PML. In patient four (D), the post-contrast image shows no enhancement of the lesions (typical of PML). A fifth patient is shown in the bottom row of images (E-G). The baseline FLAIR image (E) shows a right frontal white matter hyperintensity. Single voxel proton MR spectroscopy (F) (TE=144 msec) of the core of the lesion shows increased choline, decreased NAA, and increased lactate (see inverted lactate doublet). The repeat FLAIR image two months later (G) shows rapid progression of the lesion. In all five patients, the lack of mass effect is typical of PML.

et al., 1990a; Kioumehr, et al., 1995; Runge, et al., 1995; Bakshi, et al., 1999b; Tsuchiya, et al., 1997; Bakshi, et al., 1999c). On noncontrast conventional MRI scans uncomplicated infectious meningitis typically shows normal findings, or if the inflammation is robust, dilitation of the subarachnoid space or hyperintensity of the cisterns may be seen on proton density images. FLAIR is more sensitive than conventional MRI or CT for the evaluation of intracranial infections in the HIV/AIDS population (Thurnher, et al., 1997a; Tsuchiya, et al., 1997). Abnormalities on FLAIR images in meningitis include hyperintensity of the cerebral vessels and subarachnoid space (Kamran et al., 2004). After gadolinium administration, intravascular enhancement and homogeneous enhancement of the leptomeninges including the tentorium, convexities, basal cisterns, and falx is typically seen on MRI (Kioumehr, et al., 1995; Runge, et al., 1995; Bakshi, et al., 1999b). However, FLAIR subarachnoid hyperintensity or meningeal or intravascular enhancement is not specific for infection (Bakshi, et al., 2000; Bakshi, et al., 1999b; Bakshi, et al., 1999c; Bakshi, et al., 1999d). Neuroimaging plays a key role in the early recognition of the complications of meningitis (Bakshi, et al., 1997; Chan, et al., 2003; Johkura, et al., 2002; Chelaifa, et al., 2003; Bhojo, et al., 2002; Smith, et al., 2002) such as potential neurosurgical emergencies including ventriculitis (Bakshi, et al., 1997), hydrocephalus (Chan, et al., 2003), cerebritis/abscess (Chelaifa, et al., 2003), and subdural empyema (Smith, et al., 2002). There is hope that advanced MRI techniques such as magnetization transfer (Runge, et al., 1995) and DWI (Abe, et al., 2002; Peng, et al., 2003) may increase the sensitivity of MRI for the evaluation of meningitis and its complications. One such example includes the detection of hyperintensity of the meninges or brain parenchyma on DWI scans (Abe, et al., 2002; Peng, et al., 2003).

Fungal Infections

Fungal brain infections in immunocompromised hosts show a wide spectrum of manifestations on MRI (Figures 6, 7) (Harris, et al., 1997a; Troncoso, et al., 2002; Miszkiel, et al., 1996; Berkefeld, et al., 1999; Bazan, et al., 1991; Andreula, et al., 1993; Caldenmeyer, et al., 1997; Cox, et al., 1992; Ostrow, et al., 1994; Tien, et al., 1991; Wrobel, et al., 1992; Boes, et al., 1994). The hyphal or pseudohyphal fungi, such as mucormycosis and aspergillus (Figure 6) are angioinvasive and thus manifest on neuroimaging studies as ischemia/infarction, hemorrhage, or cerebritis. This subgroup of fungi also commonly involves the paranasal sinuses and orbits. Fungi that proliferate in yeast forms, such as histoplasmosis and cryptococcus (Figure 7), tend to present as leptomeningitis with or without cerebritis. The meningitis has a propensity to affect the basal brain regions. Fungal infections in immunocompromised hosts may also involve the spinal region through hematogenous spread extending to the leptomeninges, spinal cord, or both (Thurnher, et al., 1997b; Harris, et al., 1997a).

Tuberculosis

Intracranial tuberculosis may occur in a variety of forms on neuroimaging studies (Wasay, et al., 2003; Gupta, et al., 1988 ; Daikos, et al., 2003; Gupta, et al., 2001; Campi-de-Castro, et al., 1991; Chang, et al., 1990b; Tayfun, et al., 1996; Gupta, et al., 1999; Whiteman, 1997; Whiteman, et al., 1995), such as tuberculomas, frank abscesses, meningitis, and cerebritis (Figure 8). The meningitis commonly affects the basal cisterns disproportionately. Intracranial tuberculomas are usually isointense on T1WI and mixed hypointense and hyperintense on T2WI (Figure 8). Homogeneous or ringlike enhancement is most commonly noted after gadolinium administration (Figure 8). A growing body of evidence indicates that advanced MRI techniques such as MRS and magnetization transfer add sensitivity and specificity for the evaluation of tuberculosis (Gupta, et al., 2001; Gupta, et al., 1999). One example of the increased specificity offered by MRS is a study showing that pyogenic brain abscesses had elevated amino acids, lactate and lipids while tuberculous lesions showed only elevated lactate/lipids (Gupta, et al., 2001). Tuberculosis in the HIV/AIDS population may also affect the spine with a myriad of sites of involvement such as the bony spine, epidural region, leptomeninges, spinal cord, or nerve roots (Thurnher, et al., 1997b; Whiteman, 1997).

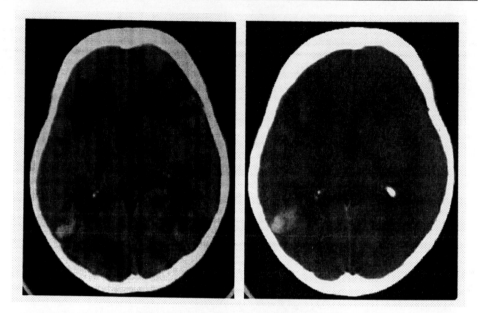

Figure 6. Aspergillus cerebritis: serial non-contrast CT in a fatal case. Bilateral intermixed hypodense and hyperdense lesions are seen in the bilateral frontal, parietal and occipital lobes. Hyperdense areas represent hemorrhage. Hypodense areas represent varying degrees of ischemia/infarction, cerebritis, and edema. The two scans are separated by three days. Note that the repeat CT (right) shows that diffuse brain edema has developed (note loss of sulcal and gray/white definition). Autopsy revealed systemic and multiorgan aspergillus infection with multiple brain abscesses, angioinvasion and hemorrhage. Reprinted with permission (Bakshi, 2004).

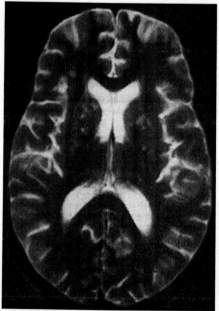

Figure 7. An axial conventional spin-echo T2WI is shown of a 27-year-old patient with a cryptococcal brain infection in AIDS. Note the multiple small bilateral hyperintense lesions in the corpus striatum (caudate and putamen). These lesions are most likely reflective in part of mucoid material secreted by the fungal organisms.

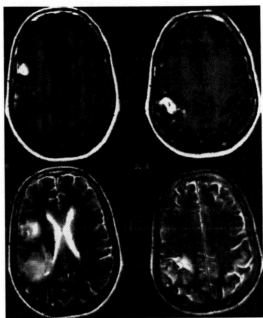

Figure 8. Tuberculosis of the brain with cerebritis and abscess (tuberculoma) formation. MRI scans of a patient are shown including post-contrast T1WI (upper row) and T2WI (lower row). Heterogeneous lesions are seen in the frontal and parietal region, involving both cortical and subcortical areas. The intermixed hypointensities on T2WI most likely represent hypercellularity, free radicals, or both. Postcontrast axial T1WI shows parenchymal and leptomeningeal enhancement, representing both meningitis and sub-pial extension.

Neurosyphilis

Intracranial neurosyphilis in immunocompromised hosts may occur as meningitis, cranial neuritis, cerebrovascular disease, or parenchymal gumma (Schiff, et al., 2002; Harris, et al., 1997b; Fox, et al., 2000; Brightbill, et al., 1995; Holland, et al., 1986; Agrons, et al., 1991). The meningitis in neurosyphilis has a propensity to affect basilar brain regions and thus affect the lower cranial nerves (Harris, et al., 1997b) (Figure 9). The cerebrovascular disease typically manifests as vasculitis (i.e. endarteritis) of medium and large arteries (Heubner's arteritis) or, less commonly, small arteries and arterioles (Nissl-Alzheimer arteritis) (Harris, et al., 1997b). Neuroimaging shows multiple areas of ischemia and infarction in syphilitic vasculitis with enhancement of basilar regions (Figure 9). Parenchymal syphilitic masses, know as gummas, range in diameter from a few millimeters to several centimeters commonly involving the cerebral cortex (Schiff, et al., 2002; Harris, et al., 1997b; Brightbill, et al., 1995; Agrons, et al., 1991). Orbital syphilis, particularly of the roof and supraorbital rim, may also occur (Harris, et al., 1997b).

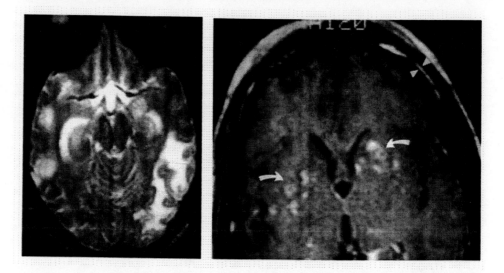

Figure 9. Meningovascular syphilis is shown in a 25-year-old man with new onset seizures and confusion. T2-weighted axial image (left) shows multiple hyperintensities in the bilateral medial temporal, bilateral lateral temporal, and left occipito-parietal lobes affecting both white and gray matter. The bilateral temporal lobe abnormalities evolved into infarctions. The patient had meningovascular syphilis with associated vasculitis. Post-contrast MRI (right) shows multiple bilateral enhancing parenchymal nodules in the basal ganglia (curved arrows), thalamus, ependymal region, and dural meninges (arrowheads). The enhancement is consistent with cerebritis and meningitis. The patient was treated with penicillin and in a follow-up MRI scan a week later the parenchymal lesions and abnormal enhancement had resolved (not shown).

Cytomegalovirus

The advent of HAART therapy has reduced the incidence of cytomegalovirus (CMV) encephalitis in patients with AIDS (Gray, et al., 2003). The most common forms of intracranial CMV infection in the immunocompromised host include multifocal white matter disease, meningoencephalitis, and ventriculitis/ependymitis (Lizerbram, et al., 1997; Luttmann, et al., 1997; Brechtelsbauer, et al., 1997; Holland, et al., 1994; Miller, et al., 1997; Vinters, et al., 1989). The most common MRI findings are brain atrophy and periventricular/subcortical multifocal and diffuse white matter hypodensities on CT scans (Figure 10) and hyperintense lesions on T2WI (Holland, et al., 1994). The noncontrast MRI findings may mimic HIV encephalitis (Miller, et al., 1997b). Ependymal involvement and enhancement on post-contrast images is also a common finding (Figure 10). The presence of subependymal or meningeal enhancement favors CMV rather than direct HIV infection (Lizerbram, et al., 1997; Holland, et al., 1994). CMV infection of the spinal cord (myelitis) usually preferentially affects the lumbar region including clumping of the intraspinal nerve roots in the lumbar thecal sac, and diffuse enhancement of the leptomeninges of the conus medullaris, cauda equina (Lizerbram, et al., 1997).

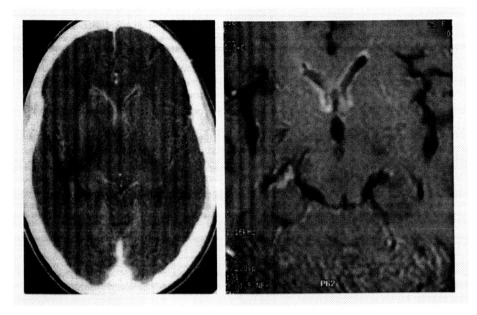

Figure 10. Cytomegalovirus encephalitis in a 26-year old woman with AIDS. Post-contrast CT (left) shows confluent hypodensities in the white matter, most prominent in the right posterior internal capsule and temporal lobe. Both the CT and post-contrast MRI (right) show bilateral enhancement of the ependyma surrounding the frontal horns of the lateral ventricles and adjacent to the temporal horn of the right lateral ventricle (see MRI scan). The findings are consistent with leukoencephalitis and ventriculitis, typical of cytomegalovirus brain infection.

Other Conditions

In this review, we have focused on neuroimaging of the most common CNS manifestations of HIV/AIDS. The reader is referred to additional reviews of neuroimaging features of HIV/AIDS, such as viral infections (Lizerbram, et al., 1997), bacterial infections (Cohen, 1997), vasculitis (Berkefeld, et al., 2000), stroke (Gillams, et al., 1997; Patsalides, et al., 2002), spinal disease (Thurnher, et al., 1997b; Quencer, et al., 1997; Thurnher, et al., 2000), and the pediatric population (States, et al., 1997).

Acknowledgments

This work was supported in part by a research grant from the National Institutes of Health (NIH-NINDS 1 K23 NS42379-01, Dr. Bakshi). We are grateful to Ms. Sophie Tamm and Ms. Erika Balajti for assistance with preparation of the manuscript.

References

Abe, M., Takayama, Y., Yamashita, H., Noguchi, M., and Sagoh, T. (2002). Purulent meningitis with unusual diffusion-weighted MRI findings. *Eur. J. Radiol, 44*, 1-4.

Agrons, G. A., Han, S. S., Husson, M. A., and Simeone, F. (1991). MR imaging of cerebral gumma. *AJNR Am. J. Neuroradiol, 12*, 80-81.

Andreula, C. F., Burdi, N., and Carella , A. (1993). CNS cryptococcosis in AIDS: Spectrum of MR findings. *J. Comput. Assist. Tomogr, 17*, 438-441.

Anneken K, Fischera M, Evers S, Kloska S, Husstedt IW. Recurrent vacuolar myelopathy in HIV infection. *J. Infect.* (in press)

Avison, M. J., Nath, A., and Berger, J. R. (2002). Understanding pathogenesis and treatment of HIV dementia: a role for magnetic resonance? *Trends Neurosci, 25*, 468-473.

Bakshi, R. (2004). Neuroimaging of HIV and AIDS related illnesses: a review. *Frontiers in Bioscience, 9*, 632-646.

Bakshi, R., Kinkel, P. R., Mechtler, L. L., and Bates, V. E. (1997). Cerebral ventricular empyema associated with severe adult pyogenic meningitis: Computed tomography findings. *Clin. Neurol. Neurosurg, 99*, 252-255.

Bakshi, R., Mazziotta, J. C., Mischel, P. S., Jahan, R., Seligson, D. B., and Vinters, H. V. (1999a). Lymphomatosis cerebri presenting as a rapidly progressive dementia: clinical, neuroimaging and pathologic findings. *Dementia Geriatr. Cogn. Disord, 10*, 152-157.

Bakshi, R., Kinkel, W. R., Bates, V. E., Mechtler, L. L., and Kinkel, P. R. (1999b). The cerebral intravascular enhancement sign is not specific: a contrast-enhanced MRI study. *Neuroradiology, 41*, 80-85.

Bakshi, R., Mechtler, L. L., Kamran, S., Gosy, E., Bates, V. E., Kinkel, P. R., and Kinkel, W. R. (1999c). MRI findings in lumbar puncture headache syndrome: abnormal dural-meningeal and dural venous sinus enhancement. *Clin. Imaging, 23*, 73-76

Bakshi, R., Kamran, S., Kinkel, P. R., Bates, V. E., Mechtler, L. L., Janardhan, V., Belani, S., and Kinkel, W. R. (1999d). Fluid-attenuated inversion-recovery MR findings in acute and subacute cerebral intraventricular hemorrhage. *AJNR Am. J. Neuroradiol, 20*, 629–636.

Bakshi, R., Caruthers, S. D., Janardhan, V. and Wasay, M. (2000). Intraventricular CSF pulsation artifact on fast fluid-attenuated inversion-recovery MR images: analysis of 100 consecutive normal studies. *AJNR Am. J. Neuroradiol, 21*, 503-508.

Bakshi, R., Ariyaratana, S., Benedict, R. H. B., and Jacobs, L. (2001). Fluid-attenuated inversion recovery magnetic resonance imaging detects cortical and juxtacortical multiple sclerosis lesions. *Arch. Neurol, 58*, 742-748.

Balakrishnan, J., Becker, P. S., Kumar, A. J., Zinreich S. J., McArthur J. C., and Bryan, R. N. (1990). Acquired immunodeficiency syndrome: Correlation of radiologic findings in the brain. *Radiographics, 10*, 201-215.

Bammer, R., Skare, S., Newbould, R., Liu, C., Thijs, V., Ropele, S., Clayton, D.B., Krueger, G., Moseley, M.E. and Glover G.H (2005). Foundations of advanced magnetic resonance imaging. *NeuroRx, 2,* 167-96

Bazan, C., Rinaldi, M. G., Rauch, R. R., and Jinkins, J. R. (1991). Fungal infections of the brain. *Neuroimag Clin. of N. Amer, 1*, 57-88.

Berger, J. R., and Sabet, A. (2002). Infectious myelopathies. *Semin. Neurol, 22*, 133-142.

Berkefeld, J., Enzensberger, W., and Lanfermann, H. (1999). Cryptococcus meningoencephalitis in AIDS: parenchymal and meningeal forms. *Neuroradiology, 41*, 129-123.

Berkefeld, J., Enzensberger, W., and Lanfermann, H. (2000). MRI in human immunodeficiency virus-associated cerebral vasculitis. *Neuroradiology, 42*, 526-528.

Bhigjee, A. I., Madurai, S., Bill, P. L., Patel, V., Corr, P., Naidoo, M. N., Gopaul, W. M., Smith, A. and York, D. (2001). Spectrum of myelopathies in HIV seropositive South African patients. *Neurology, 57*, 348-351.

Bhojo, A. K., Akhter, N., Bakshi, R., and Wasay, M. (2002). Thoracic myelopathy complicating acute meningococcal meningitis: MRI findings. *Am. J. Med. Sci, 323*, 263-265.

Boes, B., Bashir, R., Boes, C., Hahn, F., McConnell, J. R., and McComb, R. (1994). Central nervous system aspergillosis. Analysis of 26 patients. *J. Neuroimaging, 4*, 123-129.

Brechtelsbauer, D. L., Urbach, H., Sommer, T., Blumcke, I., Woitas, R., and Solymosi, L. (1997). Cytomegalovirus encephalitis and primary cerebral lymphoma mimicking Wernicke's encephalopathy. *Neuroradiology, 39*, 19-22.

Brightbill, T. C., Ihmeidan, I. H., Post, M. J., Berger, J. R., and Katz, D. A. (1995). Neurosyphilis in HIV-positive and HIV-negative patients: neuroimaging findings. *AJNR Am. J. Neuroradiol, 16*, 703-711.

Brooks DJ (2005). Positron emission tomography and single-photon emission computed tomography in central nervous system drug development. *Neuro.Rx, 2*, 226-36

Caldenmeyer, K. S., Mathews, V. P., Edwards-Brown, M. K., and Smith, R. R. (1997). Central nervous system crytococcosis: Parenchymal calcification and large gelatinous pseudocysts. *AJNR. Am. J. Neuroradio, 18*, 107-109.

Camacho, D. L. A., Smith, J. K., and Castillo, M. (2003). Differentiation of toxoplasmosis and lymphoma in AIDS patients by using apparent diffusion coefficients. *AJNR Am. J. Neuroradiol, 24*, 633-637.

Campi-de-Castro, C., and Hesselink, J. R. (1991). Tuberculosis. *Neuroimaging Clin. of N. Amer, 1*, 119-139.

Chan, K. H., Cheung, R. T., Fong, C. Y., Tsang, K. L., Mak, W., and Ho, S. L. (2003). Clinical relevance of hydrocephalus as a presenting feature of tuberculous meningitis. *QJM, 96*, 643-648.

Chang, K. H., Han, M. H., Roh, J. K., Kim, I. O., Han, M. C., and Kim, C. W. (1990a). Gd-DTPA-enhanced MR imaging of the brain in patients with meningitis: Comparison with CT. *AJNR Am. J. Neuroradiol, 11*, 69-76.

Chang, K. H., Han, M. H., Roh, J. K., Kim, I. O., Han, M. C., Choi, K. S., and Kim, C. W. (1990b). Gd-DTPA enhanced MR imaging in intracranial tuberculosis. *Neuroradiology, 32*, 19-25.

Chang, L., Miller, B. L., McBride, D., Cornford, M., Oropilla, G., Buchthal, S., Chiang, F., Aronow, H., Beck, C. K., and Ernst, T. (1995). Brain lesions in patients with AIDS: H-1 MR spectroscopy. *Radiology, 197*, 525-31.

Chang, L., and Ernst, T. (1997). MR spectroscopy and diffusion-weighted MR imaging in focal brain lesions in AIDS. *Neuroimaging Clin. N. Am, 7*, 409-426.

Chang, L., Ernst, T., Leonido-Yee, M., Witt, M., Speck, O., Walot, I., and Miller, E. N (1999). Highly active antiretroviral therapy reverses brain metabolite abnormalities in mild HIV dementia. *Neurology, 53,* 782-789.

Chang, L., Ernst, T., Leonido-Yee, M., and Speck, O. (2000). Perfusion MRI detects rCBF abnormalities in early stages of HIV-cognitive motor complex. *Neurology, 54,* 389-396.

Chelaifa, K., Bouzaidi, K., Azaiz, O., Ridene, I., Ben Messaoud, M., and Slim, R. (2003). Tuberculous meningitis with pituitary abscess. *J. Neuroradiol, 30,* 188-191.

Chinn, R. J. S., Wilkinson, I. D., Hall-Craggs, M. A., Paley, M. N. J., Miller, R. F., Kendall, B. E., Newman, S. P., and Harrison, M. J. G. (1995). Toxoplasmosis and primary central nervous system lymphoma in HIV infection: diagnosis with MR spectroscopy. *Radiology, 197,* 649-654.

Chong, J., Di Rocco, A., Tagliati, M., Danisi, F., Simpson, D. M., and Atlas, S. W. (1999). MR findings in AIDS-associated myelopathy. *AJNR Am. J. Neuroradiol, 20,* 1412-1416.

Chrysikopoulos, H. S., Press, G. A., Grafe, M. R., Hesselink, J. R., and Wiley, C. A. (1990). Encephalitis caused by human immunodeficiency virus: CT and MR imaging manifestations with clinical and pathologic correlation. *Radiology, 175,* 185-191.

Cohen, W. A. (1997). Intracranial bacterial infections in patients with AIDS. *Neuroimaging Clin. N. Am., 7,* 223-229.

Cordoliani, Y. S., Derosier, C., Pharaboz, C., Jeanbourquin, D., Schill, H., and Cosnard, G. (1992). Primary cerebral lymphoma in patients with AIDS: MR findings in 17 cases. *AJR Am. J. Roentgenol, 159,* 841-847.

Coulon, A., Lafitte, F., Hoang-Xuan, K., Martin-Duverneuil, N., Mokhtari, K., Blustajn, J., and Chiras, J. (2002). Radiographic findings in 37 cases of primary CNS lymphoma in immunocompetent patients. *Eur. Radiol, 12,* 329-340.

Cox, J., Murtagh, R., Wilfong, A., and Brenner, J. (1992). Cerebral aspergillosis: MR imaging and histopathologic correlation. *AJNR Am. J. Neuroradiol, 13,* 1489-1492.

Daikos, G. L., Cleary, T., Rodriguez, A., and Fischl, M. A. (2003). Multidrug-resistant tuberculous meningitis in patients with AIDS. *Int. J. Tuberc. Lung. Dis, 7,* 394-398.

De La Pena, R. C., Ketonen, L., and Villanueva-Meyer, J. (1998). Imaging of brain tumors in AIDS patients by means of dual-isotope thallium-201 and technetium-99m sestamibi single-photon emission tomography. *Eur. J. Nucl. Med., 25,* 1404-11.

Di Rocco, A., and Simpson, D. M. (1998). AIDS-associated vacuolar myelopathy. *AIDS Patient Care STDS, 12,* 457-461.

Drost, D. J., Riddle, W. R., and Clarke, G. D. (2002). Proton magnetic resonance spectroscopy in the brain: report of AAPM MR Task Group #9. *Med. Phys, 29,* 2177-2197.

Eggers, C. H. (2002). German Neuro-AIDS Working Group. HIV-1 associated encephalopathy and myelopathy. *J. Neurol, 249,* 1132-1136.

Flowers, C. H., Mafee, M. F., Crowell, R., Raofi, B., Arnold, P., Dobben, G., and Wycliffe, N (1990). Encephalopathy in AIDS patients: Evaluation with MR imaging. *AJNR. Am. J. Neuroradiol, 11,* 1235-1245.

Fox, P. A., Hawkins, D. A., and Dawson, S. (2000). Dementia following an acute presentation of meningovascular neurosyphilis in an HIV-1 positive patient. *AIDS, 14,* 2062-2063.

Garrels, K., Kucharczyk, W., Wortzman, G., and Shandling, M. (1996). Progressive multifocal leukoencephalopathy: Clinical and MR response to treatment. *AJNR. Am. J. Neuroradiol, 17*, 597-600.

Giglio, P., Bakshi, R., Block, S., Ostrow, P., and Pullicino, P. M. (2002). Primary central nervous system lymphoma masquerading as herpes encephalitis: clinical, magnetic resonance imaging, and pathologic findings. *Am. J. Med. Sci, 323*, 59-61.

Gillams, A. R., Allen, E., Hrieb, K., Venna, N., Craven, D., and Carter, A. P. (1997). Cerebral infarction in patients with AIDS. *AJNR Am. J. Neuroradiol, 18*, 1581-1585.

Gray, F., Chretien, F., Vallat-Decouvelaere, A. V., and Scaravilli, F. (2003). The changing pattern of HIV neuropathology in the HAART era. *J. Neuropathol. Exp. Neurol, 62*, 429-40.

Gupta, R. K., Jena, A., Sharma, A., Guha, D. K., Khushu, S., and Gupta, A. K. (1988). MR imaging of intracranial tuberculomas. *J. Comput. Assist. Tomogr, 12*, 280-285.

Gupta, R. K., Kathuria, M. K., and Pradhan, S. (1999). Magnetization transfer MR imaging in CNS tuberculosis. *AJNR Am. J. Neuroradiol, 20*, 867-875.

Gupta, R. K., Vatsal, D. K., Husain, N., Chawla, S., Prasad, K. N., Roy, R., Kumar, R., Jha, D., and Husain, M. (2001). Differentiation of tuberculous from pyogenic brain abscesses with in vivo proton MR spectroscopy and magnetization transfer MR imaging. *AJNR Am. J. Neuroradiol, 22*, 1503-1509.

Harris, D. E., and Enterline, D. S. (1997a). Neuroimaging of AIDS. I. Fungal infections of the central nervous system. *Neuroimaging Clin N. Am, 7*, 187-198.

Harris, D. E., Enterline, D. S., and Tien, R. D. (1997b). Neurosyphilis in patients with AIDS. *Neuroimaging Clin. N. Am, 7*, 215-221.

Hawkins, C. P., McLaughlin, J. E., Kendall, B. E., and McDonald, W. I. (1993). Pathological findings correlated with MRI in HIV infection. *Neuroradiology, 35*, 264-268.

Heyes, M. P., Ellis, R. J., Ryan, L., Childers, M. E., Grant. I., Wolfson, T., Archibald, S., and Jernigan, T. L. (2001). HNRC Group. HIV Neurobehavioral Research Center. Elevated cerebrospinal fluid quinolinic acid levels are associated with region-specific cerebral volume loss in HIV infection. *Brain, 124*, 1033-1042.

Hochberg, F. H., and Miller, D. C. (1988). Primary central nervous system lymphoma. *J. Neurosurg, 68*, 835-853.

Hoffmann C, Horst HA, Albrecht H, Schlote W (2003). Progressive multifocal leucoencephalopathy with unusual inflammatory response during antiretroviral treatment. *J. Neurol. Neurosurg. Psychiatry, 74*, 1142-1144

Holland, B. A., Perrett, L. V., and Mills, C. M. (1986). CT and MR findings. *Radiology, 158*, 439-442.

Holland, N. R., Power, C., Mathews, V. P., Glass, J. D., Forman, M., and McArthur, J. C. (1994). Cytomegalovirus encephalitis in acquired immunodeficiency syndrome (AIDS). *Neurology, 44*, 507-514.

Ionita, C., Wasay, M., Balos, L., and Bakshi, R. (2004). MRI in toxoplasmosis encephalitis after bone marrow transplantation: paucity of enhancement despite fulminant disease. *AJNR Am. J. Neuroradiol, 25*, 270-273.

Iranzo, A., Moreno, A., Pujol, J., Marti-Fabregas, J., Domingo, P., Molet, J., Ris, J., and Cadafalch, J. (1999). Proton magnetic resonance spectroscopy pattern of progressive multifocal leukoencephalopathy in AIDS. *J. Neurol. Neurosurg. Psychiatry, 66*, 520-523.

Issakhanian, M., Chang, L., Cornford, M., Witt, M., Speck, O., Goldberg, M., and Ernst, T. (2001). T. HIV-2 infection with cerebral toxoplasmosis and lymphomatoid granulomatosis. *J. Neuroimaging, 11*, 212-216.

Johkura, K., Nishiyama, T., and Kuroiwa, Y. (2002). Bilateral basal ganglia infarctions in a patient with Streptococcus pneumoniae meningitis. *Eur. Neurol, 48*, 123-124.

Jordan, J. and Enzmann, D. R. (1991). Encephalitis. *Neuroimag Clin. N. Am, 1*, 17-38.

Kamran, S., Bener, A.B., Alper, D., Bakshi, R (2004). Role of fluid-attenuated inversion recovery in the diagnosis of meningitis: comparison with contrast-enhanced magnetic resonance imaging. *J. Comput. Assist. Tomogr, 28*, 68-72

Kastrup, O., Maschke, M., Diener, H. C., and Wanke, I. (2002). Progressive multifocal leukoencephalopathy limited to the brain stem. *Neuroradiology, 44*, 227-229.

Keston, P., Murray, A. D., and Jackson, A. (2003). Cerebral perfusion imaging using contrast-enhanced MRI. *Clin. Radiol, 58*, 505-513.

Ketonen, L., De La Pena R, and Villanueva-Meyer, J. (1998). MR and TL-201 Spect imaging with pathologic correlation for the assessment of CNS lymphoma vs. toxoplasmosis in AIDS patients. *Journal of neuro-AIDS, 2*, 21-42.

Kioumehr, F., Dadsetan, M. R., Feldman, N., Mathison, G., Moosavi, H., Rooholamini, S. A., and Verma, R. C. (1995). Postcontrast MRI of cranial meningitis: Leptomeninigitis versus pachymeningitis. *J. Comput. Assist. Tomogr, 19*, 713-720.

Laissy, J. P., Soyer, P., Parlier, C., Lariven, S., Benmelha, Z., Servois, V., Casalino, E., Bouvet, E., Sibert, A., and Vachon, F. (1994). Persistent enhancement after treatment for cerebral toxoplasmosis in patients with AIDS: Predictive value for subsequent recurrence. *AJNR Am. J. Neuroradiol, 115*, 1773-1778.

Leclerc, X., Huisman, T. A., and Sorensen, A. G. (2002). The potential of proton magnetic resonance spectroscopy [(1)H-MRS)] in the diagnosis and management of patients with brain tumors. *Curr. Opin. Oncol, 14*, 292-298.

Lee, P.L., Yiannoutsos, C.T., Ernst, T., Chang, L., Marra, C.M., Jarvik, J.G., Richards, T.L., Kwok, E.W., Kolson, D.L., Simpson, D., Tang, C.Y., Schifitto, G., Ketonen, L.M., Meyerhoff, D.J., Lenkinski, R.E., Gonzalez, R.G., Navia, B.A. and HIV MRS Consortium (2003). A multi-center 1H MRS study of the AIDS dementia complex: validation and preliminary analysis. *J. Magn. Reson. Imaging, 17*, 625-633

Lin, A., Ross, B.D., Harris, K., Wong, W (2005). Efficacy of proton magnetic resonance spectroscopy in neurological diagnosis and neurotherapeutic decision making. *NeuroRx, 2*, 197-214

Lizerbram, E. K., and Hesselink, J. R. (1997). Neuroimaging of AIDS. I. Viral infections. *Neuroimaging Clin. N. Am, 7*, 261-280.

Luft, B. J., Hafner, R., Korzun, A. H., Leport, C., Antoniskis, D., Bosler, E. M., Bourland, D. D. 3rd Uttamchandani, R., Fuhrer, J., Jacobson, J., Morlat, P., Vilde, J. L., and Remington, J. S. (1993). Toxoplasmic encephalitis in patients with the acquired immunodeficiency syndrome. *N. Engl. J. Med, 329*, 995-1000.

Luttmann, S., Husstedt, I. W., Lugering, N., Heese, C., Stoll, R., Domschke, W., Evers, S., Kuchelmeister, K., and Gullotta, F. (1997). Cytomegalovirus encephalomyelomeningoradiculitis in acquired immunodeficiency syndrome (AIDS). *J. Infect, 35*, 78-81.

Miller, R. F., Lucas, S. B., Hall-Craggs, M. A., Brink, N. S., Scaravilli, F., Chinn, R. J., Kendall, B. E., Williams, I. G., and Harrison, M. J. (1997). Comparison of magnetic resonance imaging with neuropathological findings in the diagnosis of HIV and CMV associated CNS disease in AIDS. *J. Neurol. Neurosurg. Psychiatry, 62*, 346-351.

Miszkiel, K. A., Hall-Craggs, M. A., Miller, R. F., Kendall, B. E., Wilkinson, I. D., Paley, M. N., and Harrison, M. J. (1996). The spectrum of MRI findings in CNS cryptococcosis in AIDS. *Clin. Radiol, 51*, 842-850.

Naddaf, S. Y., Akisik, M. F., Aziz, M., Omar, W. S., Hirschfeld, A., Masdeu, J., Donnenfeld, H., and Abdel-Dayem, H. M. (1998). Comparison between 201Tl-chloride and 99Tc(m)-sestamibi SPET brain imaging for differentiating intracranial lymphoma from non-malignant lesions in AIDS patients. *Nucl. Med. Commun, 19*, 47-53.

Navia, B. A., and Gonzalez, R. G. (1997). Functional imaging of the AIDS dementia complex and the metabolic pathology of the HIV-1 infected brain. *Neuroimaging Clin. N. Am, 7*, 431-445.

Olsen, W. L., Longo, F. M., Mills, C. M., and Norman, D. (1988). White matter disease in AIDS: Findings at MR imaging. *Radiology, 169*, 445-448.

Ostrow, T. D., and Hudgins, P. A. (1994). : Magnetic resonance imaging of intracranial fungal infections. *Top. Magn. Res. Imag, 6*, 22-31.

Patsalides, A. D., Wood, L. V., Atac, G. K., Sandifer, E., Butman, J. A., and Patronas, N. J. (2002). Cerebrovascular disease in HIV-infected pediatric patients: neuroimaging findings. *AJR. Am. J. Roentgenol, 179*, 999-1003.

Peng, S. S., Tseng, W.Y., Liu, H. M., Li, Y. W., and Huang, K. M. (2003). Diffusion-weighted images in children with meningoencephalitis. *Clin. Imaging, 27*, 5-10.

Pomara, N., Crandall, D. T., Choi, S. J., Johnson, G., and Lim, K. O. (2001). White matter abnormalities in HIV-1 infection: a diffusion tensor imaging study. *Psychiatry Res, 106*, 15-24.

Pomper, M. G., Constantinides, C. D., Barker, P. B., Bizzi, A., Dobgan, A. S., Yokoi, F., McArthur, J. C., and Wong, D. F. (2002). Quantitative MR spectroscopic imaging of brain lesions in patients with AIDS: correlation with [11C-methyl]thymidine PET and thallium-201 SPECT. *Acad. Radiol, 9*, 398-409.

Porter, S. B., and Sande, M. A. (1992). Toxoplasmosis of the central nervous system in the acquired immunodeficiency syndrome. *N. Engl. J. Med, 327*, 1643-1648.

Post, M. J. D., Tate, L. G., Quencer, R. M., Hensley, G. T., Berger, J. R., Sheremata, W. A., and Maul, G. (1988). CT, MR, and pathology in HIV encephalitis and meningitis. *AJNR. Am. J. Neuroradiol*, 469-476.

Post, M. J., Yiannoutsos, C., Simpson, D., Booss, J., Clifford, D. B., Cohen, B., McArthur, J. C., and Hall, C. D. (1999). Progressive multifocal leukoencephalopathy in AIDS: are there any MR findings useful to patient management and predictive of patient survival? *AJNR. Am. J. Neuroradiol, 20*, 1896-1906.

Power, C., Nath, A., Aoki, F. Y., and Bigio, M. D. (1997). Remission of progressive multifocal leukoencephalopathy following splenectomy and antiretroviral therapy in a patient with HIV infection. *N. Engl. J. Med, 336*, 661-662.

Quencer, R. M., and Post, M. J. (1997). Spinal cord lesions in patients with AIDS. *Neuroimaging Clin. N. Am, 7*, 359-373.

Ramsey, R., and Gean, A.D. (1997). Neuroimaging of AIDS I. Central nervous system toxoplasmosis. *Neuroimaging Clin. N. Am, 7*, 171-186.

Revel, M. P., Grey, F., Brugieres, P., Geny, C., Sobel, A., and Gaston, A. (1992). Hyperdense CT foci in treated AIDS toxoplasmosis encephalitis: MR and pathologic correlation. *J. Comput. Assist. Tomogr, 16*, 372-375.

Rosas, M. J., Simoes-Ribeiro, F., An, S. F., and Sousa, N. (1999). Progressive multifocal leukoencephalopathy: unusual MRI findings and prolonged survival in a pregnant woman. *Neurology, 52*, 657-659.

Rottnek, M., Di Rocco, A., Laudier, D., and Morgello, S. (2002). Axonal damage is a late component of vacuolar myelopathy. *Neurology, 58*, 479-481.

Ruiz, A., Ganz, W. I., Post, M. J., Camp, A., Landy, H., Mallin, W., and Sfakianakis, G. N. (1994). Use of thallium-201 brain SPECT to differentiate cerebral lymphoma from toxoplasma encephalitis in AIDS patients. *AJNR. Am. J. Neuroradiol, 15*, 1885-1894.

Ruiz, A., Post, M. J. D., Bundschu, C., Ganz, W. I., and Georgiou, M. (1997). Primary central nervous system lymphoma in patients with AIDS. *Neuroimaging Clin. N. Am, 7*, 281-296.

Runge, V. M., Wells, J. W., Williams, N. M., Lee, C., Timoney, J. F., and Young, A. B. (1995). Detectability of early brain meningitis with magnetic resonance imaging. *Invest. Radiol, 30*, 484-495.

Sartoretti-Schefer, S., Blattler, T., and Wichmann, W. (1997). Spinal MRI in vacuolar myelopathy, and correlation with histopathological findings. *Neuroradiology, 39*, 865-869.

Schiff, E., and Lindberg, M. (2002). Neurosyphilis. *South. Med. J, 95*, 1083-1087.

Shapiro, R. A., Mullane, K. M., Camras, L., Flowers, C., and Sutton, S. (2001). Clinical and magnetic resonance imaging regression of progressive multifocal leukoencephalopathy in an AIDS patient after intensive antiretroviral therapy. *J. Neuroimaging 11*, 336-339.

Sidtis, J. J., and Price, R. W. (1990). Early HIV-1 infection and the AIDS dementia complex. *Neurology, 40*, 323-326.

Simone, I. L., Federico, F., Tortorella, C., Andreula, C. F., Zimatore, G. B., Giannini, P., Angarano, G., Lucivero, V., Picciola, P., Carrara, D., Bellacosa, A., and Livrea, P. (1998). Localised 1H-MR spectroscopy for metabolic characterisation of diffuse and focal brain lesions in patients infected with HIV. *J. Neurol. Neurosurg. Psychiatry, 64*, 516-523.

Smith, T. L., and Nathan, B. R. (2002). Central nervous system infections in the immune-competent adult. *Curr. Treat. Options. Neurol, 4*, 323-332.

Sorensen, A. G, Buonnanno, F. S., Gonzalez, R. G., Schwamm, L. H., Lev, M. H., Huang-Hellinger, F. R., Reese, T. G., Weisskoff, R. M., Davis, T. L., Suwanwela, N., Can, U., Moreira, J. A., Copen, W. A., Look, R. B., Finkelstein, S. P., Rosen, B. R., and Koroshetz W. J. (1996). Hyperacute stroke: evaluation with combined multisection diffusion-weighted and hemodynamically weighted echo-planar MR imaging. *Radiology, 199*, 391-401.

States, L. J., Zimmerman, R. A., and Rutstein, R. M. (1997). Imaging of pediatric central nervous system HIV infection. *Neuroimaging Clin. N. Am, 7*, 321-339.

Sugahara, T., Korogi, Y., Shigematsu, Y., Hirai, T., Ikushima, I., Liang, L., Ushio, Y., and Takahashi, M. (1999). Perfusion-sensitive MRI of cerebral lymphomas: a preliminary report. *J. Comput. Assist. Tomogr, 23*, 232-237.

Suwanwelaa, N., Phanuphak, P., Phanthumchinda, K., Suwanwela, N. C., Tantivatana, J., Ruxrungtham, K., Suttipan, J., Wangsuphachart, S., and Hanvanich, M. (2000). Magnetic resonance spectroscopy of the brain in neurologically asymptomatic HIV-infected patients. *Magn. Reson. Imaging, 18*, 859-865.

Taiwo, B. O. (2000). AIDS-related primary CNS lymphoma: A brief review. *AIDS Read, 10*, 486-491.

Tayfun, C., Ucoz, T., Tasar, M., Atac, K., Ogur, T., and Yinanc, M. A. (1996). Diagnostic value of MRI in tuberculous meningitis. *Neuroradiology, 6*, 380-386.

Thurner, M.M, Thurner, S. A., Fleischmann, D., Steuer, A., Rieger, A., Helbich, T., Trattnig, S., Scindler, E., and Hittmair, K. (1997a). Comparison of T2-weighted and fluid-attenuated inversion-recovery fast spin-echo MR sequences in intracerebral AIDS-associated disease. *AJNR. Am. J. Neuroradiol, 18*, 1601-1609.

Thurnher, M. M., Jinkins, J. R., and Post, M. J. (1997b). Diagnostic imaging of infections and neoplasms affecting the spine in patients with AIDS. *Neuroimaging Clin. N. Am., 7*, 341-357.

Thurnher, M. M., Post, M. J., and Jinkins, J. R. (2000). MRI of infections and neoplasms of the spine and spinal cord in 55 patients with AIDS. *Neuroradiology, 42*, 551-563.

Thurnher, M. M., Rieger, A., Kleibl-Popov, C., Settinek, U., Henk, C., Haberler, C., and Schindler, E. (2001). Primary central nervous system lymphoma in AIDS: a wider spectrum of CT and MRI findings. *Neuroradiology, 43*, 29-35.

Tien, R. D., Chu, P. K., Hesselink, J. R., Duberg, A., and Wiley, C. (1991). Intracranial cryptococcosis in immunocompromised patients: CT and MR findings in 29 cases. *AJNR. Am. J. Neuroradiol, 12*, 283-289.

Tracey, I., Hamberg, L.M., Guimaraes, A.R., Hunter, G., Chang, I., Navia, B.A. and Gonzalez, R.G. (1998). Increased cerebral blood volume in HIV-positive patients detected by functional MRI. *Neurology, 50*, 1821-1826

Troncoso, A., Fumagalli, J., Shinzato, R., Gulotta, H., Toller, M., and Bava, J. (2002). CNS cryptococcoma in an HIV-positive patient. *J. Int. Assoc. Physicians AIDS Care, 1*, 131-133.

Trotot, P. M., and Gray, F. (1997). Neuroimaging of AIDS I. Diagnostic imaging contribution in the early stages of HIV infection of the brain. *Neuroimaging Clin. N. Am, 7*, 243-260.

Tsuchiya, K., Inaoka, S., Mizutani, R., and Hachiya, J. (1997). Fast fluid-attenuated inversion-recovery MR of intracranial infections. *AJNR. Am. J. Neuroradiol,18*, 909-913.

Villringer, K., Jager, H., Dichgans, M., Ziegler, S., Poppinger, J., Herz, M., Kruschke, C., Minoshima, S., Pfister, H. W., and Schwaiger, M. (1995). Differential diagnosis of CNS lesions in AIDS patients by FDG-PET. *J. Comput. Assist. Tomogr, 19*, 532-536.

Vinters, H. V., Kwok, M. K., Ho, H. W., Anders, K. H., Tomiyasu, U., Wolfson, W. L., and Robert, F. (1989). Cytomegalovirus in the nervous system of patients with the acquired immune deficiency syndrome. *Brain, 112*, 245-268.

Vyas, R., and Ebright, J. R. (1996). Toxoplasmosis of the spinal cord in a patient with AIDS: case report and review. *Clin. Infect. Dis, 23*, 1061-1065.

Walot, I., Miller, B. L., Chang, L., and Mehringer, C. M. (1996). Neuroimaging findings in patients with AIDS. *Clin. Infect. Dis, 22*, 906-919.

Wasay, M., Kheleani, B. A., Moolani, M. K., Zaheer, J., Pui, M., Hasan, S., Muzaffar, S., Bakshi, R., and Sarawari, A. R. (2003). Brain CT and MRI findings in 100 consecutive patients with intracranial tuberculoma. *J. Neuroimaging, 13*, 240-247.

Whiteman, M. L., Post, M. J., Berger, J. R., Tate, L. G., Bell, M. D., and Limonte, L. P. (1993). Progressive multifocal leukoencephalopathy in 47 HIV-seropositive patients: Neuroimaging with clinical and pathologic correlation. *Radiology, 187*, 233-240.

Whiteman, M., Espinoza, L., Post, M. J., Bell, M. D., and Falcone, S. (1995). Central nervous system tuberculosis in HIV-infected patients: clinical and radiographic findings. *AJNR. Am. J. Neuroradiol, 16*, 1319-1327.

Whiteman, M. L. (1997). Neuroimaging of central nervous system tuberculosis in HIV-infected patients. *Neuroimaging Clin. N. Am, 7*, 199-214.

Wrobel, C. J., Meyer, S., Johnson, R. H., and Hesselink, J. R. (1992). MR findings in acute and chronic coccidioidomycosis meningitis. *AJNR Am. J. Neuroradiol, 13*, 1241-1245.

Xavier, A. R., Qureshi, A. I., Kirmani, J. F., Yahia, A. M., and Bakshi, R. (2003). Neuroimaging of stroke: a review. *South. Med. J, 96*, 367-379.

In: Neuro-AIDS
Editors: A. Minagar and P. Shapshak, pp. 225-245

ISBN: 1-59454-610-X
© 2006 Nova Science Publishers, Inc.

Chapter X

Molecular Basis for Opioids and AIDS Virus Interactions

Ronald Y. Chuang, Linda F. Chuang and Roy H. Doi

Department of Medical Pharmacology and Toxicology, School of Medicine and Section
of Molecular and Cellular Biology, University of California, Davis, California 95616

Abstract

Illicit drug users constitute a large proportion of the patient population contracting AIDS.
The purpose of our research is to determine the mechanism by which drugs such as
opioids attenuate host immune function. The Simian AIDS (SAIDS) model is among the
best available animal model systems for studying human AIDS. Using the SAIDS model,
we have found that monkeys chronically treated with morphine and infected with simian
AIDS virus have a faster rate of viral replication and mutation and a shorter life span
than infected monkeys that have not been treated with morphine. Mechanistic studies
have shown that opiates modulate simian AIDS progression by (i) stimulating the
expression of chemokine receptor CCR5, a co-receptor on immune cells for HIV/SIV
entry and (ii) slowing down the apoptosis of SIV-infected cells, permitting the
persistence and survival of the virus.

Key words: Morphine, simian AIDS, SIV, CCR5, apoptosis

Introduction

A variety of events occur following the establishment of opioid dependency. Whatever
cellular events make up the tolerant state, it is assumed that the tolerant state can be
maintained in a stable condition with the continued maintenance of the body burden of
opioid(s). Dole and Nyswander (1983) pointed out that the pharmacokinetics of the opioid
was important for stabilizing both the tolerant state and the wellbeing of the subject. They

compared heroin, morphine, and methadone effects in humans and concluded that the pharmacokinetics of heroin and morphine precluded the maintenance of a "stable" tolerant state. They also reported the swinging or cycling of a constellation of effects that make up the components of behavior. Underlying mechanisms must include swings in internal milieu as controlled by the autonomic nervous system, the endocrine system, and the immune system. Methadone, via its cascade of metabolites (Pierce et al., 1992), was able to stabilize the dependent state and all aspects of behavioral fluctuation (Batki, 1988; Sees et al., 2000).

Acquired Immunodeficiency Syndrome (AIDS) is a cellular immune disorder found in patients infected by HIV. At the end of the December 2002, the US Center for Disease Control and Prevention (CDC) estimates that 384,906 persons were living with AIDS in America. Of the 298,248 men (13 years or older) who were living with AIDS, 31% were injection drug users and of the 82,764 adult, adolescent women with AIDS, 36% were exposed through injection drug use (Center for Disease Control and Prevention Report, 2002:14). However, among drug users, needle-sharing alone cannot explain the reportedly high levels of infectivity, since the blood volumes transferred by shared needles are rather small (<0.75 μl according to Gaughwin et al., 1991). Opioid addicts who did not share needles also showed substantial rates of seropositivity to HIV (Marmor, 1987). Opioids have thus been considered a cofactor contributing to an individual's susceptibility to HIV infection and to the high incidence of secondary opportunistic infections among AIDS patients (see Review, Friedman and Eisenstein, 2004).

To investigate the effect of opioids on AIDS progression, we resorted to a rhesus macaque model. The simian immunodeficiency virus (SIV), a simian counterpart of the human AIDS virus, infects rhesus macaques with clinical symptoms similar to those of HIV infection in man, though the onset of simian AIDS (SAIDS) is much more rapid (within three months, Desrosiers, 1990). Through the use of SIVmac239-infected monkeys, our laboratory has shown that morphine enhances the pathogenesis of SAIDS. Within 17 months post-infection, the occurrence of secondary infections and diseases such as Giardiasis, enterocolitis, amyloidosis, cholecystitis, and lymphoma leading to expiration of the animals was more frequent and occurred much more rapidly in morphine-treated monkeys than in similarly infected monkeys not exposed to morphine (Chuang et al., 1993c; 1997a), which, in contrast, have survived an average of 18-22 months after infection with the virus. A recent study done in the laboratories of Kumar and Donahoe (Kumar et al., 2004) substantiated our findings by demonstrating that morphine-injected, SIV-infected rhesus macaques had a greater loss in CD4+ T cells and a higher plasma viral replication, as compared to non-morphine treated animals. It thus appears that laboratory investigation has confirmed the results of epidemiological studies which indicate that morphine has an unequivocal role in causing immune dysfunction and promoting the AIDS epidemic. One would naturally ask the following questions: do cells of the immune system possess classical opioid receptors? How do opioids or opioid receptors affect AIDS virus infection?

While there is some controversy in the literature (see review, Rouveix, 1992), the weight of the evidence suggests the existence of brain-like opioid receptors on immune cells (Madden et al., 1987; Sibinga and Goldstein, 1988; Heagy et al., 1990, Rouveix, 1992). With the availability of the gene sequence of opioid receptor cDNA from brain cells, our laboratory presented the evidence, and later confirmed by others, that opioid receptor genes (for all three types of receptors, *delta, kappa* and *mu*) are indeed transcribed and translated in cells of the immune system (Chuang et al., 1994b; 1995a; 1995c; Gaveriaux-Ruff et al., 1995; Sedqi et al., 1995; Wick et al., 1996; Sharp et al., 1998; Pampusch et al., 1998; Alicea et al., 1998; Suzuki et al., 2000; 2001). The discoveries of the existence of classical opioid receptor transcripts and their corresponding proteins on cells of the immune system have therefore provided a direct link between opioid effect and immune dysfunction.

Neutrophils and monocytes/macrophages, the phagocytic cells of the immune system, constitute the first line of defense mechanism of the host's immune response. One important function of monocytes and neutrophils is their migration from the blood to the site of infection in response to inflammatory mediators such as chemokines in a process called chemotaxis. Once inside an inflammatory site, these host cells eliminate many pathogens by phagocytosis. Chemokines consist of four related but distinct groups: CC and CXC chemokines, lymphotactin and neurotactin (Kelvin et al., 1993; Wang et al., 1993; Hedrick and Zlotnik, 1997; Pan et al., 1997). We have shown that addition of opioid agonists to CC or CXC chemokines would reduce the chemotactic activities of monocytes or neutrophils (Choi et al., 1999; Miyagi et al., 2000b), suggesting that the presence of opioids during SIV/HIV infection alters leukocyte-mediated immune functions. In other words, opioids can disrupt the body's first line of defense against harmful external pathogens such as SIV/HIV. These observations may provide an indirect mechanism to explain why primates or humans dependent upon intravenous drug administration have a higher probability of developing into a full-blown disease than non-drug users when exposed to a viral challenge.

The questions remain: (i) do opioids such as morphine have a direct effect on the susceptibility of immune cells to SIV/HIV infection? and (ii) once the virus enters its target cells, do opioids affect viral propagation? To further search for the molecular basis for opioid-virus interactions, we have performed both *in vitro* (tissue culture cell) and *in vivo* (animal) studies and found (i) opioid receptors form an oligomeric protein complex with chemokine receptor CCR5 on the cell membrane of immune cells; the activation of opioid receptors by morphine simultaneously induces the expression of CCR5, a co-receptor of HIV/SIV infection, allowing more virus to enter the target cell; and (ii) the activation of opioid receptors by morphine delays SIV-triggered cell lysis (or apoptosis), facilitating the intracellular survival, propagation and persistence of the AIDS virus. These studies are illustrated as follows:

Morphine Induces Expression of CCR5, a Coreceptor for SIV/HIV Entry

It has been hypothesized that chemokines such as RANTES, MIP-1α and MIP-1β may inhibit the replication of different strains of HIV-1, HIV-2 and SIV (Cocchi et al., 1995; Bostik et al., 1998). Chemokine receptor CCR5 (the cellular receptor for RANTES, MIP-1α and MIP-1β) is considered an indispensable cofactor for SIV/HIV entry (Feng et al., 1996; Marcon et al., 1997; Liao et al., 1997; Farzan et al., 1997; Kirchhoff et al., 1997; Deng et al., 1997; Yi et al., 1999; Kedzierska et al., 2003). In a study to quantify virus production in CEM x174, a lymphocytic cell line susceptible to SIVmac239 infection, we found that addition of morphine to CEM x174 cell cultures significantly increases the replication of SIVmac239 (Chuang et al., 1993b). To determine which coreceptor is responsible for the observed morphine effect, we first undertook the task of determining coreceptor densities on CEM x174 cells. Plasmids containing segments of CCR5, BOB and BONZO, and plasmids containing CCR5, BOB and BONZO segments with 96 bp (CCR5), 63 bp (BOB) and 125 bp (BONZO) deletions were constructed. Plasmids with deleted segments were used in quantitative RT/PCR as external controls for quantifying the expression of chemokine receptor genes in CEM x174 (Miyagi et al., 2000a). The results showed that in addition to BOB and BONZO, CEM x174 cells express CCR5 at the levels of fg quantity per μg of total cellular RNA. To further establish that the CCR5 transcripts detected in CEM x174 cells are translated into receptor proteins, we performed both flow cytometry and western blot analysis using fluorescein-conjugated mouse monoclonal anti-human CCR5 (for flow cytometry) and rabbit polyclonal anti-human CCR5 (for western blot). Both procedures confirmed the presence of CCR5 molecules on CEM x174 cells (Miyagi et al., 2000a). To investigate the effect of morphine treatment on the gene expression of CCR5, BOB and BONZO, the amount of cDNA amplified by competitive RT-PCR from cells treated with morphine was compared with that of untreated cells. Morphine treatment, if used, was either 10 μM or 10 nM; these are physiological morphine concentrations in morphine-dependent individuals (Liu et al. 1992). Samples were taken 0, 12, 24 and 36 hr post morphine treatment for analysis. It was found that at 12 hr post-treatment, 10 μM morphine increased CCR5 expression 207% whereas 10 nM morphine induced a 240% increase of CCR5 by 24 hr post-morphine treatment. On the contrary, morphine treatment did not affect the expression of BOB or BONZO, two other chemokine receptors on CEM x174 cells not involved in SIV entry (Fig. 1). Further experiments showed that the morphine-induced increase in CCR5 expression correlated with the amount of CCR5 proteins on the cell surface as revealed by both FACS and Western blot analyses (Miyagi et al., 2000a) and that the effect was opioid receptor-mediated, since it could be completely abolished when cells were pre-treated with naloxone, a *mu* opioid receptor antagonist (Fig. 2). It was also demonstrated that the induction of CCR5 by morphine results in an increased SIVmac239 production (Table 1) and a similar morphine effect was not observed on CEM x174 infected with SRV (simian retroviruses), which do not depend on CCR5 for entry (Table 1).

Table I. Morphine enhances the propagation of SIVmac239, but not SRV-1.
The reverse transcriptase activity was assayed using standard [^{32}P]dTTP incorporation.
The mean cpm for the cells alone was 167. The mean cpm for the scintillation fluid was
20. Data were reproducible in three independent experiments

Virus	Morphine Concentrations							
	0 μm		0.4 μm		4.0 μm		10.0 μm	
	Day 6	Day 8	Day 6	Day 8	Day 6	Day 8	Day 6	Day 8
SIVmac 239[a]	266 (1.0)[b]	568 (1.0)	603 (2.3)	2310 (4.1)	699 (2.6)	3674 (6.5)	1168 (4.4)	2885 (5.1)
SRV-1[c]	256 (1.0)	454 (1.0)	225 (0.9)	389 (0.9)	228 (0.9)	444 (1.0)	221 (0.9)	338 (0.7)

[a] The p value is < 0.0001 by analysis of variance, considered highly significant.
[b] CPM ratio between sample and no-morphine control.
[c] The p value is >0.1 by analysis of variance, considered not significant.

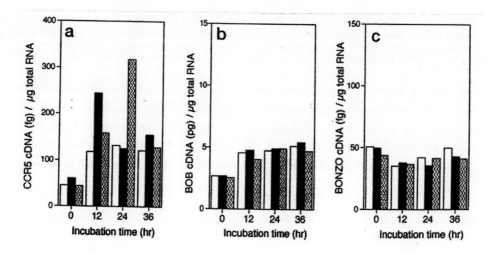

Figure 1. Morphine induces the expression of CCR5, but not BOB or BONZO. The amount of (a) CCR5, (b) BOB or (c) BONZO expressed in CEM x174 cells was determined by the competitive RT-PCR after treatment of the cells with 10 μM (solid column) or 10 nM (wavy column) morphine sulfate for the indicated time. Control (clear column), H₂O-treated cells.

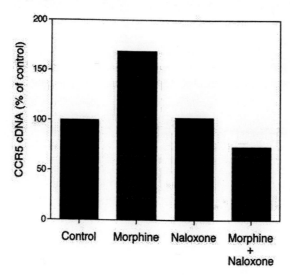

Figure 2. Effect of naloxone on morphine-induced CCR5 expression. The amount of CCR5 expressed in CEM x174 cells was determined by the competitive RT-PCR after treatment of the cells for 12 hrs with 10 nM morphine, 10 nM naloxone or a combination of naloxone and morphine (10 nM each).

When monkey peripheral blood mononuclear cells (PBMC) were isolated and cultured in the presence of morphine, a similar morphine effect was observed. As shown in Fig. 3, CCR5 expression on PBMC showed a time-responsive increase at both 10 μM and 10 nM morphine. The phenomenon of an elevated CCR5 expression in morphine-treated PBMC correlated with our findings that plasma viremia was increased in morphine-dependent monkeys (Suzuki et al., 2002b). In practice, the isolation of HIV or SIV from PBMC of infected humans or animals relies on a cocultivation procedure: PBMC are cultured *in vitro* in the presence of T cells of an immortalized cell line (e.g., Hut 78 or CEM x174). Without cocultivation, the virus load in infected PBMC is below the threshold of detection by conventional assays and cannot sustain continuous replication. In our study, however, it was found that SIV could be detected in the morphine-dependent, SIVmac239-infected animals' PBMC without cocultivation with an immortalized tissue culture cell line. In contrast, virus titers from the PBMC of saline-treated, morphine-naïve SIVmac239-infected animals remained undetectable in the absence of cocultivation (Suzuki et al., 2002b). These studies further establish the unequivocal role of opioids as a risk factor in promoting the propagation of AIDS virus. These studies and their significance were later confirmed by others who showed that (a) treatment of human astrocyte cultures with morphine enhanced the expression of CCR5 gene (Mahajan et al., 2002); (b) morphine enhanced HIV R5 strain infection of macrophages through the upregulation of CCR5 expression (Guo et al., 2002; Ho et al., 2003) and (c) morphine enhanced both CXCR4 and CCR5 expression and subsequently increased both X4 and R5 HIV-1 infection (Steele et al., 2003).

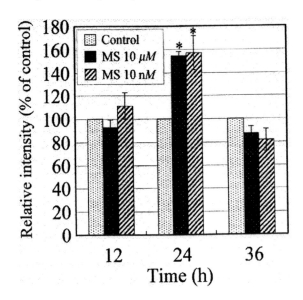

Figure 3. Effect of morphine on expression of CCR5 protein by monkey peripheral blood mononuclear cells (PBMC). PBMC were isolated from four morphine-naïve, non-SIVmac239-infected monkeys and cultured *in vitro* for indicated time in the presence of 10 μM or 10 nM morphine sulfate (MS) as indicated. Protein was isolated from cultured PBMC, separated on a 10% SDS/polyacrylamide gel, blotted onto a nitrocellulose filter, and incubated with rabbit anti-CCR5-NT. % Intensity, intensity of Western blot signals compared with that of no morphine treatment control. Statistical analysis was performed on duplicate experiments using mean values from four monkeys (#28305, #28378, #28474 and #28717). Bar, standard error. $*p<0.05$.

Opioid Receptors and Chemokine Receptor CCR5 Form an Oligomeric Protein Complex on Cell Surface

Since chemokine receptor CCR5 stands out in our studies – it can be induced by morphine and it serves as an entry co-receptor for SIV/HIV-- we began to analyze the structure and subcellular functions of CCR5 and its relationship with opioid receptors. Polymorphisms in CCR5 genes have been implicated in HIV disease progression, resistance or non-progressive infection. For example (Huang et al., 1996), a 32-bp deletion in the CCR5 coding region (CCR5 δ32) protects a CCR5 δ32 homozygote from infection and delays the disease progression in a CCR5 δ32 heterozygous individual. Multiple CCR5 transcripts and mRNA diversity have also been described. The generation of multiple CCR5 transcripts has consequences for the regulation of CCR5 gene expression. In spite of all these studies, multiple forms of CCR5 protein have not been described. In one of our studies (Suzuki et al., 2002d), we presented evidence to show that two distinct forms of CCR5 protein, 62 kDa and 42 kDa, are present in human lymphocytic cells and monkey PBMC. The ratio of these two forms of CCR5 changes with cell growth. Morphine induces the formation and expression of both forms of CCR5 whereas RANTES, MIP-1α or MIP-1β inhibits them. Localization studies indicated that the 62 kDa CCR5 resides mainly on the cell membrane and the 42 kDa CCR5 is present solely in the cytoplasm of the cells (Fig. 4). We subsequently demonstrated by immunoprecipitation, electrophoresis and crosslinking studies that the 62 kDa CCR5, the membrane CCR5, is in close proximity and forms an oligomeric complex with opioid receptors on the cell membrane and this complex formation modulates receptor functions.

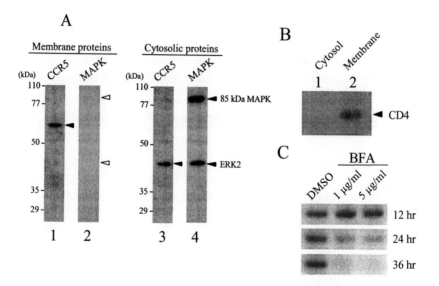

Figure 4. Cellular localization of the 42 kDa and the 62 kDa CCR5. (A) Membrane and cytosolic CCR5. Membrane and cytosolic proteins of CEM x174 cells were prepared separately and a 10-μg protein sample was subjected to 10 % SDS/PAGE followed by Western blot analysis using anti-CCR5-NT (lanes 1 and 3) or anti-MAPK (lanes 2 and 4) as immunodetection probe. Closed arrows, immunoreactive signals of CCR5 (lanes 1 and 3), 85 kDa MAPK (lane 4) or ERK2 (lane 4). Open arrows, the expected positions of the 85 kDa MAPK and ERK2. The positions of molecular size markers are indicated on the left. (B) Western blot analysis of cytosolic (lane 1) or membrane (lane 2) CD4 glycoprotein using anti-CD4 antibody. (C) Effect of BFA treatment on the transport of CCR5 to cell membrane. CEM x174 cells were treated with DMSO (as control), 1 μg/ml BFA or 5 μg/ml BFA for the indicated times. Membrane proteins (10 μg) were isolated from the treated cells and subjected to 10% SDS/PAGE followed by Western blot analysis using anti-CCR5-NT. Brefeldin A (BFA) was used here to monitor protein transport to cell membrane. The data show that BFA treatment reduced the amount of the 62 kDa CCR5 on cell membrane, further supporting the notion that the cell membrane of CEM x174 cells possesses a unique form of CCR5.

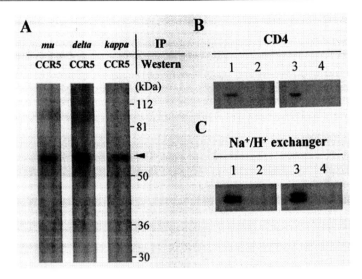

Figure 5. Co-immunoprecipitation of CEM x174 membrane protein with opioid receptors. (A) Detection by anti-CCR5 antibodies. Total protein from CEM x174 was isolated and immunoprecipitated with antibodies against *mu* (lane 1), *delta* (lane 2) or *kappa* (lane 3). The immunoprecipitated materials were subjected to a 10% SDS/PAGE and blotted onto a PVDF membrane. Immunodetection was performed on each blot using anti-CCR5-NT as a probe. The arrow indicates the position of a 62 kDa CCR5 band. The positions of SDS/PAGE molecular weight size markers are indicated on the right. (B) Detection by anti-CD4 antibodies. Total protein (20 μg, lane 1 or 3) or protein immunoprecipitated with antibodies against *mu* (lane 2) or against *delta* (lane 4) was subjected to SDS/PAGE and analyzed using anti-CD4 antibodies as immuno-probes. (C) Detection by anti-Na^+/H^+ exchanger antibodies. Total protein (20 μg, lane 1 or 3) or protein immunoprecipitated with antibodies against *mu* (lane 2) or against *delta* (lane 4) was subjected to SDS/PAGE and analyzed using anti-Na^+/H^+ exchanger antibodies as immuno-probes. IP, immunoprecipitation.

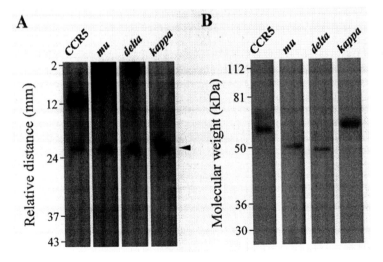

Figure 6. Detection of a receptor complex by non-denaturing PAGE. (A) Western blot analysis on non-denaturing PAGE showing a single polypeptide band. CEM x174 protein (75 μg) was loaded onto a 6% non-denaturing PAGE and electro-transferred onto a PVDF membrane. Western blot analyses with antibodies against CCR5 (lane 1), *mu* (lane 2), *delta* (lane 3) or *kappa* (lane 4) opioid receptors were performed, showing an identical immunoreactive band (arrow). The numbers on the left indicate the relative migration of molecular weight size markers during electrophoresis (millimeters). (B) Extraction and analysis of the

immunoreactive protein identified in the non-denaturing gel showing the single band in (A) contains CCR5, mu, delta and kappa. The immunoreactive band (shown by arrow) in Fig. 6A was excised from the gel and protein extracted. The protein extract was subjected to 10% SDS/PAGE and western blot analysis with antibodies against CCR5 (lane 1), *mu* (lane 2), *delta* (lane 3) or *kappa* (lane 4) opioid receptors. The numbers on the left indicate the positions of SDS/PAGE molecular weight size markers.

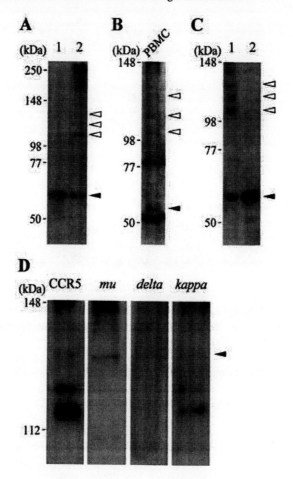

Figure 7. Crosslink of a receptor complex by glutaraldehyde. The membrane fraction of CEM x174 cells (A, C and D) or monkey PBMC (B) was treated with 0.05% glutaraldehyde. Protein was isolated from the treated samples and an aliquot of the isolated protein solution (10 μg protein) was subjected to a 10% (A-C) or 4.5% (D) SDS/PAGE followed by western blot analysis using anti-CCR5-NT (A-C and lane 1 of D), anti-MOR-1 (lane 2 of D), anti-DOR-1 (lane 3 of D) or anti-kappa-opioid receptor antibodies (lane 4 of D) as immunodetection probes. (A) Glutaraldehyde crosslink of CEM x174. The amount of CCR5 monomers (62 kDa, closed arrow) in untreated samples (lane 1) was decreased after crosslinking (lane 2), resulting in three upper bands of molecular masses of 113, 118 and 124 kDa (open arrows). (B) Glutaraldehyde crosslinking of monkey PBMC, showing results similar to CEM x174 crosslink samples (lane 2 of A). (C) Glutaraldehyde crosslink of CEM x174 membrane protein isolated with RIPA lysis buffer. Protein was first isolated from the membrane fraction of CEM x174 cells using RIPA lysis buffer and then subjected to a glutaraldehyde crosslink reaction. Lane 1, control: glutaraldehyde crosslinking of membrane proteins as in lane 2 of A; lane 2, isolation of membrane protein by RIPA lysis buffer prior to glutaraldehyde treatment, indicating that crosslinking did not occur. Open arrows indicate the expected positions of 113, 118 and 124 kDa polypeptides, if present; closed arrow indicates the position of the 62 kDa CCR5 monomers. (D) Western blot analyses of the CEM x174 crosslinked proteins using antibodies against both CCR5 and opioid receptors. The results indicate that the 124 kDa protein (arrow) was immunoreactive not only with anti-

CCR5-NT (lane 1), but also with antibodies against the three subtypes of opioid receptors (lanes 2-4). The numbers on the left indicate the positions of SDS/PAGE molecular weight size markers run in a parallel lane. These results represent reproducible data from at least three independent experiments. Other experiments with crosslinking agent BS^3 suggested that the intermolecular distance between opioid receptors and CCR5 is less than 11.4Å.

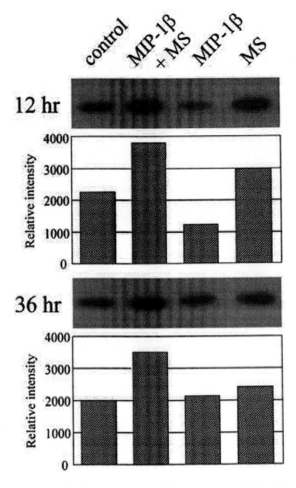

Figure 8. Effect of morphine and MIP-1β treatment on CCR5 expression. CEM x174 cells were treated with 10 nM morphine or 250 ng/ml MIP-1β or morphine (10 nM) plus MIP-1β (250 ng/ml) for 12 or 36 h. Total protein (20 μg) was isolated from the treated samples and subjected to 10% SDS/PAGE followed by western blot analysis using anti-CCR5-NT as an immunodetection probe. The graph below each autoradiograph picture corresponds to the relative intensity of CCR5 expression of each gel lane calculated by densitometry scanning. The data presented were for the 42 kDa CCR5 and were representatives of reproducible results from four independent experiments. Similar results were obtained for the 62 kDa CCR5. MS, morphine. Statistical analyses (student's *t*-test): For the 12 hr data, the values of MIP-1β+MS or MS only were significantly greater than that of control ($p<0.05$) and the value of MIP-1β was significantly lower than that of control ($p<0.05$). For the 36 hr data, the value of MIP-1β plus MS was significantly greater than that of control ($p<0.05$).

Immunoprecipitation experiments in the study showed that CCR5 (62 kDa), but not CD4 nor Na$^+$/H$^+$ exchanger, coprecipitates with all three subtypes (*mu, delta* and *kappa*) of opioid receptors (Fig. 5). In addition, a single protein band immunoreactive with antibodies against both the CCR5 and the three opioid receptors was identified after electrophoresis on non-denaturing polyacrylamide gels (Fig. 6). Chemical cross-linking experiments using glutaraldehyde or BS^3 indicate that these receptors are closely situated on the cell membrane with an intermolecular distance of less than 11.4 Å (Fig. 7). Functional studies revealed that a combination treatment of cells with morphine, an agonist for *mu*, and MIP-1β, a ligand for CCR5, suppresses the inhibitory effect of MIP-1β and increases the stimulatory effect of morphine on CCR5 expression (Fig. 8). These results suggest that oligomerization of chemokine receptor CCR5 with opioid receptors on the cell membrane of human or monkey lymphocytes may further modulate receptor functions. The implication of this study may explain at a cellular level the higher prevalence of HIV-1 infection among IV drug users (Suzuki et al., 2002c).

Morphine Protects Human Lymphocytic Cells and Monkey PBMC from Apoptosis

In an effort to determine possible signal transduction pathways that morphine may use to effect its immunomodulatory action, we used a reverse transcription-polymerase chain reaction-based differential display technique (RT-PCR DD) coupled with a hybridization procedure to compare gene expression patterns of morphine-treated cells with those of control cells. Using this technique, we identified novel specific genes, mRNAs and proteins that we had no previous knowledge of and whose expression in immune cells was regulated by the presence of morphine. Through assiduous screening efforts, ten positive gene segments including two morphine down-regulated genes and eight morphine up-regulated genes were identified in CEM x174 lymphocytes (Suzuki et al., 2003a). Among these genes, two apoptosis/cell growth-related genes (PNAS-133 and Krüppel-like factor 7) were revealed. PNAS-133 (apoptosis) gene was found to be down-regulated by morphine whereas Krüppel-like factor 7 (KLF7), a zinc finger transcription factor, was up-regulated by morphine. The up-regulation of KLF7 by morphine was noted to be present at both the transcriptional and translational levels (Fig. 9). The morphine effect could be reversed by naloxone, indicating an opioid receptor-mediated event (Suzuki et al., 2003a). These findings suggest a unique role for morphine in the regulation of cell proliferation and apoptosis in lymphocytes. In HIV-infected humans or SIV-infected animals, apoptosis plays a role in eliminating infected and/or uninfected CD4+ lymphocytes (Cotton et al., 1996; Ansari 2004; Bouzar et al., 2004). We further defined the role of morphine in the cell's apoptotic process after the cell was triggered to undergo apoptosis in response to an extracellular signal (e.g. actinomycin D, HIV/SIV, etc.). The addition of morphine was found to suppress the expression of active (Ser^{15} phosphorylated) p53 (Fig. 10), possibly through activation of the MAPK pathway (Chuang et al., 1997b; Ritchie et al., 1999). Blockade of p53 phosphorylation/activation was noted to induce down-regulation of *Bax* (an apoptosis-promoter) and up-regulation of *Bcl-2* (an apoptosis -inhibitor), thus increasing the ratio of *Bcl-2* to *Bax* in mitochondria (Fig. 11). Hence, the death signaling, possibly through the caspase (also known as CPP32) pathway we previously identified in CEM x174 cells (Rought et al., 2000), might be transiently suppressed by changes in the ratio of *Bcl-2/Bax* in mitochondria, leading to increased cell growth and an arrest in apoptosis (Suzuki et al.,

2003b). Our studies have therefore provided a mechanism (as illustrated in Fig. 12) to account for the delayed apoptosis and prolonged SIV infection in morphine-treated cells that we had previously observed in both CEM x174 lymphocytic cells (Chuang et al., 1993b) and monkey PBMC (Chuang et al., 1993b; Suzuki et al., 2002b).

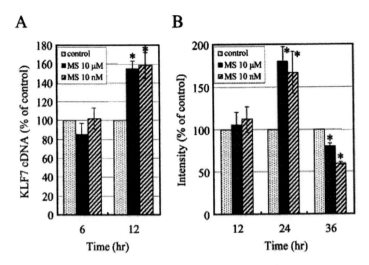

Figure 9. Effect of morphine on KLF7 gene and protein expression. CEM x174 cells were treated with 10 μM or 10 nM morphine sulfate (MS) or with H_2O as control. After incubation at the indicated time, total RNA and protein were isolated from the cells. (A) KLF7 gene expression. The amount of KLF7 transcripts as expressed by KLF7 cDNA was determined by competitive RT-PCR and the data were calculated as the percentage of control. Bar, standard error (n=5). * $p < 0.05$, compared with control (Student's t-test). (B) KLF7 protein expression. Western blot analysis was performed to determine the relative amount of KLF protein expressed. The intensity of band reacted with anti-GKLF was measured and calculated as the percentage of control. Bar, standard error (n=4). * $p < 0.05$, compared with control (Student's t-test).

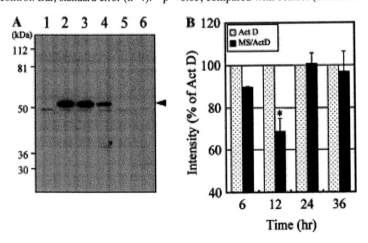

Figure 10. Effect of morphine on actinomycin D-induced p53 activation. (A) CEM x174 cells were pretreated with 10 μM (lane 3) or 10 nM (lane 4) morphine sulfate for 18 hr followed by treatment of the cell culture with 0.5 μg/ml actinomycin D. Protein was isolated 12 hr post actinomycin D treatment and subjected to SDS/PAGE and Western blot analysis using anti-p53 (phosphorylated Ser-15) antibody as an immuno-detection probe. Lane 1, control cells with no drug treatment. Lane 2, cells treated with actinomycin D only. Lane 5 and lane 6, cells treated with 10 μM or 10 nM morphine sulfate, respectively, in the absence of actinomycin treatment. The positions of SDS/PAGE molecular weight size markers are indicated on the left.

The arrow indicates the position of activated p53. (B) The intensities of the immunoreactive signals of activated p53 of cells treated with 10 nM morphine sulfate followed by actinomycin D treatment (MS/ActD) were measured by densitometry scanning and calculated as a percentage of the intensities obtained from the cells treated with actinomycin D alone (ActD, as 100%). Bar, standard error (n=4). * p < 0.05, compared with ActD treatment.

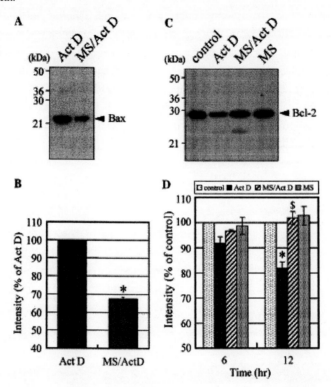

Figure 11. Effect of morphine on *Bax* and *Bcl-2* expression. CEM x174 cells were pretreated with 10 nM morphine for 18 hrs followed by treatment with 0.5 µg/ml actinomycin D. Protein was isolated 36 hrs post actinomycin D treatment for western blot analysis of *Bax* expression (A and B). For western blot analysis of *Bcl-2* expression (C and D), protein was isolated 6 hr (D) or 12 hr (C and D) post actinomycin D treatment. The arrows indicate the position of *Bax* (A) and *Bcl-2* (C). The positions of SDS/PAGE molecular weight size markers are indicated on the left. The intensities of the immunoreactive signals of *Bax* and *Bcl-2* were measured by densitometry scanning; relative intensities were calculated as a percentage of ActD (B) or of control (D). Act D, cells received actinomycin D only. MS/Act D, cells received both morphine sulfate and actinomycin D. MS, cells received morphine sulfate only. Bar, standard error (n=3). B, * $p < 0.05$ compared with actinomycin D treatment. D, * $p < 0.05$ compared with control; $ $p < 0.05$ compared with actinomycin D treatment.

Conclusion

Individuals infected with human immunodeficiency virus (HIV) vary in the rate of development to AIDS, suggesting that co-factors other than the virus itself are involved in influencing the rate of disease progression. Opioid addicts make up a significant proportion of the AIDS population. The above studies determine whether, and by what mechanism, opioids attenuate host immune function and in turn alter AIDS disease progression. Using the simian immunodeficiency virus (SIV)-infected rhesus monkey as an animal model to

Ronald Y. Chuang, Linda F. Chuang and Roy H. Doi

investigate the effect of opioids on the pathogenesis of AIDS, we have revealed that morphine-treated animals had faster rates of SIV replication and mutation and a shorter life span than morphine-naïve cohorts (Chuang et al., 1993a; 1994a; 1995b; 1997a). These results have also led to our discovery of the expression of brain-like opioid receptors on lymphocytes, the cells of the immune system. By studying lymphocyte opioid receptors, we found that morphine may exert diverse mechanisms to promote SIV infection: firstly, morphine may increase SIV entry into cells by increasing CCR5, a co-receptor for SIV infection; secondly, after the virus has entered the cells, morphine may delay cell apoptosis, thus augmenting viral replication. These studies may provide fundamental insight in regard to consideration of the specific receptors as potential therapeutic targets as well as initiators in promoting the development of specific regimens for the treatment and prevention of AIDS, especially in the drug abuse population.

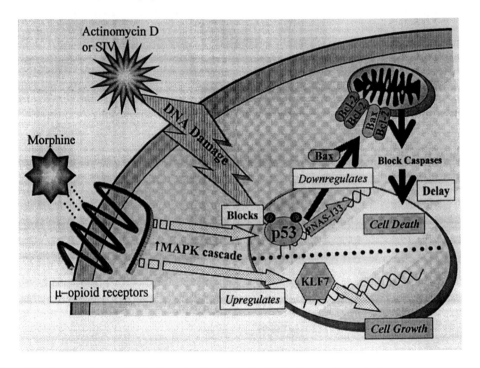

Figure 12. A hypothetical model for the role of morphine in SIV-induced cell apoptosis.

Suggestions for Future Research

The above studies demonstrated that morphine has a direct role in promoting AIDS virus infection and disease progression. The Office of National Drug Control Policy estimates that among the large population of chronic opiate users in the United States, the major treatment modality for opiate addiction is currently methadone maintenance programs (Kreek and Vocci, 2002). In fact, methadone is used worldwide for the treatment of morphine/heroin addiction (Salsitz et al., 2000; Sees et al., 2000; Chan and Lee, 2004). In 1990, an age and sex-matched cohort study reported that methadone maintenance patients had a 6-fold reduction in death rate as compared to untreated addicts (7.2% vs. 1.4%) (Kreek and Vocci, 2002). Methadone is a synthetic opiate receptor agonist that is rapidly absorbed and slowly eliminated from the plasma (Wolff et al., 1993). That a decline in rates of arrest and criminal convictions for both HIV-positive and HIV-negative patients on methadone treatment was reported (Stenbacka et al., 2003; Keen et al., 2003). Although there is little known about the effects of methadone on immune function in AIDS patients, studies on street heroin addicts and addicts undergoing methadone treatment show an apparently better functioning immune system among the methadone patients (Falek et al., 1986; Lazzarin et al., 1984; Grass et al., 2003), suggesting that methadone may have a different effect on AIDS progression than morphine/heroin (Beck et al., 2002). While methadone maintenance therapy for treatment of opiate abuse has been suggested in the U.S. as a cost-effective intervention for slowing the spread of AIDS among drug users (Gibson et al., 1999; Sorensen and Copeland, 2000), conflicting results in Amsterdam and Thailand have been reported (Langendam et al., 1999; Vanichseni et al., 2001). HIV-1 transmission risk remains high among Bangkok IDUs despite methadone treatment and other current prevention strategies (Vanichseni et al., 2001). Our *in vitro* (tissue culture) studies have shown that like morphine, methadone is able to stimulate the expression of chemokine receptor CCR5, a co-receptor for HIV/SIV entry, and enhance SIV replication (Suzuki et al., 2002a). Methadone was also found to inhibit chemokine-mediated chemotaxis of monkey monocytes and neutrophils (Choi et al., 1999). Therefore, questions remain: (i) will these immunotoxic properties of methadone stultify the methadone treatment program? (ii) will methadone countervail or, in fact, facilitate the detrimental effects of morphine or heroin on the immune system? (iii) what makes the methadone maintenance program effective in slowing the spread of AIDS, or (iv) can methadone treatment indeed halt the transmission of the AIDS disease? While our previous *in vivo* (animal) studies strived to model the effects of opiate use on AIDS patients in the field, future studies may focus on delineating mechanisms behind the safety and validity of treating opiate-addicted AIDS patients with methadone in clinics. A systematical study using the SAIDS animal model system comparing the effect of methadone treatment with that of morphine treatment on the expression of opioid receptors, chemokine receptors and simian AIDS progression will be able to answer many important and timely questions.

Acknowledgment

This work was supported by NIH research grants DA 05901 and DA 10433 from the National Institute on Drug Abuse.

References

Alicea C, Belkowski SM, Sliker JK, Zhu J, Liu-Chen LY, Eisenstein TK, Adler MW, and Rogers TJ. (1998) Characterization of kappa-opioid receptor transcripts expressed by T cells and macrophages. *J. Neuroimmunol.* 91:55-62.

Ansari AA. (2004) Autoimmunity, anergy, lentiviral immunity and disease. *Autoimmun. Rev.* 3:530-540.

Batki SL. (1988) Treatment of intravenous drug users with AIDS: the role of methadone maintenance. *J. Psychoactive Drugs* 20:213-216.

Beck M, Mirmohammadsadegh A, Franz B, Blanke J, and Hengge UR. (2002) Opioid receptors on white blood cells: effect of HIV infection and methadone treatment. *Pain* 98:187-194.

Bostik P, Villinger F, Brice GT, Chikkala NF, Brar SS, Cruikshank WW, Adams JW, Hillyer CD and Ansari AA. (1998) Expression and in vitro evaluation of rhesus macaque wild type (wt) and modified CC chemokines. *J. Med. Primatol.* 27:113-120.

Bouzar AB, Villet S, Morin T, Rea A, Genestier L, Guiguen F, Garnier C, Mornex JF, Narayan O and Chebloune Y. (2004) Simian immunodeficiency virus Vpr/Vpx proteins kill bystander noninfected CD4+ T-lymphocytes by induction of apoptosis. *Virol.* 326: 47-56.

Chan MK, and Lee SS. (2004) Can the low HIV prevalence in Hong Kong be maintained? *AIDS Educ. Prev.* 16:18-26.

Choi Y, Chuang LF, Lam KM, Kung H-F, Wang JM, Osburn BI, and Chuang RY. (1999) Inhibition of chemokine-induced chemotaxis of monkey leukocytes by μ-opioid receptor agonists. *In Vivo* 13:389-396.

Chuang AJ, Killiam KF, Jr., Chuang RY, Rice WG, Schaeffer CA, Mendeleyev J, and Kun E. (1993a) Inhibition of the replication of native and 3'-azido-2',3'-dideoxy-thymidine (AZT)-resistant simian immunodeficiency virus (SIV) by 3-nitrosobenzamide. *FEBS Letter* 326:140-144.

Chuang LF, Blackbourn DJ, Chuang AJ, Killam KF Jr, Liu X, Li Y, Kung HF, and Chuang RY. (1994a) Emergence of antigenic variants of simian immunodeficiency virus (SIVmac) in a seronegative macaque after SIVmac239 infection. *Cellular and Molecular Biology Research* 40:661-669.

Chuang LF, Chuang TK, Killam KF Jr, Chuang AJ, Kung HF, Yu L, and Chuang RY. (1994b) Delta opioid receptor gene expression in lymphocytes. *Biochem. Biophys. Res. Commun.* 202:1291-1299.

Chuang LF, Chuang TK, Killam KF Jr, Qiu Q, Wang XR, Lin JJ, Kung HF, Sheng W, Chao C, Yu L, and Chuang RY. (1995a) Expression of kappa opioid receptors in human and monkey lymphocytes. *Biochem. Biophys. Res. Commun.* 209:1003-1010.

Chuang LF, Killam KF Jr, and Chuang RY. (1993b) Increased replication of simian immunodeficiency virus in CEM x174 cells by morphine sulfate. *Biochem. Biophys. Res. Commun.* 195:1165-1173.

Chuang LF, Killam KF Jr, and Chuang RY. (1993c) Effect of chronic opioid treatment on simian immunodeficiency virus infection in rhesus monkeys. NIDA Res. *Monograph: Problems of Drug Dependence* 141:419.

Chuang LF, Killam KF Jr, and Chuang RY. (1997a) SIV infection of macaques: a model for studying AIDS and drug abuse. *Addiction Biol.* 2:421-430.

Chuang LF, Killam LF Jr, and Chuang RY. (1997b) Induction and activation of mitogen-activated protein kinases of human lymphocytes as one of the signaling pathways of the immunomodulatory effects of morphine sulfate. *J. Biol. Chem.* 272:26815-26817.

Chuang RY, Chuang LF, Li Y, Kung H-F, and Killam KF Jr. (1995b) SIV mutations detected in morphine-treated *Macaca mulatta* following SIVmac239 infection. *Adv. Exp. Med. Biol.* 373, 175-181.

Chuang TK., Killam KF Jr, Chuang LF, Kung HF, Sheng WS, Chao CC, Yu L, and Chuang RY. (1995c) Mu opioid receptor gene expression in immune cells. *Biochem. Biophys. Res. Commun.* 216:922-930.

Cocchi F, DeVico AL, Garzino-Demo A, Arya SK, Gallo RC, and Lusso P. (1995) Identification of RANTES, MIP-1α, and MIP-1β as the major HIV-suppressive factors produced by CD8+ T cells. *Science* 270:1811-1815.

Cotton MF, Cassella C, Rapaport EL, Tseng PO, Marschner S, and Finkel TH. (1996) Apoptosis in HIV-1 infection. *Behring Inst. Mitt.* 97:220-231.

Deng HK, Unutmaz D, Ramani VNK, and Littman DR. (1997) Expression cloning of new receptors used by simian and human immunodeficiency viruses. *Nature* 388:296-300.

Desrosiers RC. (1990) The simian immunodeficiency viruses. *Annu. Rev. Immunol.* 8:557-578.

Dole VP, and Nyswander ME. (1983) Pharmacological treatment of narcotic addiction. Proc. Comm. Probl. Drug Dependence: *NIDA Res. Monogr.* 43:5-9.

Falek A, Madden JJ, Shafer DA, and Donahoe RM. (1986). Individual differences in opiate-induced alterations at the cytogenetic, DNA repair, and immunologic levels: opportunity for genetic assessment. In: Braude, M.C. and Chao, H.M. (eds.). Genetic and Biological Markers in Drug Abuse and Alcoholism. *NIDA Res. Monog.* 66, pp. 11-24, Rockville, Maryland.

Farzan M, Choe H, Martin K, Marcon L, Hofmann W, Karlsson G, Sun Y, Barrett P, Marchand N, Sullivan N, Gerard N, Gerard C, and Sodroski J. (1997) Two orphan seven-transmembrane segment receptors which are expressed in CD4-positive cells support simian immunodeficiency virus infection. *J. Exp. Med.* 186:405-411.

Feng Y, Broder CC, Kennedy PE, and Berger EA. (1996) HIV-1 entry cofactor: functional cDNA cloning of a seven-transmembrane, G protein-coupled receptor. *Science* 272:872-875.

Friedman H, and Eisenstein TK. (2004) Neurological basis of drug dependence and its effects on the immune system. *J. Neuroimmunol.* 147:106-108.

Gaughwin MD, Gowans E, Ali R, and Burrell C. (1991) Bloody needles: the volumes of blood transferred in simulations of needlestick injuries and shared use of syringes for injection of intravenous drugs. *AIDS* 5:1025-1027.

Gavériaux-Ruff C, Peluso J, Simonin F, Laforet J, and Kieffer B. (1995) Identification of κ- and δ-opioid receptor transcripts in immune cells. *FEBS Lett.* 369:272-276.

Gibson DR, Flynn NM, and McCarthy JJ. (1999) Effectiveness of methadone treatment in reducing HIV risk behavior and HIV seroconversion among injecting drug users. *AIDS* 13:1807-1818.

Grass H, Behnsen S, Kimont HG, Staak M, and Kaferstein H. (2003) Methadone and its role in drug-related fatalities in Cologne 1989-2000. *Forensic Sci. Int.* 132:195-200.

Guo CJ, Li Y, Tian S, Wang X, Douglas SD, and Ho WZ. (2002) Morphine enhances HIV infection of human blood mononuclear phagocytes through modulation of beta-chemokines and CCR5 receptor. *J. Investig. Med.* 50:435-442.

Heagy W, Laurance M, Cohen E, and Finberg R. (1990) Neurohormones regulate T cell function. *J. Exp. Med.* 171:1625-1633.

Hedrick JA, and Zlotnik A. (1997) Lymphotactin: a new class of chemokine. *Methods in Enzymol.* 287:206-215.

Ho W-Z, Guo C-J, Yuan C-S, Douglas SD, and Moss J. (2003) Methylnaltrexone antagonizes opioid-mediated enhancement of HIV infection of human blood mononuclear phagocytes. *J. Pharmacol. Exp. Ther.* 307:1158-1162.

Huang Y, Paxton WA, Wolinsky SM, Neumann AU, Zhang L, He T, Kang S, Ceradini D, Jin Z, Yazdanbakhsh K, Kunstman K, Erickson D, Dragon E, Landau NR, Phair J, Ho DD, and Koup RA. (1996) The role of a mutant CCR5 allele in HIV-1 transmission and disease progression. *Nat. Med.* 2:1240-1243.

Kedzierska K, Crowe SM, Turville S, and Cunningham, AL. (2003) The influence of cytokines, chemokines and their receptors on HIV-1 replication in monocytes and macrophages. *Rev. Med. Virol.* 13:39-56.

Keen J, Oliver P, Rowse G, and Mathers N. (2003) Does methadone maintenance treatment based on the new national guidelines work in a primary care setting? *Br. J. Gen Pract.* 53: 461-467.

Kelvin DJ, Michiel DF, Johnston JA, Lloyd AR, Sprenger H, Oppenheim JJ, and Wang JM. (1993) Chemokines and serpentines: the molecular biology of chemokine receptors. *J. Leukocyte Biol.* 54:604-612.

Kirchhoff F, Pohlmann S, Hamacher M, Means RE, Kraus T, Uberla K, and di Marzio P. (1997) Simian immunodeficiency virus variants with differential T-cell and macrophage tropism use CCR5 and an unidentified cofactor expressed in CEMx174 cells for efficient entry. *J. Virol.* 71:6509-6516.

Kreek MJ, and Vocci FJ. (2002) History and current status of opioid maintenance treatment: blending conference session. *J. Subst. Abuse Treat.* 23:93-105.

Kumar R, Torres C, Yamamura Y, Rodriguez I, Martinez M, Staprans S, Donahoe RM, Kraiselburd E, Stephens EB, and Kumar A. (2004) Modulation of viral set point by morphine in rhesus macaques infected with SIV and SHIV. Manuscript. Also, Abstract: Kumar R et al. (2004) Effect of morphine-dependence on viral replication and host-induced immune responses in macaque model of AIDS. The *10th Annual Meeting on Neuroimmune Circuits and Infectious Diseases*, Santa Fe, New Mexico, p. 50.

Langendam MW, van Brussel GHA, Coutinho RA, and van Ameijden EJC. (1999) Methadone maintenance treatment modalities in relation to incidence of HIV: results of the Amsterdam cohort study. *AIDS* 13:1711-1716.

Lazzarin A, Mella L, Trombini M, Uberti-Foppa C, Franzetti F, Mazzoni G, and Galli M. (1984) Immunological status in heroin addicts: effects of methadone maintenance. *Drug and Alcohol Dependence* 13:117-123.

Liao F, Alkhatib G, Peden KWC, Sharma G, Berger EA, and Farber JM. (1997) STRL33, a novel chemokine receptor-like protein, functions as a fusion cofactor for both macrophage-tropic and T cell line-tropic HIV-1. *J. Exp. Med.* 185:2015-2023.

Liu Y, Blackbourn DJ, Chuang LF, Killam KF Jr., and Chuang RY. (1992) Effects of *in vivo* and *in vitro* administration of morphine sulfate upon rhesus macaque polymorphonuclear cell phagocytosis and chemotaxis. *J. Pharmacol. Exp. Ther.* 263:533-539.

Madden JJ, Donahoe RM, Zwemer-Collins J, Shafer DA, and Falek A. (1987) Binding of naloxone to human T lymphocytes. *Biochem. Pharmacol.* 36:4103-4109.

Mahajan SD, Schwartz SA, Shanahan TC, Chawda RP, and Nair MP. (2002) Morphine regulates gene expression of alpha- and beta-chemokines and their receptors on astroglial cells via the opioid mu receptor. *J. Immunol.* 169:3589-3599.

Marcon L, Choe H, Martin KA, Farzan M, Ponath PD, Wu L, Newman W, Gerard N, Gerard C, and Sodroski J. (1997) Utilization of C-C chemokine receptor 5 by the envelope glycoproteins of a pathogenic simian immunodeficiency virus, SIVmac239. *J.Virol.* 71:2522-2527.

Marmor M, Des Jarlais DC, Cohen H, Friedman SR, Beatrice ST, Dubin N, El-Sadr W, Mildvan D, Yancovitz S, Mathur U, and Holzman R. (1987) Risk Factors for Infection with Human Immunodeficiency Virus among Intravenous Drug Abusers in New York City. *AIDS* 1:39-44.

Miyagi T, Chuang LF, Doi RH, Carlos MP, Torres JV, and Chuang RY. (2000a) Morphine induces gene expression of CCR5 in human CEMx174 lymphocytes. *J. Biol. Chem.* 275:31305-31310.

Miyagi T, Chuang LF, Lam KM, Kung H-F, Wang JM, Osburn BI, and Chuang RY. (2000b) Opioids suppress chemokine-mediated migration of monkey neutrophils and monocytes – an instant response. *Immunopharmacol.* 47:53-62.

Pampusch MS, Osinski MA, Serie JR, Murtaugh MP, and Brown DR. (1998) Opioid receptor gene expression in the porcine immune system. *Adv. Exp. Med. Biol.* 437: 59-65.

Pan Y, Lloyd C, Zhou H, Dolich S, Deeds J, Gonzalo J-A, Vath J, Gosselin M, Ma J, Dussault B, Woolf E, Alperin G, Culpepper J, Gutierrez-Ramos JC, and Gearing D. (1997) Neurotactin, a membrane-anchored chemokine upregulated in brain inflammation. *Nature* 387:611-617.

Pierce TL, Murray AG, and Hope W. (1992) Determination of methadone and its metabolites by high performance liquid chromatography following solid-phase extraction in rat plasma. *J. Chromatographic Sci.* 30:443-447.

Ritchie A, Braun SE, He J, and Broxmeyer HE. (1999) Thrombopoietin-induced conformational change in p53 lies downstream of the p44/p42 mitogen activated protein kinase cascade in the human growth factor-dependent cell line M107e. *Oncogene* 18:1465-1477.

Rought SE, Yau PM, Guo XW, Chuang LF, Doi RH, and Chuang RY. (2000) Modulation of CPP32 activity and induction of apoptosis in human CEM X174 lymphocytes by heptachlor, a chlorinated hydrocarbon insecticide. J. Biochem. Mol. Toxicol. 14:42-50.

Rouveix B. (1992) Opiates and immune function. *Therapie* 47:503-512.

Salsitz EA, Joseph H, Frank B, Perez J, Richman BL, Salomon N, Kalin MF, and Novick DM. (2000) Methadone medical maintenance (MMM): treating chronic opioid dependence in private medical practice – a summary report (1983-1998). *Mount Sinai J. Med.* 67:388-397.

Sedqi M, Roy S, Ramakrishnan S, Elde R, and Loh HH. (1995) Complementary DNA cloning of a μ-opioid receptor from rat peritoneal macrophages. *Biochem. Biophys. Res. Commun.* 209:563-574.

Sees KL, Delucchi KL, Masson C, Rosen A, Clark HW, Robillard H, Banys P. and Hall SM. (2000) Methadone maintenance vs. 180-day psychosocially enriched detoxification for treatment of opioid dependence. *JAMA* 283:1303-1310.

Sharp BM, Roy S, and Bidlack JM. (1998) Evidence for opioid receptors on cells involved in host defense and the immune system. *J. Neuroimmunol.* 83:45-56.

Sibinga NES, and Goldstein A. (1988) Opioid peptides and opioid receptors in cells of the immune system. *Ann. Rev. Immunol.* 6:219-249.

Sorensen JL, and Copeland AL. (2000) Drug abuse treatment as an HIV prevention strategy: a review. *Drug and Alcohol Dependence* 59:17-31.

Steele AD, Henderson EE, and Rogers TJ. (2003) Mu-opioid modulation of HIV-1 coreceptor expression and HIV-1 replication. *Virology* 309:99-107.

Stenbacka M, Leifman A, and Romelsjo A. (2003) The impact of methadone treatment on registered convictions and arrests in HIV-positive and HIV-negative men and women with one or more treatment periods. *Drug Alcohol Rev.* 22:27-34.

Suzuki S, Carlos MP, Chuang LF, Torres JV, Doi RH and Chuang RY. (2002a) Methadone induces CCR5 and promotes AIDS virus infection. *FEBS Lett.* 519:173-177.

Suzuki S, Chuang AJ, Chuang LF, Doi RH, and Chuang RY. (2002b) Morphine promotes simian acquired immunodeficiency syndrome virus replication in monkey peripheral mononuclear cells: Induction of CC chemokine receptor 5 exrpession for viral entry. *J. Infect. Dis.* 185:1826-1829.

Suzuki S, Chuang LF, Doi RH, Bidlack JM, and Chuang RY. (2001) *kappa*-opioid receptors of human lymphocytic cell line: morphine-induced upregulation as evidenced by competitive RT-PCR and indirect immunofluorescence. *Int'l Immunopharmacol.* 1:1733-1742.

Suzuki S, Chuang LF, Doi RH, and Chuang RY. (2003a) Identification of opioid-regulated genes in human lymphocytic cells by differential display: up-regulation of Krüppel-like factor 7 by morphine. *Exp. Cell Res.* 291:340-351.

Suzuki S, Chuang LF, Doi RH, and Chuang RY. (2003b) Morphine suppresses lymphocyte apoptosis by blocking p53-mediated death signaling. *Biochem. Biophys. Res. Commun.* 308:802-808, 2003.

Suzuki S, Chuang LF, Yau P, Doi RH, and Chuang RY. (2002c) Interactions of opioid and chemokine receptors: oligomerization of mu, kappa and delta with CCR5 on immune cells. *Exp. Cell Res.* 280:192-200.

Suzuki S, Miyagi T, Chuang LF, Yau PM, Doi RH, and Chuang RY. (2002d) Chemokine receptor CCR5: polymorphism at protein level. *Biochem. Biophys. Res. Commun.* 296:477-483.

Suzuki S, Miyagi T, Chuang TK, Chuang LF, Doi RH and Chuang RY (2000) Morphine upregulates *mu* opioid receptors of human and monkey lymphocytes. *Biochem. Biophys. Res. Commun.* 279:621-628.

Vanichseni S, Kitayaporn D, Mastro T D, Mock PA, Raktham S, Des Jarlais DC, Sujarita S, Srisuwanvilai L, Young NL, Wasi C, Subbarao S, Heyward WL, Esparza J, and Choopanya K. (2001) Continued high HIV-1 incidence in a vaccine trial preparatory cohort of injection drug users in Bangkok, Thailand. *AIDS* 15:397-405.

Wang JM, Sherry B, Fivash MJ, Kelvin DJ, and Oppenheim JJ. (1993) Human recombinant macrophage inflammatory protein-1α and -1β and monocyte chemotactic and activating factor utilize common and unique receptors on human monocytes. *J. Immunol.* 150:3022-3029.

Wick MJ, Minnerath SR, Roy S, Ramakrishnan S, and Loh HH. (1996) Differential expression of opioid receptor genes in human lymphoid cell lines and peripheral blood lymphocytes. *J. Neuroimmunol.* 64:29-36.

Wolff K, Hay AW, Raistrick D, and Calvert, R. (1993) Steady-state pharmacokinetics of methadone in opioid addicts. *Eur. J. Clin. Pharmacol.* 44:189-194.

Yi Y, Isaacs SN, Williams DA, Frank I, Schols D, De Clercq E, Kolson DL, and Collman RG. (1999) Role of CXCR4 in cell-cell fusion and infection of monocyte-derived macrophages by primary human immunodeficiency virus type 1 (HIV-1) strains: two distinct mechanisms of HIV-1 dual tropism. *J. Virol.* 73:7117-7125.

Index

A

acceptance, 125, 126, 127, 131

access, 24, 127, 148, 166

accounting, 58

accumulation, 10, 56, 69

accuracy, 207

acetylcholine, 99, 156

acid, 5, 43, 45, 57, 58, 71, 77, 83, 89, 108, 132

acquired immunodeficiency syndrome, ix, 40, 68, 96, 181, 183, 196, 199, 218, 220, 244

ACTH, 135, 136, 137, 145, 146, 151

activation, 6, 8, 17, 25, 30, 42, 43, 44, 45, 46, 48, 49, 50, 52, 53, 54, 55, 56, 57, 58, 61, 64, 71, 75, 78, 79, 82, 85, 86, 87, 88, 89, 95, 102, 132, 135, 136, 139, 140, 154, 164, 201, 227, 235, 236, 240

active transport, 29

acute infection, 17, 18, 20, 21, 22, 23

adaptation, viii, 95, 121, 129, 130, 145

ADC, 8, 74, 200

addiction, 91, 238

adenosine, 7

adhesion, 7, 27, 58, 70, 71, 86, 90

adipocyte, 135

adipose, 139, 200

adjustment, 128, 167

adolescents, 155, 186, 188, 195

adrenal insufficiency, 136, 137

adrenoceptors, 132

adrenocorticotropic hormone, 135

adults, 27, 39, 65, 82, 100, 139, 155, 157, 161, 179, 180, 186, 188, 190, 195, 196, 197

advocacy, 127

affect, 5, 50, 61, 78, 84, 86, 95, 131, 140, 202, 204, 210, 212, 226, 227, 228

Afghanistan, 127

Africa, 126, 149, 163, 180, 189

African Americans, 122

age, ix, 3, 19, 47, 114, 123, 133, 138, 145, 165, 167, 170, 174, 185, 186, 187, 202, 208, 238

agent, 5, 50, 128, 188, 234

aggregates, 159

aging, 133, 139, 174, 187

aging population, 187

agonist, 87, 93, 98, 135, 235, 239

AIDS, i, iii, v, vi, vii, viii, ix, 1, 2, 3, 4, 5, 8, 10, 11, 12, 13, 16, 19, 20, 26, 29, 31, 32, 33, 34, 35, 36, 37, 38, 39, 40, 42, 47, 63, 65, 66, 68, 70, 72, 73, 74, 75, 76, 77, 81, 83, 85, 92, 93, 94, 95, 96, 97, 98, 99, 101, 103, 115, 116, 117, 118, 119, 121, 122, 123, 124, 125, 126, 127, 131, 132, 133, 135, 136, 137, 138, 140, 141, 142, 143, 144, 145, 146, 147, 149, 151, 152, 153, 154, 155, 156, 157, 158, 159, 160, 161, 162, 163, 164, 166, 167, 170, 173, 174, 177, 178, 179, 180, 181, 182, 183, 185, 186, 187, 188, 189, 190, 191, 193, 194, 195, 196, 197, 198, 199, 200, 201, 203, 204, 205, 206, 207, 208, 209, 211, 213, 214, 215, 216, 217, 218, 219, 220, 221, 222, 223, 225, 226, 227, 230, 237, 238, 240, 241, 242, 243, 244

albumin, 192

alcohol, viii, 81, 83, 93, 94, 95, 97, 99, 100, 128

alcohol abuse, 83, 97, 100

alcohol use, 93, 100

alcoholics, 84

alcoholism, 17, 84, 88, 94, 96

alertness, 122

alienation, 125, 129

allele, 11, 63, 70, 242

alpha interferon, 149

alternative, 90, 126, 146

alters, 7, 32, 33, 36, 38, 60, 76, 92, 140, 147, 227

M

O

P

T